Making Babies in Early Modern England

Early modern English people were obsessed with making babies. In this fascinating new history, Leah Astbury traces this preoccupation through manuscript letters, diaries, recipe books and almanacs, revealing its centrality to family life. Information was plentiful in guides on the burgeoning fields of domestic conduct and midwifery, as well as in the many satirical ballads focused on sex, marriage and family. Astbury utilises this broad source base to explore all aspects of early modern childbearing, from conception to the months after delivery. She demonstrates that, while religious and cultural ideals dictated that women carry out all of this work, men were engaged in its practice through directing medical decisions. With the entire household including servants, wetnurses and other unexpected actors included in the project, childbearing can be situated within the histories of gender, medicine, social status, family and record-keeping. This title is also available as open access on Cambridge Core.

LEAH ASTBURY is a Lecturer in Health History at the University of Bristol.

Making Babies in Early Modern England

Leah Astbury
University of Bristol

CAMBRIDGE
UNIVERSITY PRESS

CAMBRIDGE
UNIVERSITY PRESS

Shaftesbury Road, Cambridge CB2 8EA, United Kingdom

One Liberty Plaza, 20th Floor, New York, NY 10006, USA

477 Williamstown Road, Port Melbourne, VIC 3207, Australia

314–321, 3rd Floor, Plot 3, Splendor Forum, Jasola District Centre, New Delhi – 110025, India

103 Penang Road, #05–06/07, Visioncrest Commercial, Singapore 238467

Cambridge University Press is part of Cambridge University Press & Assessment, a department of the University of Cambridge.

We share the University's mission to contribute to society through the pursuit of education, learning and research at the highest international levels of excellence.

www.cambridge.org
Information on this title: www.cambridge.org/9781009602860

DOI: 10.1017/9781009602846

First published 2025

Cover image: A. Marsh, The Ten Pleasures of Marriage (London: 1682), p. 188, The Huntington Library, San Marino, California.

A catalogue record for this publication is available from the British Library

A Cataloging-in-Publication data record for this book is available from the Library of Congress

ISBN 978-1-009-60286-0 Hardback

For Mum and Dad.

Contents

Figures

Acknowledgements

This book has taken a long time and I have accrued many debts.

I am eternally grateful to Lauren Kassell whose exemplary scholarship and mentorship have been from the beginning, and will continue to be, a model of academic practice to me. This book grew out of my PhD thesis, which Lauren supervised, and Laura Gowing and Mary E. Fissell examined. Both Mary and Laura have provided ongoing guidance and comments that have shaped this book and my research career more broadly. Elizabeth Foyster was an important source of moral and intellectual encouragement in my journey to become a historian. I am very grateful to Sasha Handley for allowing me the time to finish parts of the manuscript whilst working as a postdoc at the University of Manchester.

I have been fortunate to have received several grants over my research career that have given me the luxury of time to write and research, and in particular, have allowed me to travel to collect the rich manuscript paperwork that is the backbone of this book. Thank you to the Oxford Research Centre in the Humanities (TORCH) and the Society of Renaissance Studies. The 2017/18 Molina Fellowship at the Huntington Library provided invaluable space to gestate this book. I am particularly grateful to the group of long-term fellows at the Huntington, especially Allison Margaret Bigelow, Andrew Lipman, Mary E. Mendoza, Catherine Roach and Amanda Vickery. Thanks to Steve Hindle, Joel L. Klein and Vanessa Wilkie for their comments on papers that eventually became chapters, directing me to sources and providing me with the opportunity to be part of the southern Californian academic community.

I am extremely grateful to the Department of History and Philosophy of Science (HPS) at the University of Cambridge. It was the ideal home in which to grow, flourish and be challenged as a scholar, especially as part of the Generation to Reproduction project. For memorable conversations at HPS I thank Salim Al-Gailani, Jenny Bangham, Christoffer Basse Eriksen, Christina Benninghaus, Riana Betzler, Boyd Brogan, Sarah Bull, Margaret Carlyle, Pippa Carter, Silvia De Renzi, Jo Edge, Seb Falk, Rebecca Flemming, Susannah Gibson, Meira Gold, Jessica Hamel-Akré, Nick Hopwood, Peter

Murray Jones, Natalie Kaoukji, Elaine Leong, Dániel Margócsy, Katrina Maydom, Richard McKay, Dmitriy Myelnikov, Lea T. Olsan, Jesse Olszynko-Gryn, Carolin Schmitz, Tillmann Taape, John Young and Gabriella Zuccolin. For administrative support, thank you to Toby Bryant, Tamara Hug, Agnieska Lanucha, Louisa Russell and David Thompson. During Covid and beyond, Andrew Clarke and Dmitriy Myelnikov provided much solace and kinship through joint writing sessions.

I would like to extend my sincere gratitude to new colleagues at the University of Bristol in particular Kenneth Austin, Victoria Bates, Gonzalo Velasco Berenguer, Mark Hailwood, Stephen Mawdsley, Zahra Shah, Kate Skinner and James Thompson.

At conferences, seminars and through fellowships I have been fortunate to have met and had formative conversations with David Cressy, Isabel Davis, Catherine Evans, Lisa Forman Cody, Sarah Fox, Kate Gibson, Stefan Hanss, Karen Harvey, Stephanie Howard-Smith, Emily May Vine, Lisa Smith, Rebecca Whiteley and Amanda Vickery. Olivia Weisser has been tremendously generous to me in her guidance both in writing this book as well as in navigating academia more generally. Special thanks to Elaine Leong and Hannah Murphy who have at different points provided the encouragement and advice necessary to finish this project.

Parts of Chapter 4 were published in '"Ordering the Infant": Caring for Newborns in Early Modern England' in Sandra Cavallo and Tessa Storey (eds.), *Conserving Health in Early Modern Culture* (Manchester: Manchester University Press, 2017). An earlier version of Chapter 5 was published in *Social History of Medicine* as 'Being Well, Looking Ill: Childbirth and the Return to Health in Seventeenth-century England', 30, no. 3 (2017): 500–519.

The Wellcome Trust generously funded this research [088708 and 205358/Z/16/Z]. At Wellcome, I thank Tom Bray, Chris Hassan, Sophie Hutchinson and Dan O'Connor for all of their support.

It has been a privilege and an honour to work with Lucy Rhymer and the editorial team at Cambridge University Press. I am indebted to the anonymous reviewers for carefully reading the entire book and for their advice. Any remaining errors or deficiencies are my responsibility.

My utmost gratitude to the archivists at the Cheshire Archives and Local Studies Centre, the Huntington Library and the University of Glasgow for allowing me to reproduce images of items in their collections.

Thank you to my parents for always encouraging my intellectual and creative pursuits. Their support and love have been the greatest asset. The final stages of writing this book were quite different from the early stages. It was completed despite the best efforts of Juno the Pup, and as I learnt afresh the importance of neighbourhood, family and kinship. Thank you to John for swiping right and making me happier than I ever could have imagined.

Abbreviations

BL	British Library, London
CB	*The Casebooks of Simon Forman and Richard Napier, 1596–1634: A Digital Edition*, Lauren Kassell et al. (eds.)
EBBA	English Broadside Ballad Archive
EBBO	Early English Books Online
HEH	Huntington Library, San Marino, CA
KHLC	Kent History and Library Centre, Maidstone
ODNB	Oxford Dictionary of National Biography
OED	Oxford English Dictionary
WL	Wellcome Library, London

Introduction

In the summer 1695, a masked woman hurried into a house on Little Queen Street in Piccadilly in London and upstairs to an apartment she had rented by the day. She was accompanied by three women: her maid, Dinah Alsop; a midwife, Mrs Richardson; and a nurse, Mrs Pleasant. That night, as London bustled beneath her, still masked, she went into labour. As she cried out in pain, her mask slipped, revealing her identity. She was Anne Gerard, the Countess of Macclesfield, wife of Charles Gerard, a prominent army officer, who had recently been released from the Tower on suspicion for his involvement in the treasonous Rye House plot of 1683 and Monmouth Rebellion of 1685. Between two and three o'clock in the morning she gave birth to a baby girl she named after herself, Anne. That evening, while she lay in the front room recovering, her baby was hastily christened in the back room.

As the House of Lords would later hear, the baby was not her husband's. The father was a 'tall Gent' that had frequented Beaufort House from time to time (the residence in Chelsea that she had been living in alone, separated from her husband for a decade). He was rumoured to be Richard Savage, an army officer and fourth Earl Rivers.[1] Mother and baby remained in Little Queen Street for three or four days before Mrs Richardson took little Anne to Walthamstow to look after her at her own house while the countess returned to Beaufort House as if nothing had happened. Baby Anne was not given the last name Mason (the countess' maiden name) nor Gerard (the countess' married name) but Savage.[2] Two years later, the countess gave birth to another baby, a little boy called Richard, in almost identical circumstances, although this time, his last name was written in the baptism register as Smith. Although the playwright and poet Richard Savage later claimed to be Anne and Richard's illegitimate offspring, Anne kept their paternity a secret until her death and claimed both had died as babies.

[1] ODNB.

[2] 'An Act for dissolving ye Marriage betweene Charles Earle of Maclesfeld, and Anne his Wife and to Illegitimate the Children of the said Anne', Parliamentary Archives, Palace of Westminster, London, HL/PO/JO/10/1/496/1197.

We know about Anne and her clandestine births because her husband, Charles, petitioned parliament to disinherit the countess and her 'spurious Issue'. He was granted a bill of divorce, the first of its kind, in January 1698, allowing him to marry again and ensuring that she and her children lost the title of Macclesfield. The case captured the imaginations of early modern writers. The sordid details of the disastrous marriage and the countess' infidelity were broadcast in a court case that called on servants, midwives, nurses and even the minister that baptised the children to give testimonies. This, in turn, became the subject of numerous sensationalist pamphlets that were eagerly consumed by literate Londoners. Childbearing was of great interest in early modern England at all levels of society.

Although Charles' case and resulting divorce might at first glance seem to herald the beginning of what has been perceived as a dissolution or disintegration of marriage and family from the seventeenth century onwards, in the form of divorce, it is in fact quite the opposite. The case enshrined in law an expectation that women would carry out the work of childbearing exhaustively and intensively solely for their husband's name and family and they would do so with just the right amount of fuss. Beneath the vitriolic insults that Charles and his supporters hurled at her was another complex and longstanding notion that the material benefits of marriage for women were entirely conditional on the performance of this procreative work. This was called generation in early modern England, a term that pre-dates our modern 'reproduction' and refers to all the stages of making babies.[3] This kind of capacious terminology is apparent in the titles of childbearing guides of the period that were addressed to 'teeming' or 'breeding' women.

The Macclesfields' court case lays bare for the historian the profound instability of the system of generation that had huge stakes for the entire family of a couple but was a process that mothers were very often represented (inaccurately) as the sole workers in. Generation redounded to family name, and by extension the stability of households and the Church, but it could not be easily or effortlessly managed, however much some authorities might have wished otherwise. Anne through her 'open Adultery', getting pregnant by another man but also more importantly 'using vile Practices to have her spurious Issue imposed and obtruded upon him [Charles]', or in other words, dragging the family name through the mud, had endangered the orderly performance of gendered domestic labour, inheritance and lineage.[4] In a

[3] Nick Hopwood, Rebecca Flemming and Lauren Kassell, 'Reproduction in History', in *Reproduction: Antiquity to the Present Day* (Cambridge: Cambridge University Press, 2018), 4.

[4] Anonymous, *Reasons for the Earl of Maclesfeld's Bill in Parliament for Dissolving the Marriage between him and his wife, and illegitimating their spurious issue* (1697).

1685 letter to Anne, Charles described how he had tolerated her 'youth and folly' initially, but once she taunted him by saying she would never have his children, pretended to get pregnant every time he went out of town and spoke about Charles and *his* family with 'scorn and contempt', he resolved to leave her. Within this we can see a cultural assumption that some parts of having babies ought to be made public and celebrated – through announcing pregnancy to family and friends and including them in the rituals of delivery, Christening and Churching (the ceremony after birth in which a newly delivered woman went to Church to give thanks) – and some parts kept just between a couple. Poor male sexual performance or infertility, for example, was to be shrouded from even close family members and shared only between husbands and wives. Anne violated this norm.

The fact that the countess had given birth and christened her babies secretly was taken as incriminating evidence that she been unfaithful *and* she had deliberately sought to pass off her illegitimate children as legitimate. When Elizabeth Wiget, one of the women present at the birth of Richard, was asked why she thought the woman she had attended was not of 'Quality', or of good means and repute, she remarked 'I thought she would have had soem Woman friend with her & not have trusted to a stranger.' John Smith, when questioned about Richard's baptism, noted that he assumed the infant was 'base born' because there was no one else there, alluding to the sinfulness of his conception as well as his perceived lowly social status. For middling and elite individuals in England during the seventeenth and early eighteenth centuries there was an expectation that birth would be an event witnessed by others and documented in family paperwork. The tension between displaying certain parts of domestic life for the good of family name and status, and the insistence that women keep other bits secret, can, through careful work, be parsed out in all kinds of documentary evidence in family archives. This book shows that these cultural and social expectations shaped the experience of having babies even whilst the minds and bodies of men and women might not live up to these lofty ideals.

Prior to the Enlightenment, historians have argued that women were wholly in control of childbirth and that this took place away from family interests and incursion. This is because the chambers that women gave birth in were usually female-only. When 1970s sociologists and historians started being interested in women's experiences in the past, parturition seemed an obvious focus and case study for understanding the experience of being a woman. Having babies was represented as uniquely central to women's social and biological selves in the past and present. The moment at which men entered the birthing chamber in the eighteenth century as man-midwives was represented as a turning point where women irrevocably lost bodily agency, a trend that was reified and intensified by the formation of lying-in institutions in the eighteenth century and then the rise of hospital birth at the end of the nineteenth century.[5] By attending births, men supposedly disrupted the feminine, supportive, intuitive and importantly, private, ceremony of childbirth.[6] In some accounts, male practitioners literally killed off their competitors by accusing female midwives of being witches.[7] Whereas previous accounts posit the eighteenth century as the moment at which science, medicine and rationality replaced superstition and ignorance, these feminist accounts of birth configured these developments as harbingers of patriarchal intrusion and interference.[8]

Making Babies in Early Modern England takes a long frame that considers not just the moment of delivery but the ways that family members shaped and made the experience of generation from conception to after-birth care. The book examines the paperwork that early modern families created that documented this process (albeit in tellingly fragmented or selective ways). These records reveal that making babies was a lengthy, complex and fluid process that men were far more active in directing and producing than has previously been accounted for. Despite this, women *and* men sought to write about childbearing in ways that showed their household as mirroring the prevailing ideals of domestic labour, which were neatly and discretely gendered where men provided and women laboured to birth, heal, clothe and feed family members. Women were expected and compelled to do the majority of the work of bearing children, including the difficult and attentive medical work and care involved in the months after birth. Although this laborious work was not always properly credited, as Anne's case reveals, it was not inevitable that women would take on this work gladly for their husband's family and name. This was one reason why making babies was such a preoccupation of early modern households.

Whilst this book finds that having babies embedded women literally and figuratively within family structures, other historians have suggested that generation allowed them to circumvent domestic expectations and worlds. Rachel Weil summarises that because women knew more about having babies than men in the period, they could 'speak authoritatively on a matter of political importance' to raise questions about power, privilege and property

[5] For a summary of scholarship, see: Salim Al-Gailani, 'Hospital Birth', in Hopwood, Kassell and Flemming, ed., *Reproduction*; Ann Oakley, *The Captured Womb: A History of the Medical Care of Pregnant Women* (Oxford: Basil Blackwell, 1984), is a particularly notable feminist critque of institutionalised maternity care.

[6] Lisa Forman Cody, *Birthing the Nation: Sex, Science, and the Conception of Eighteenth-Century Britons* (Oxford: Oxford University Press, 2005), 23.

[7] Barbara Ehrenreich and Deirdre English, *Witches, Midwives, and Nurses: A History of Women Healers* (Oyster Bay, NY: Glass Mountain Pamphlets, 1971).

[8] See, for example: Oakley, *The Captured Womb*.

rights.[9] Adrian Wilson pithily claims that 'Before childbirth belonged to medicine, it belonged to women', distinguishing between the social practices of delivery that were attended by only women and the involvement of men as necessarily making it more scientific and medical. The majority of medical encounters in the period were at the outset domestic.[10] These worlds of professional and domestic medicine, this book finds, were far from distinct. Linda Pollock and Laura Gowing who have cautioned that the delivery room was not unconditionally supportive, still see it as a female world, albeit not necessarily a peaceable one.[11] Midwives and other women attending a birth might police and enforce certain practices and behaviours and the social rituals of childbirth like gossips (female friends, neighbours and family members who assisted and accompanied women while they laboured) and feasting were denied to those who were unmarried.

Single pregnant women were poked, prodded, inspected and often forced to give birth outside. Anne too of course was forced to rent a room away from the marital home in order to give birth to her illegitimate child. This option of renting a room was not available to most unwed mothers. In these accounts, getting pregnant within wedlock offered women privacy and agency, and was an experience that at least temporarily removed them from the family. Elite married women most certainly had a more positive experience of childbearing than the impoverished and unmarried women that have been central in other accounts, but this book shows the ways in which women's extraordinary and exhaustive labour was often subsumed within broader familial narratives rather than attributed to them as individuals. In doing so, it resists the distinction that has been present in previous accounts between parts of family life that were political, public and almost exclusively male and those that were domestic, private and almost exclusively female. The analogies that reformers and others made between the family and the state – that the disorder of the former would lead to the disarray of the latter – were ideological and artificial rather than structural and organic. This framework allowed those furthering a certain social and political agenda to link those hierarchies to a substantially less

9 Rachel J. Weil, 'The Politics of Legitimacy and the Warming-Pan Scandal', in *Political Passions: Gender, the Family and Political Argument in England* (Manchester: Manchester University Press, 1999), 87.

10 Adrian Wilson, 'The Ceremony of Childbirth and Its Interpretation', in *Women as Mothers in Pre-Industrial England: Essays in Memory of Dorothy McLaren*, ed. Valerie Fildes (London: Routledge, 1990), 70.

11 Linda A. Pollock, 'Childbearing and Female Bonding in Early Modern England', *Social History* 22, no. 3 (1997): 286–306; Laura Gowing, *Common Bodies: Women, Touch and Power in Seventeenth-Century England* (New Haven, CT: Yale University Press, 2003); Laura Gowing, 'Secret Births and Infanticide in Seventeenth-Century England', *Past & Present* 156 (1997): 87–115.

contested and more familiar patriarchal order.[12] The family, it appears, was constantly shifting and contested but nevertheless an important force in identity, community, religion and governance. As the Macclesfields' case indicates, law alone was not sufficient to clarify the complexities of the early modern family project of proper and godly procreation. The domestic world was central to male positioning and fashioning, but not always in ways that were commensurate or even compatible with women's labour.

This book considers childbearing even, or perhaps especially, within domestic spaces to be as much a medical experience as a social one, and in doing so, frames these efforts as 'work', or as Mary Fissell has suggested 'bodywork'.[13] It becomes clear that generation required the input of more than simply a mother and more than a father too. Making and reproducing one (elite) family often drew on the work and effort of others who were not related by blood but nevertheless considered part of the 'family' when it was advantageous to employers. Early modern people commonly referred to those who lived in the same confines as them 'family', even, and perhaps especially, if they were servants.[14] Whilst this has often been raised in relation to the subject of affect, this terminology is accidentally revealing. Servants were very often physically and emotionally involved in sustaining and furthering their employers' lineage. As Sarah Knott has noted, we can learn much from the work of anthropologists on 'shadow mothers', 'care chains' and 'alloparenting'.[15] *Making Babies in Early Modern England* is not just about what we now might term biological parents but about nurses, servants, friends and midwives, even though which tasks and activities made up their work as individuals is often unclear. Although it may have been more favourable for families to represent babies as exclusively raised by their mothers, this was rarely the case. It is important to note that although this book uses the term 'woman' to describe those who got pregnant and gave birth to babies because those are the terms that early modern people used, it simultaneously acknowledges that not all mothers birth and not all people who give birth are female. Assuming the opposite, however, was (and continues to be) a powerful thread in normative representations of making babies.

[12] Susan D. Amussen, 'Gender, Family and the Social Order, 1560–1725', in *Order and Disorder in Early Modern England*, ed. Anthony Fletcher and John Stevenson (Cambridge: Cambridge University Press, 1985), 196–217.

[13] For more on 'bodywork' and its intersection with women's (especially medical) work more broadly, see: Mary E. Fissell, 'Women, Health, and Healing in Early Modern England', *Bulletin of the History of Medicine* 82, no. 1 (2008), 10–12.

[14] Naomi Tadmor, *Family and Friends in Eighteenth-Century England: Household, Kinship and Patronage* (Cambridge: Cambridge University Press, 2001).

[15] Sarah Knott, 'Theorizing and Historicizing Mothering's Many Labours', *Past & Present* 246, no. Supplement 15 (2020): 1–24.

The Politics of Generation

Having babies was a veritable obsession in the seventeenth century and intersected with a variety of political, religious and social hierarchies. Protestant Reformers advocated godly marriage as an appropriate and pious route to salvation in contrast to celibacy, which was lauded by the pre- and counter-Reformation Church. Bearing children was 'a thing so much needful to all mankind', the authors of a 1656 guide to giving birth, *The Compleat Midwifes Practice*, explained.[16] Robert Barret reminded readers in his 1699 *A Companion for Midwives* that the 'whole World is govern'd by' the womb's 'fertile product'.[17] John Oliver, a churchman and the president of Magdalen College, Oxford, wrote in the epistle of his 1663 *A Present for Teeming Women* that 'much of the comfort of the present generation, and the honour of God, and future being of his Church in succeeding generations, is concerned in those Infants un-borne.'[18] In 1571, the second tome of sermons by the Church of England to be preached in church every Sunday instructed parishioners in the 'Homily on the State of Matrimony' that marriage would help individuals 'avoid Fornication' and bring 'forth fruit'. These children were blessings from God and ought to be 'brought up' by godly parents 'in the knowledge of Gods word.' This would ensure that 'the knowledge of God and true Religion might be delivered by Succession from one to another.'[19] Martin Luther preached that Eve, and by extension women, had caused the Fall, and that they could be sanctified by bearing children.[20] Childbirth was therefore intertwined not only with the survival of the Church but with the practice and experience of devotion in early modern England.

Early modern people had plenty of obvious models of the devastating consequences of childlessness. Henry VIII's literally deadly attempts to secure an heir indirectly caused the Reformation. After the Restoration in 1660, childlessness again dominated the conversation around Charles II's throne

[16] Thomas Chamberlayne, *The Complete Midwife's Practice Englarged, In the most Weighty and High Concernments of the Birth of Man Containing a perfect Directory, or Rules for Midwives and Nurses* (London: 1656), 1.

[17] Robert Barret, *A Companion for Midwives, Child-bearing Women, and Nurses Directing them how to Perform their Respective Offices: Together with an Essay, Endeavouring to Shew the Influence of Moral Abuses upon the Health of Children* (London: 1699), 59.

[18] John Oliver, *A Present for Teeming Women, or, Scripture-directions for Women with Child How to Prepare for the Houre of Travel. Written first for the private use of a Gentlewoman of Quality in the West, and now Published for the Common Good* (London: 1663), sig. A2v.

[19] 'An Homylee of the state of Matrimonie', in *Certaine sermons or homilies appoynted to be read in churches in the time of the late Queene Elizabeth of famous memory and now reprinted for the use of private families, in two parts. The second Tome of Homilees, of such matters as were promised, and instituted in the former part of Homilees* (London: 1571), 476.

[20] Ulinka Rublack, 'Pregnancy, Childbirth and the Female Body in Early Modern Germany', *Past & Present* 150, no. 1 (1996): 84–110.

and lack of heir. His wife, Catherine of Braganza, had three miscarriages. He was succeeded by his brother, James II, who also struggled to produce heirs. His wife, Mary of Modena, similarly suffered a series of miscarriages and still births, which were gossiped about in court and in pamphlets that speculated about an attempted Catholic coop of the British crown. When Mary gave birth to a living, healthy baby boy in 1688, James II's enemies fostered a conspiracy that she had in fact had a stillborn child that was swapped out for a 'pretender' in a warming-pan. The details of Mary's pregnancy and birth became central parts of public discourse, and the scandal a key contributor to the Glorious Revolution.[21] Queen Anne's eighteen pregnancies, which ended either in miscarriage, stillbirth or premature death between 1684 and 1700, intersected with her father's own fertility troubles and her childlessness and associated poor health was an omnipresent part of her reign from 1702 onwards. Conception and birth were not only practically essential to the perpetuation of political stability but used to contextualise and understand civic events. Tales of babies born with missing heads, as animals, in multiples of 365 or with deformities were common in pamphlets and ballads exploring the diabolical and disorderly, and parliamentary and religious factionalism. What could go wrong in generation provided a model for thinking about what might go wrong in Heaven and on Earth.[22]

These contexts fed into a pervasive fear that fertility was flagging and the population dwindling in the period. Satirical pamphlets such as the 1643 *The Mid-wives just Petition* fretted about the 'naturall depopulation of towns and Cities', especially in London, which would become 'very thin of people'.[23]

[21] Mary E. Fissell, *Vernacular Bodies: The Politics of Reproduction in Early Modern England* (Oxford: Oxford University Press, 2004), 230–243; Corrine Harol, 'Misconceiving the Heir: Mind and Matter in the Warming Pan Propaganda', in *Vital Matters: Eighteenth-Century Views of Conception, Life and Death*, ed. Helen Deutsch and Mary Terrall, UCLA Clark Memorial Library Series (Toronto: University of Toronto Press, 2012), 130–147; Weil, 'The Politics of Legitimacy and the Warming-Pan Scandal'.

[22] Kathryn M. Brammall, 'Monstrous Metamorphosis: Nature, Morality, and the Rhetoric of Monstrosity in Tudor England', *Sixteenth Century Journal* 27, no. 1 (1996): 3–21; David Cressy, 'Monstrous Births and Credible Reports: Portents, Texts, and Testimonies', in *Travesties and Transgressions in Tudor and Stuart England: Tales of Discord and Dissension* (Oxford: Oxford University Press, 1999), 29–50; Harriet Lyon, 'The Fisherton Monster: Science, Providence, and the Politics in Early Restoration England', *The Historical Journal* 60, no. 2 (2016): 333–362; Alexandra Walsham, '"Tongues of Heaven": Prodigies, Portents, and Prophets', in *Providence in Early Modern England* (Oxford: Oxford University Press, 2001), 167–218.

[23] *The Mid-wives just Petition or, A complaint of divers good Gentlewomen of that faculty. Shewing to the whole Christian world their just cause of their sufferings in these distracted Time, for their want of Trading* (London: 1643), sig. A2r. Reprinted in Lisa Forman Cody, ed., *The Early Modern Englishwoman: A Facsimile Library of Essential Works. Printed Writings, 1641–1700: Part I. Writings on Medicine*, vol. 4, II (Aldershot: Ashgate, 2002). Doreen Evenden has argued that the *Petition* is a serious proposal to parliament made by London midwives, but Cody notes that the satirical tone suggests it was a spoof, xvii.

Couples should make love not war, the petition written by a (real or imagined) company of midwives proposed. It blamed recent conflicts on the number of women who lay 'in their beds like cold marble images cut out by some Artificers hand' rather than having passionate sex with their husbands.[24] This was not unfounded. Despite a rise in the English population in the sixteenth and early seventeenth centuries, in the seventeenth century, the population began to fall.[25] Generation was at once simultaneously a profoundly quotidian and individual experience, as well as interwoven into the most fundamental questions about the perpetuation of humankind, economic prosperity, the meaning of life and the nature of God in early modern England.

Sources and Methodology

When I began this project, I assumed I would mostly be spending my time reading women's letters and diaries. I got very good at spotting the looser and less stylised handwriting of women in the reams of paper bundled together in stout boxes of 'family papers' that I was ordering to reading rooms in local record offices and national libraries. I expected I would find a lot of letters between mothers and daughters imparting knowledge gained through experience and hearsay. I also imagined the advice that pregnant or newly delivered women might receive would be gentle and sympathetic. I thought I would really have to hunt for information about sex, menstruation, labour and breastfeeding, for surely it would have been indecorous to write openly about such things in the period? One reason I made these assumptions is because archivists themselves have often sought to separate out 'personal' from 'official' or 'political' correspondence in the paperwork left by families, which often fall largely along gendered lines. Archives are always subjective and are co-created by historical actors, archivists and historians.[26] Nineteenth-century editors of many early modern diaries and letters were disinterested in what was deemed corporeal and scatological. Birth often fell into this category. When Alice Thornton's three volumes of writings were bequeathed to the British Library in 2013 after being held in a private, and therefore inaccessible,

[24] *Ibid.*, sig. A4r.

[25] E. A. Wrigley and R. S. Schofield, *The Population History of England 1541–1871: A Reconstruction* (London: Edward Arnold, 1981), 161–162; Sarah Toulalan, *Imagining Sex: Pornography and Bodies in Seventeenth-Century England* (Oxford: Oxford University Press, 2007), 63–64.

[26] Kathryn Burns, *Into the Archive: Writing and Power in Colonial Peru* (Durham, NC: Duke University Press, 2010); Alexandra Walsham, 'The Social History of the Archive: Record-Keeping in Early Modern Europe', *Past & Present* 230, no. 11 (2016): 9–48; Elizabeth Yale, 'The History of Archives: The State of the Discipline', *Book History* 18 (2015): 332–359.

collection for years prior, I discovered that the 1875 'transcriber' Charles Jackson had left out more than half the material on giving birth.[27]

Sitting in archives amongst these papers, however, I quickly discovered that literate middling and elite men as well as women were obsessed with some of the details of generation and what women's bodies felt and looked like in early modern England. They wrote in their letters, diaries, almanacs, account books, commonplace books and spiritual meditations about their own and others' conceptions with candour. They weighed in with their own advice, contradicted the due dates pregnant women proffered and freely blamed them for causing miscarriage by not eating properly or being too sad. They were also not always polite, but often admonishing and sometimes cruel in a way that made it very quickly apparent to me that family members perceived women to be labouring for them and their interests rather than for the couple or the community. Families kept recipe books stuffed with culinary and medicinal recipes to increase fertility, increase milk supply and intensify labour pains.

Many families kept lists of the birth (and death) dates of their children, sometimes continued across many generations. Recipe books, account books or bibles were often filled with the birth (and death) dates of their children, sometimes continued across many generations. Just to cite a few, Dorothy Frances Feilding recorded the birthdays of her children in the beautifully bound book of poetry, select reflections, biblical passages and medical recipes.[28] Anne Glyd wrote 'A memorial of our childrens births', beginning with her son John Glyd on 22 September 1650, and on another page when her daughter, also called Anne, married and when her grandsons were born (Figure I.1). Francis Witton copied out his wedding day and the birth and death dates of his seventeen children, including two listed as stillborn on a piece of paper kept with other family papers of the non-conformist Henry family.[29] These papers survive not by chance but because families thought it said something important about them and their identity. Families were made and remade through the process of bearing and raising children. Over the course of researching this book, I had to write to surviving family members to request permission to use the documents in their archives: these collections continue to

[27] Raymond A. Anselment's new edition, Alice Thornton, *My First Booke of My Life: Alice Thornton*, ed. Raymond A. Anselment (Lincoln: University of Nebraska Press, 2014), is a more faithful transcription. Cordelia Beattie has recently discovered the 'lost' fourth volume of Thornton's meditations now held in Durham Cathedral Library and Archives, 'Thornton's Memoirs', Comber 7. See: Cordelia Beattie, 'The Discovery of Two Missing Alice Thornton Manuscripts', *Notes and Queries* 66, no. 4 (2019): 547–553. This is the basis for a digital edition of Thornton's works (https://thornton.kdl.kcl.ac.uk, last accessed 10/03/2025).

[28] Feilding family, 'Commonplace book c. 1684', Beinecke Rare Book and Manuscript Library, Osborn b226.

[29] 'Notes of Marriage of Francis Witton and Sarah Sergeant on 6 April, 1675, and of Birthdays of Family members', Cheshire Record Office, Chester, ZDBAS/12.

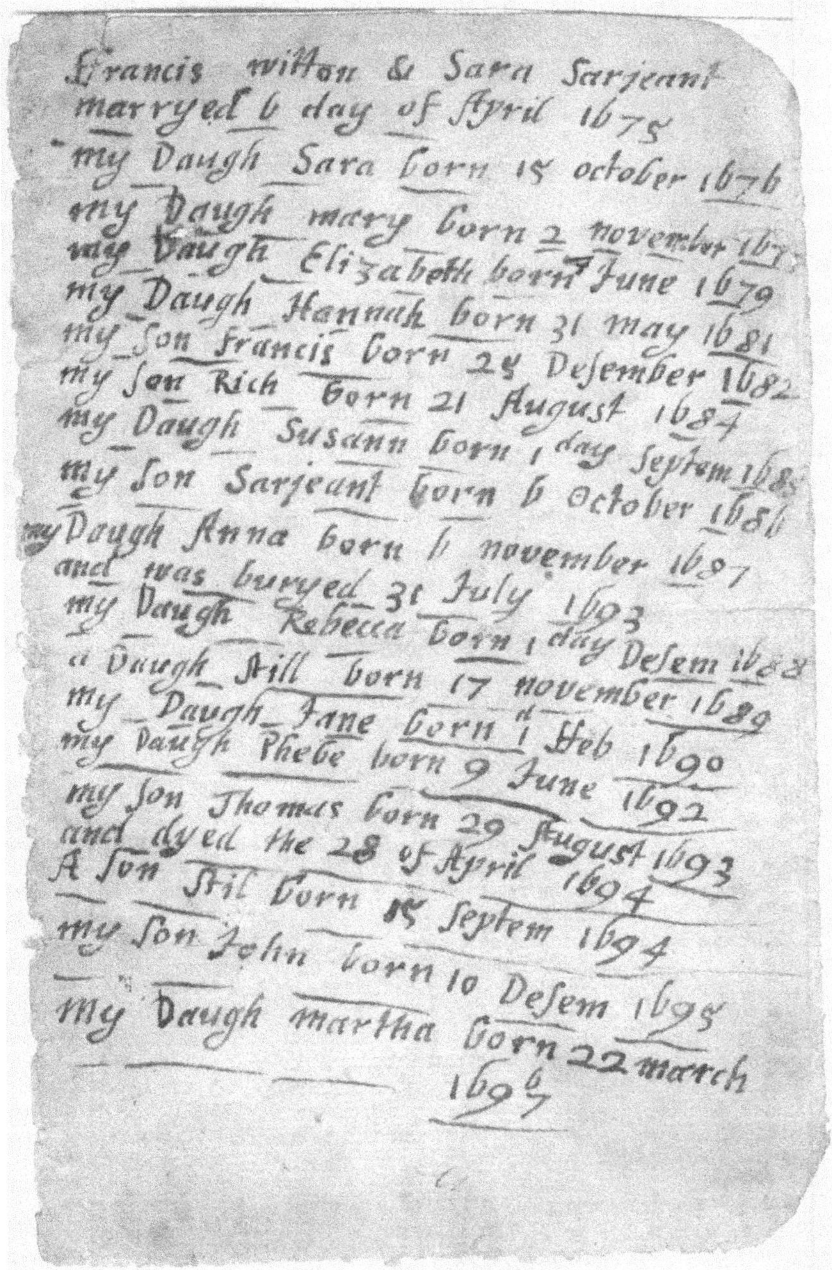

Francis witton & Sara Sarjeant
marryed 6 day of April 1675
my Daugh Sara born 15 october 1676
my Daugh mary born 2 november 1677
my Daugh Elizabeth born 7 June 1679
my Daugh Hannah born 31 may 1681
my Son Francis born 28 Desember 1682
my Son Rich born 21 August 1684
my Daugh Susann born 1 day Septem 1685
my Son Sarjeant born 6 October 1686
my Daugh Anna born 6 november 1687
and was buryed 31 July 1693
my Daugh Rebecca born 1 day Desem 1688
a Daugh Still born 17 november 1689
my Daugh Jane born 1d Feb 1690
my Daugh Phebe born 9 June 1692
my Son Thomas born 29 August 1693
and dyed the 28 of April 1694
A Son Stil born 15 Septem 1694
my Son John born 10 Desem 1695
my Daugh martha born 22 march 1696/7

Figure I.1 'Notes of Marriage of Francis Witton and Sarah Sergeant on 6 April, 1675, and of Birthdays of Family members', Cheshire Archives and Local Studies. Reproduced with the permission of Cheshire Archives and Local Studies and the owner/depositor to whom copyright is reserved.

represent and embody the status and reputation of what were once prominent aristocratic families. The revived interest in genealogy and family history shows that many people still feel that lineage and reproduction is central to understanding oneself.

Of course, it was not just childbirth that families wrote about in early modern England. Although the majority of people were not literate in this period, elite and middling sort families wrote things down for all kinds of purposes. Men and women kept notebooks, journals and commonplace books; scribbled in the blank spaces of almanacs; and kept track of their spending in account books and wrote out useful culinary and medicinal recipes. Letters were important tools in negotiating business, managing the household and maintaining the connection between separated friends, spouses and family members, and sometimes all three at once. These sources have often been understood as 'life-writing' or 'ego-literature' and connected to a Protestant imperative to self-examine and self-define.[30] Writing helped individuals fashion and display their credit and status, which intersected in complex and not always obvious ways with wealth.[31] The records that individuals and families kept on paper might not conform to an obvious genre and might present multiple perspectives and narratives at once.[32] Women *and* men wrote letters, diaries and account books, but women, historians have shown, were particularly active in keeping genealogical records.[33] Keeping 'house' and reciprocal accounts was central to the performance and construction of men's economic

[30] Michael Maschuch, *Origins of the Individualist Self: Autobiography and Self-Identity in England, 1591–1791* (Cambridge: Cambridge University Press, 1996); Alex Ryrie, *Being Protestant in Reformation Britain* (Oxford: Oxford University Press, 2013); Matthew Kadane, *The Watchful Clothier: The Life of an Eighteenth-Century Protestant Capitalist* (New Haven, CT: Yale University Press, 2013); Jason Scott-Warren, 'Early Modern Bookkeeping and Life-Writing Revisited: Accounting for Richard Stonley', *Past & Present* 230, no. supplement 11 (2016): 151–170.

[31] Craig Muldrew, *The Economy of Obligation: The Culture of Credit and Social Relations in Early Modern England* (Basingstoke: Palgrave, 1998); Alexandra Shepard, *Accounting for Oneself: Worth, Status, and the Social Order in Early Modern England* (Oxford: Oxford University Press, 2015); K. Tawny Paul, 'Accounting for Men's Work: Multiple Employments and Occupational Identities in Early Modern England', *History Workshop Journal* 85 (2018): 26–46.

[32] Andrew Cambers, 'Reading, the Godly, and Self-Writing in England, circa 1580–1720', *Journal of British Studies* 46, no. 4 (2007): 796–825; Adam Smyth, *Autobiography in Early Modern England* (Cambridge: Cambridge University Press, 2010); Sheila Ottway, 'Autobiography', in *A Companion to Early Modern Women's Writing*, ed. Anita Pacheco, Blackwell Companions to Literature and Culture (Oxford: Blackwell, 2002), 231–247.

[33] Katharine Hodgkin, 'Women, Memory and Family History in Seventeenth-Century England', in *Memory before Modernity: Practices of Memory in Early Modern Europe*, ed. Ericka Kuijpers et al. (Leiden: Brill, 2013), 297–313; Megan Matchinske, *Women Writing History in Early Modern England* (Cambridge: Cambridge University Press, 2009); Mihoko Suzuki, 'Anne Clifford and the Gendering of History', *Clio* 30, no. 2 (2001): 195–229.

and political identity too.[34] These two imperatives converged in middling and elite family paperwork.

While much of this scholarship has focused on how writing and keeping records facilitated the emergence of a sense of self, others have highlighted that keeping records on paper could be done on behalf of others and as part of a collective project, which this book draws on and contributes to. Brodie Waddell notes that the writings of middling-sort literate individuals such as the tradesman Joseph Bufton indicate many individuals recorded theirs and others' not for self-exploration but to create an account for the community at large.[35] Recipe books, in particular, were constantly revised and added to by multiple generations of family members.[36] I borrow the term 'paperwork' from Elaine Leong's work on recipe books because it usefully captures the ways in which the stuff of family archives evade classification and often collaboratively compiled and curated.[37] Generation sat comfortably alongside other aspects of the everyday and extraordinary that people wrote about in these texts.

These families were the kinds of people who could afford the increasingly numerous books on conduct, medicine, philosophy, religion and other subjects available in the seventeenth century. They could also afford the services of medical practitioners of various kinds and levels. They thus make an ideal case study for examining the ways in which prescription interacted with practice in the period. This book uses family paperwork and medical and conduct books to ask how families defined their experiences in relation to prescriptive frameworks and norms. The casebooks of medical practitioners provide yet another glimpse into the ways individuals understood their bodies and what being healthy meant to them. Finally, ballads, pamphlets and other cheap print were similarly obsessed with generation in the period. These texts reached a far more socially diverse audience than relatively expensive childbearing guides, and thus they offer a window into the assumptions, fears and humour of the

[34] Joanne Bailey, *Unquiet Lives: Marriage and Marriage Breakdown in England, 1660–1800* (Cambridge: Cambridge University Press, 2003); Hannah Barker, 'Soul, Purse and Family: Middling and Lower-Class Masculinity in Eighteenth-Century Manchester', *Social History* 33, no. 1 (2008): 12–35; Karen Harvey, *The Little Republic: Masculinity and Domestic Authority in Eighteenth-Century Britain* (Oxford: Oxford University Press, 2012).

[35] Brodie Waddell, 'Writing History from Below: Chronicling and Record-Keeping in Early Modern England', *History Workshop Journal* 85, no. Spring (2018): 239–264.

[36] Elaine Leong, *Recipes and Everyday Knowledge: Medicine, Science, and the Household in Early Modern England* (Chicago: University of Chicago Press, 2018); Sara Pennell, 'Perfecting Practice? Women, Manuscript Recipes and Knowledge in Early Modern England', in *Early Modern Women's Manuscript Writing: Selected Papers from the Trinity/Trent Colloquium*, ed. Victoria Burke and Jonathan Gibson (Aldershot: Ashgate, 2004), 237–258; Jennifer K. Stine, 'Opening Closets: The Discovery of Household Medicine in Early Modern England' (PhD dissertation, Stanford University, 1996).

[37] Leong, *Recipes and Everyday Knowledge*.

people that elite families often employed to assist in making and remaking their families. The book begins in the second half of the sixteenth century with the rise of vernacular medical print and the raft of childbearing guides that were aimed at literate householders. It ends in the early eighteenth century where other histories of 'reproduction' begin with the institutionalisation of a pro-natalist state.

Book Structure

Making Babies in Early Modern England is structured in a way that mirrors the layout of early modern childbearing guides, beginning with efforts to conceive and ending with descriptions of how to 'order' mother and child after birth that set out an idealised vision of what to expect while expecting. Procreation was an experience that, despite the best efforts of authors, medical practitioners and interested family members, was often unpredictable and unknowable, however much families tried to impose order and make it seem easy in their paperwork. The structure of the book reflects an expectation or hope that rarely adequately described experience.

Chapter 1 asks how early modern people managed fertility at home. Conception and pregnancy were a source of fascination and gossip for elite families. Men and women both had to take on work to ensure they were fertile, and yet male procreative responsibility was minimised in paperwork. Historians have noted that despite the abundance of references to increasing lust and fertility in printed medical and popular texts, there is limited evidence of the diagnosis and treatment of barrenness, especially of men. Examining recipe books, casebooks and correspondence suggests men understood themselves to be potentially responsible for childlessness. Added to this, wives were represented as being in charge of diagnosing and remedying infertility for both themselves and their husbands, meaning that evidence of male treatment is often treated discreetly within records of medical practice.

Chapter 2 examines how women and their families deduced, or decided, they were pregnant. Childbearing guides of the period told women and their families that they might and indeed should know they were pregnant very soon after sex and connected this to sexual and moral continence. Women were encouraged to keep 'accounts' of their bodies to pinpoint conception reliably. These records, in turn, became part of other sorts of family paperwork that inscribed legitimacy and ascendancy. Writing about conception and pregnancy sought to impose certainty on what was otherwise an unknowable experience.

Chapter 3 looks at the social and material preparations that households made for an impending birth. Family members were fascinated by the look and size of women's bellies. Married women's 'big bellies' were celebrated: they displayed the fruitfulness of the family. The process of buying and borrowing things for childbirth including linens, baby clothes and birthing stools have often been represented as hallmarks of a celebratory and extravagant female culture. The process of imagining the unborn child alongside material preparations was instead a family affair that men were intimately involved in in ways that complemented the written accounts that families made.

Chapter 4 focuses on the choices that families made about who would deliver babies and where women would give birth. From the eighteenth century in England, man-midwives dominated the delivery of babies. Historians' accounts have suggested that this incursion was a dramatic and transformative moment in which men wrestled control of childbirth from women. This chapter suggests that this trend in practice was only the more obvious and tangible reflection of a broader pattern in which men and the family directed and controlled childbearing. Although the birthing chamber may have been female-only, women often travelled to their father or father-in-law's house to give birth. When man-midwives entered the birthing room, this chapter suggests they might not have seen it as the haven of female sociability that some historians have represented it as.

Chapter 5 examines early modern expectations of delivery and recovery from childbirth by women. Medical manuals expected women would give birth painfully but without complication, stay in bed (or 'lie in') for a month, go to church to give thanks to God for their survival and then the return to their normal selves. This chapter shows that although this ideal helped to frame women's experiences of delivery and recovery, it rarely captured the reality of the emotional and bodily difficulties they faced.

Chapter 6 asks how newborns were cared for and charts the formulaic regimen of getting babies to cry, watching them change colour, cutting their navel cord, searching their bodies for impediment, bathing them, swaddling them, putting them down to sleep and, finally, suckling them. Authors often expressed the expectation that mothers would do this work or if they were unable, nurses and servants, although these latter figures are rarely named or credited in the same ways. A great many families hired or retained nurses and servants during the period of childbearing who became temporary members of the family and carried out this care. Wet nursing is the most powerful example of elite families getting servants to prioritise their employers' family over their own. Asking someone who was close to or already part of the household meant families could maintain their control and authority over childrearing. Making babies was a family project, albeit one in which family members did not have equal stakes and one in which mothers' and other women's procreative work was often subsumed within everyday expectations of domestic labour.

The findings of this book – that although it was convenient to represent childbearing as unchallenging and women's work, it was actually central to the family as a whole and very complicated and laborious – unpick the cultural, social, medical and bodily threads that were the fabric of early modern life. As well as revealing the ways in which people understood medicine, health and generation in early modern England, placing the household centre stage when examining childbirth helps to dismantle a pervasive yet popular stereotype that birthing in the past was somehow more intuitive, natural and unbidden. Not only were parents and other family members constantly seeking to optimise the health of their unborn children, but they also saw the way women conceived, carried and raised children as mirroring and reflecting their own place in the world and their family, the status of their soul and whether they would be welcomed into the Kingdom of Heaven. Making babies was a way of enacting, displaying and proving piety and rectitude of self, family and community and brought together a myriad of religious, medical and domestic traditions and practices.

1 Fertility, Fruitfulness and Anxious Families

Paternoster Row next to St Paul's Cathedral in late sixteenth-century London was a hive of printers and book sellers. On any given day someone who had the disposable cash might be able to buy a play by William Shakespeare or Christopher Marlowe; an instructional text on music; a history of the conflicts in France, Portugal and Ireland; or a plethora of medical books.[1] Amongst the titles for sale was *The Child-birth or Womans Lecture,* written by the staunchly Puritan minister and physician Christopher Hooke. It was supposedly 'very necessarie to bee read and knowne of all young married and teeming [pregnant] Women, and not unprofitable for men of all sortes'. Someone standing in the cathedral yard leafing through the *Lecture* would have learned that difficulties in childbearing such as struggling to conceive, miscarrying, having sickly or short-lived children, or birthing 'monsters' could be divine punishment for 'rebelliously transgress[ing]' God's wishes. Being 'a fruiteful vine' was not simply about being capable of conception but having a succession of healthy, beautiful children. The pain and peril of procreation was necessary and redemptive. If one was to live piously, they would be rewarded by God with a 'quiver full' of children. In turn perpetuating the family would make believers even more full of admiration and praise for God. It was a cyclical process in which bodies mirrored the soul.[2] Childbearing was central to the practice of individual, domestic and parishioners' piety.

In this ideal model, the godly husband and wife's 'table' would groan with 'branches' from their 'vine'. Fertility was understood in early modern England as both easy and hard: it was as simple and impossible as living a godly life. It is notable that Hooke was a physician as well as a cleric. His instructional text interwove religious exegesis with medical instruction. These were not distinct bodies of knowledge or practice in early modern England. In just the same way that the *Lecture* framed fertility as related to piety, the authors of regimens described how the maintenance of health through food, drink, exercise, sleep and regulating one's emotions was not just a medical task, but one of embodied devotion too. These two genres were related in yet another way as

1 EEBO search of books sold and printed in Paternoster Row.

2 Christopher Hooke, *The Child-birth or Womans Lecture* (London: 1590), sig. B3r.

well. Both childbearing and the performance of everyday medical care were envisioned to be part of female domestic labour within the household. The fact that the *Lecture* was on sale alongside other household management guides and medical texts in St Paul's churchyard quite literally displayed the domestic expectations placed upon women in the period. Conduct authors set out how men were meant to provide the financial means necessary to provide raw materials and women ought to work to clothe, nourish and heal family members. In this system, fertility was perceived as something women were meant to manage alongside a myriad of other care work. Procreation was represented as the chief purpose of marriage, a key route to religious salvation and the way in which property, faith and power were transmitted.

The stakes could not have been higher. Being fruitful was not just about producing an heir but redounded to both male and female reputation. It is no surprise that conception, pregnancy and birth were a veritable obsession for early modern people and provoked considerable anxiety for husbands, wives, the wider family, Church and state. One might assume then that early modern English family paperwork was awash with references to very specific measures to increase the likelihood of conception, in the same way that, as we shall see, printed medical guides were. And yet, although correspondents were happy to pressure newly married couples for information about whether they were pregnant or to make spurious predictions about when it might happen, they were much quieter about specific instances in which women and men took medical measures to remedy infertility. They were especially taciturn about instances in which men might be considered physiologically responsible for childlessness. This chapter mines family paperwork for hints about how elite families understood infertility and how they might have sought to remedy it. In doing so it reveals a deep-seated discomfort with the idea that men might have to put effort into perpetuating the family whilst also uncovering hints that they regularly did so. Whilst people were desperate for tardy conception to be seen as the result of women's bodily frailty, this was not always possible. Infertility could be caused by male impotence or weakness of seed, or by a lacklustre match, all explanations that sat at odds with ideals of domestic order, fruitfulness and male mastery that were core values of godly and ascendant families. Families wrote about men's and women's bodies in notably different ways that foregrounded evidence of wifely submission and male strength. The politics of getting pregnant were unstable and fraught with disruption, but also had great significance in the construction of narratives about family identity. These findings support those of historians of medicine that have been keen to point out that men were involved in household medicine.[3] Likewise, histories

[3] A Bray, 'To Be a Man in Early Modern Society: The Curious Case of Michael Wigglesworth', *History Workshop Journal* 41, no. 1 (1996): 155–165; Raewyn Connell, *Masculinities*

of early modern masculinity have highlighted how domestic spaces and material culture defined and, at times, threatened the construction and representation of male identity.[4] These two literatures encourage us to look beyond the representation of separate male and female spheres of knowledge and practice, and appreciate the ways in which normative and prescriptive models of work and expertise conditioned cultural scripts that did not always map on to the experience of gender and everyday life. Men were often involved in the practice of increasing fertility within households and outside them, and they were often thought to be physiologically and emotionally responsible for childlessness, although they and others sought to minimise or even scrub these facts out of family paperwork.

Longing to Be Fruitful

At first glance, cheap and prescriptive material would seem to suggest that everyone wanted to have children in early modern England. Added to this, elite families consistently placed a high value on conceiving in correspondence, although sometimes they wrote about childlessness in abstract terms that refrained from speculating about who or why a couple might not have had issue. A 1685 ballad described how women who were childless were constantly reminded of this fact by their neighbours' births and had to woefully attend countless christenings that rubbed salt in the wound. The ballad told the story of a *Female Doctress* who touted a medicine developed in her sixty years of practice that could cure barrenness, but was really scamming couples out of their hard-earned money.[5] The 1621 *A Discourse of the Married and Single Life* commiserated with husbands, who would live in 'great discontent' without children, believing themselves to be 'in hatred with God & nature'.[6] The sight of 'other mens children' would 'greeveth' them and they would wish that

(Cambridge: Polity, 1995); Alexandra Shepard, *Meanings of Manhood in Early Modern England*, Oxford Studies in Social History (Oxford: Clarendon Press, 2003); John Tosh, 'What Should Historians Do with Masculinity? Reflections on Nineteenth-Century Britain', *History Workshop Journal* 38 (1994): 179–202; Amanda Vickery, 'Golden Age to Separate Spheres? A Review of the Categories and Chronology of English Women's History', *The Historical Journal* 36, no. 2 (1993): 383–414.

4 For example: Elaine Leong, 'Collecting Knowledge for the Family: Recipes, Gender and Practical Knowledge in the Early Modern English Household', *Centaurus* 55, no. 2 (2013): 81–103; Lisa W. Smith 'The Relative Duties of a Man: Domestic Medicine in England and France, ca. 1685–1740', *Journal of Family History* 31, no. 3 (2006): 237–256.

5 *The Female Doctress, or, Mothers Midnights cure for Barrenness in Women, Being A True Relation of a Woman that pretended to Cure Women of Barrenness; Especially in the Mint in Southwark* (London, 1685).

6 *A Discourse of the Married and Single Life Wherein, by Discovering the Misery of the One, is Plainely Declared the Felicity of the Other* (London: 1621), 25.

even the 'worst of them were his'.[7] A glut of ballads in the seventeenth century mocked men who were cuckolded by their wives and thought that they were fathers only to discover they were raising another man's child. The midwife Jane Sharp noted in her popular 1671 *The Midwives Book* that conceiving a child was 'the earnest desire if not of all[,] yet of most women'.[8] Nicholas Culpeper, author of *A Directory for Midwives* (1656) assumed that 'All men and women desire to be fruitful'.[9] The books that literate couples kept on shelves in their home, the drinking songs that men would have encountered in ale houses, the plays they went and saw, the sermons they heard in Church and the passages from religious, medical or philosophical texts that may have been read out, all would have impressed upon couples the importance of getting pregnant quickly after marriage.

It is no wonder then that people expressed a deep longing to be fruitful, and when they did not conceive quickly became distressed. A woman called Jane Shrewsbury, who remains otherwise unknown in the historical record, wrote a 'fervent' prayer about her unrequited desire to have a baby. She told God how she and 'the world' had 'long expected to heare tydings of my safe deliverie' of a child. Would God let this 'expectation vanish into smoke?' she asked.[10] Alice Woodward sought the help of the astrologer-physician Richard Napier in 1604 because had had taken 'much guilt' and could not 'quiet her mind' because 'she hath not the fortune other women haue' after enduring six stillbirths. She had one surviving child.[11] Forty-four people asked Simon Forman and his protégé, Richard Napier, explicitly about fertility a total of fifty-two times between 1569 and 1620. But this figure obscures the larger number of women who asked the practitioners whether they were pregnant. When the woman in question was not 'with child', determined according to the stars, the case notes habitually turned to the wider problem of why the individual had not got pregnant. Elizabeth Amon, for example, asked whether she was pregnant in 1596. Forman failed to record a judgement, but thought she was 'troubled with the mother' (suffocation of the womb) and 'stopt in the stomack' and this was why she had not had a baby.[12]

In correspondence, the expectation of family members that newly married couples would get pregnant immediately after getting married was positively relentless. The tone of such letters was often humorous and yet below this veneer one senses the collective anxiety of wondering whether the family

[7] *A Discourse of the Married and Single Life*, 26.

[8] Jane Sharp, *The Midwives Book Or the Whole Art of Midwifry Discovered*, ed. Elaine Hobby, Women Writers in English 1350–1850 (Oxford: Oxford University Press, 1999), 75.

[9] Nicholas Culpeper, *A Directory for Midwives, or, A Guide for Women* (London: 1656), 74.

[10] Jane Shrewsbury, 'A fervent prayer for the obtaining of a childe', in 'Theological tracts', BL, Harley MS 6828, fols 481v–483v.

[11] CASE21091, CB. [12] CASE39, CB.

name would be continued, and what this might say about the lineage's providential destiny if it was not. John Molyneaux wrote to Alice Kenyon, a Lancashire gentlewoman, in 1674 expecting 'to hear y[o]u are w[i]th child'.[13] In 1656 the Earl of Northampton wrote to his daughter-in-law's father celebrating that his daughter, Frances, was finally pregnant. 'I am extreamly glad to heare that wee are likely to have more of y[ou]r breede by my most fertill Mistress.'[14] A later letter praised Frances for continuing 'her virtuous qualitie of Multiplying in the world'.[15] Yet another letter asked whether she 'daily encreaseth', a reference to her burgeoning belly.[16] A year after Mary Sackville, daughter of the fifth Earl of Dorset, and Roger Boyle, an Irish peer and Member of Parliament, had been married and still not had a baby, their families freely expressed their anxieties. When Sackville finally conceived, Boyle's father wrote to Mary's father, Richard, confessing that he had been 'almost asham[e]d to hear' that Richard had 'gotten' his own wife pregnant 'befor[e] my son had gotten y[ou]r Daugther with Childe'. Now that she was pregnant, he had 'Redeemed himself'. This happy outcome, he noted, was hardly surprising because Mary and Roger were a 'Coupl[e] descended from two such fruitfull families'. They would never have been long in 'Imitating their Ancestors'.[17]

Frances Widdrington wrote to her sister, Mary Arthington, both of the Yorkshire landowning Fairfax family, to say that she was sorry that she was 'not yet breeding'. Apparently Mary's husband, Henry, was convinced that Frances herself was pregnant but 'I would not have you fully to beleeve him'.[18] Joan Ellyot heard from her 'sister Bowes' that the wife of Simonds D'Ewes, the Suffolk parliamentarian and antiquarian, was pregnant and asked him for confirmation in the 1640s.[19] Another letter admonished him for not writing more regularly about the progress of 'sister Buckenham' and her pregnancy, in a way that suggests that within families pregnant or potentially pregnant women's bodies were seen as intensively, and at times exclusively, of interest.[20] News of the conception and pregnancies of family members and peers was a constant source of gossip in the correspondence of elite individuals. John Mordaunt, a politician from Warwickshire, wrote to his wife to tell her that Mistress Lucy was 'breeding' and that 'wee are now like to have

13 John Molyneux to Alice Kenyon, 28 April 1674, Lancashire Record Office, Preston, DDke 9/92/56.
14 Earl of Northampton to Richard, 5th Earl of Dorset, 28 April 1656, KHLC, U269/C86/2.
15 Earl of Northampton to Earl of Dorset, 12 January 1656, KHLC, U269/C86/3.
16 Earl of Northampton to Earl of Dorset, 21 September 1663, KHLC, U269/C86/5.
17 Lord Orrery to Richard, 5th Earl of Dorset, 2 March 1666, KHLC, U269/C19/3.
18 Frances Widdrington to Mary Arthington, 11 December 1639, 'Letter book c. 1680–1700', Bodleian Library, Oxford, MS Add A 119, fols 9r–v.
19 Joan Ellyot to Simonds D'Ewes, 12 September c. 1643, BL, Harley 382, fol. 26.
20 Joan Ellyot to Simonds D'Ewes, 22 September c. 1643, BL, Harley 382, fol. 29.

A fertile Neighbourhood'. He had heard the news from '[th]e Women yesterday'.[21] Anne Chaytor wrote to her brother, William, in 1673 in Croft near Darlington to tell him that a brewer's wife had been 'brought to bed', meaning given birth, to six babies at once – it was a 'healthy tyme hear [here] and frutfull'.[22]

This network of information about other people's fertility and sexual practices created a thick and tense environment in which elite men and women must have felt considerable anxiety. Mary Rich, the Countess of Warwick, described retrospectively in her memoirs how whilst initially her and her husband and been happy with two children, when they died, she was 'very desirous' of more and 'sought to God' to 'keep up the honour of that noble house' by conceiving. While previous generations of the family had been plentiful, she worried that the line 'grew so thin, that the name was like to sink'.[23] Her lack of issue might be the downfall of the whole family. As well as being key to the survival of the Church and to personal and familial piety, having babies was also crucial to inheritance and lineage, a question that was particularly pressing for these elite families. The repercussions of not having children for powerful families was most obviously and dramatically indicated by royal precedent – succession was a consistent concern for the English monarchy over the medieval and early modern period. Childbearing, therefore, far from being a purely domestic concern sat at the very heart of the experience of family and public life.

Although cheap print of the period was awash with instances of couples using food and medicine to bolster fertility, family correspondence was not as vocal about these cures. Furthermore, family members often refrained from speculating about the possible physiological or emotional causes of a couple's childlessness, especially when this pertained to men. Given the stakes, the candour with which correspondents discussed conception in rather public paperwork, and the ubiquity of childbearing and sex in cheap print, the absence of specific references to fertility aids is notable. Jennifer Evans has suggested that despite this relative silence in family correspondence and in practitioners' casebooks, the fact that medical, magical and practical cures for infertility were so widespread in printed medical texts and practitioners' advertisements means that fertility remedies must have been commonplace in early modern English homes.[24] In printed casebooks, particularly of

[21] John Mordaunt to Penelope Mordaunt, 1 October 1701, Warwickshire Record Office, Warwick, CR 1368, vol. 1, fol. 17.

[22] Anne Chaytor to William Chaytor, 22 July 1673, North Yorkshire Record Office, Northallerton, 9/3/11.

[23] Mary Rich, 'Some Specialties in the Life of M Warwicke', BL, Add MS 27357, fols 32v–34r.

[24] Jennifer Evans, *Aphrodisiacs, Fertility and Medicine in Early Modern England*, Studies in History (Woodbridge: Boydell & Brewer, 2014), 3.

surgeons, she shows that male patients were treated for genitourinary conditions that were thought to impact on infertility but that writers did not always linger on these ramifications, 'perhaps as a means of reassuring male readers that these outcomes were not a forgone conclusion'.[25]

Daphna Oren-Magidor similarly suggests that people, and particularly women, were embarrassed to visit a physician for conditions relating to sex and birth. Female practitioners may have offered more discretion in treating infertility, but they also rarely kept written records of their practice, and this might be why there are limited records of treatment.[26] This may very well have been true with regards to practitioners' casebooks but does not explain the tentativeness in family correspondence. The silences in this material are important in what they reveal about the place of women and their bodies within households. Male fragility or lack of virility threatened domestic order as well as the family name, and it was this familial priority that drove these absences or at times the destruction of evidence of men being physiologically responsible for childlessness. Male status within families generally was dependant on the appearance of a normative and orderly domestic realm whilst simultaneously needing to be seen as largely separate from this world and the labours that it entailed. Families then prioritised public stories of quick, easy and inevitable conception, and they sought consolation when their experiences did not live up to this ideal by explaining childlessness as women's fault and additionally their responsibility to (secretly) remedy. Reading against the grain in correspondence and recipe books reveals the subtle ways that early modern families navigated this conundrum of outcome versus appearance. It certainly did not stop men representing the victory as all theirs when women eventually conceived.

Strutting About

When men wrote to their friends and family about conception, they were keen to represent themselves as virile, and showed little interest in maternal effort. When Walter and Barbara Bagot of the prominent Staffordshire aristocratic family had a baby in 1725, Barbara's father, William, wrote to Walter commiserating that although it would have been better if the child was a boy, 'Sir Walter it is Pla[i]n you can get, and your wife can Bring children.' The birth

[25] Jennifer Evans, *Men's Sexual Health in Early Modern England*, Gendering the Late Medieval and Early Modern World (Amsterdam: Amsterdam University Press, 2023), 62.

[26] Daphna Oren-Magidor, *Infertility in Early Modern England*, Early Modern History: Society and Culture (London: Palgrave, 2017), 132–133; Daphna Oren-Magidor, 'Literate Laywomen, Male Medical Practitioners and the Treatment of Fertility Problems in Early Modern England', *Social History of Medicine* 29, no. 2 (2016): 290–310.

had made Walter an exceedingly 'happy' grandfather.[27] In 1727, when the wife of George Legge, Viscount Lewisham, gave birth to a 'fine chop[p]ing lad', he wrote to Walter, who was his brother-in-law, that he was 'vastly happy in it' and 'they say I strut about' the streets of London '& look like the Prince of Candee'.[28] In 1672, Lord Parry gossiped to his wife, Katharine, that Sir Edward Nicolls had loudly boasted to all his friends that he had 'but 2 bouts' of sex with his wife and the baby 'came'. It had also been reported that when he was told that his wife had given birth to a big healthy baby, he was so incredulous that he could be the father that he sought confirmation from the women who were with his wife during delivery.[29] As Nicolls' initial bravado and Parry's derision reveals, not everyone was convinced when men claimed to have conceived easily. This is clear in an exchange between Sir William fifth Lord Paget, a politician and Buckinghamshire landlord, and his steward, John Jone's wife, Mary, in the 1630s. He wrote to say that he was disappointed to hear that she was *still* not pregnant. The fault, he was adamant, was with her husband, 'for I thinke you very fruitful were you well handled'. He told her that he would be at his house by Michaelmas, 'where if I finde you still barren, I will take some paines with you myselfe'.[30] Conception was often represented as related to male sexual skill, or as William said of his son, down to men getting women pregnant and women bringing it to fruition. Men merely had to 'handle' women well. It is unclear how serious Paget's threats to have sex with his employee's wife were. The rate of illegitimate pregnancy in domestic servants attests to the liberty that masters took with female members of the household.[31] Underpinning the humour in Paget's letter, was clearly a reality that the Jones' childlessness reflected poorly on John, and more broadly on his employer, Paget, too.

Men felt and expressed shame, sadness and fear when they were unable to get their wives pregnant. Dudley Ryder, the future Chief Justice, fretted in his diary in 1715 when he was twenty-five that he would struggle to get a future wife 'with child'. He worried that he was not 'very powerful that way' and that

[27] William Legge to Walter Bagot, n.d. 1725, Madgalen College Library, Oxford, MC: P287/C5/10.

[28] George Legge, Viscount Lewisham, to Sir Walter Bagot, 1 August 1727, Magdalen College Library, Oxford, MC: P287/C3/47. George was apparently comparing himself to the Prince of Candia, described in Urbain Chevreau's *The Mirror of Fortune, or, The true characters of fate and destiny* (1676) as the most fortunate, beautiful, witty and intelligent man that he was 'the admiration of all the earth', 134. I am thankful to Andrew Zurcher for pointing me towards this reference.

[29] Lord Parry to Katharine Parry, 13 May 1672, Northamptonshire Record Office, Northampton, Isham MS IC/749.

[30] William Paget to Mary Jones, c. 1636, Staffordshire Record Office, Stafford, Paget MS D603/K/2/1.

[31] Laura Gowing, 'Secret Births and Infanticide in Seventeenth-Century England', *Past & Present*, no. 156 (1997): 87–115.

a future spouse would 'have reason to complain'. He even doubted whether he should marry at all but could not imagine how he might be happy without a wife.[32] There was also of course the very real threat of a marriage having to be annulled if a husband was unable to perform sexually. Lord Orrery, if we recall, told his son he was 'almost asham[e]d' of him that he had taken so long to get his wife pregnant. That his wife's parents had had a child since the young couple married only made things more humiliating. Roger only 'Redeem[e]d himself' when Mary got pregnant in 1666.[33] The conception was all thanks to the advice that Orrery had given him, which he, in turn, had passed on to Lord Powerscort, his brother-in-law, which would mean he was the 'next that Gits his Wif with Child'.[34] Sadly this advice has been lost or, more likely, was never kept, owing to its potentially mortifying content, but points to a far less visible network of men writing to share advice about conception and fertility, albeit one that made discretion paramount. Failing to conceive, particularly when the cause was lack of male vigour or virility, was not something one wanted to feature prominently in the family archive.

An equally shameful cause of childlessness was the possibility that a couple was an incompatible match. In yet another example of the ways in which families could control the evidence attesting to their fertility and reputation, when Theophilus, seventh Earl of Huntingdon sent his uncle Arthur a letter in 1672 confessing that he was unable to consummate his marriage to Elizabeth Lewis, he insisted that his uncle burn it on receipt. The only reason we know of its existence is that Arthur's letter containing advice survives. The couple had been married for six months, provoking Theophilus to ask his uncle for advice, but not without asking him first to burn the request for help upon receipt. The problem, Arthur was relieved to read, was not Theophilus' 'member', which the newly married man assured him was 'stiffe standing'. The couple had already visited two doctors. One had given Elizabeth an electuary, the other, called Dr Duchon, recommended Theophilus refrain from masturbating. It would be easier to 'gett yr P: in to her' when she had her 'flowers', or was menstruating. This was because 'those parts are most apt to delate and widen when she is in that condition'.[35] This was one area in which practice appears to have differed from prescription. Childbearing guides of the period were adamant that having sex while a woman was menstruating was ungodly and could lead to a host of infant illnesses or deformities, especially leprosy. Sharp, in her midwifery guide, for example, detailed how babies might be unhealthy if

[32] Dudley Ryder, 19 July 1716, *The Diary of Dudley Ryder 1715–1716*, ed. William Matthews (London: Methuen & Co., 1939), 279.

[33] Lord Orrery to Earl of Dorset, 2 March 1666, KHLC, U269/C19/3.

[34] Lord Broghill to Earl of Dorset, 6 April 1666, KHLC, U269/C18/3.

[35] Arthur Stanhope to Theophilus, Earl of Huntingdon, 1672, HEH, Hastings family papers, Box 33, MS HA 12503.

conceived while a woman was menstruating, but acknowledged that some couples might prefer sex at this time because the 'membranes are so dilated by the moisture of those parts that the pain is far less'.[36] This belief clearly motivated the other pieces of advice that Duchon and Arthur proposed – to keep a bottle of oil by the bedside as lubricant and Elizabeth to take a glister, or laxative, 'before you have some hopes and intend to enter her', there would be 'roome a nuffe that ye head of your pindle may enter' and there would be 'otian [ocean] a nuffe, too deepe your rudder to feele the bottom againe as it is'.

As Stanhope's letter makes clear, men being physiologically responsible for childlessness was categorically more embarrassing than blaming women, in this case, Elizabeth. But this also raised the possibility that it was not only that she was not being 'well handled', in Lord Paget's words, but that she did not love her husband. Arthur reassured Theophilus that Elizabeth loved him 'most passionately'.[37] A later letter hints at a troubled relationship. Two years and three months after Arthur's advice, Elizabeth gave birth to a son. Bridget Croft, Theophilus' godmother, reflected that they should have called the baby 'peace-maker' because 'as his first beginning in ye womb did begin in better agreement' between the couple. She hoped his birth would 'so unight your hartes in affection as nothing shall ever separate yin'.[38] This puts Arthur's cajoling that Theophilus and Elizabeth would be the 'fondest and lovingest couple in the world' when the young man's 'P: has beene up to the hilts in her C' into context, and explains why his uncle warned him against visiting a prostitute. There were clearly rumours circulating about the couple already and Arthur told him not to bother with those 'trattles and lyes that you heare'. Stanhope said he would rather his nephew was dead than shamed the family by being unfaithful to his wife and giving her the 'pox'.[39]

It was not just men that sought to conceal their own infertility, but women were encouraged to also be discreet about lack of male virility. Wives who exposed their husband's sexual frailty were severely criticised. Thus, in 1693, the *Athenian Mercury,* an early advice column that printed questions from supposed readers and answers from a (probably fictional) team of experts, printed the story of a 'very personable Gentleman' who had been happily

[36] Sharp, *The Midwives Book Or the Whole Art of Midwifry Discovered*, 44.

[37] Arthur Stanhope to Theophilus, Earl of Huntingdon, 1672, HEH, MS HA 12503.

[38] Bridget Croft to Theophilus, Earl of Huntingdon, 1674, HEH, MS HA 1779.

[39] Arthur Stanhope to Theophilus, Earl of Huntingdon, 1672, HEH, MS HA 12503. For a discussion of the shame of venereal disease, see: Kevin P. Siena, *Venereal Disease, Hospitals and the Urban Poor: London's 'Foul Wards', 1600–1800*, Rochester Studies in Medical History (Rochester, NY: University of Rochester Press, 2004) and Olivia Weisser, 'Poxed and Ravished: Venereal Disease in Early Modern Rape Trials', *History Workshop Journal* 91, no. 1 (2021): 51–70.

married to a 'fine young Lady' for three years without having any children. He knew that the fault was his. After she died, he married a woman of substantial fortune but failed to tell her he was unable to have children. His first wife's mother visited his new marital home and exposed his infertility, berating him for marrying again 'when he knew himself not qualified for a Husband'. The gentleman in question was so ashamed and horrified by the public discussion of his incapacity that 'he immediately went up stairs, and ript up his Belly' and died. When asked for its 'Sentiments' on the episode and the 'Opinion of the two Wives', the publication responded that the first wife who 'Conceal'd her Husband's Infirmity' was a 'Subject for Admiration' and the second wife was also not to blame. The mother-in-law, however, had exposed his secret, and that was worthy of condemnation.[40] The editor of the *Mercury*, John Dunton, remained childless himself and his barrenness and 'no-performance at home' was mocked in a play of the same year, 1693, by Elkanah Settle.[41] Dunton may very well have been the author of the response, and, if as Helen Berry suggests, many of the stories in the *Mercury* were manufactured, he was also possibly the author of the initial question. The impacts of being known as being generatively challenged could be devastating for men, and women were expected to be complicit in upholding this aspect of male and familial honour.

Discreet wives emerge as a theme in accounts of couples struggling to conceive. When the marriage of Robert Devereux, the third Earl of Essex, and Frances Howard, was annulled in 1613, Frances was adamant that she had kept her husband's inability to consummate their marriage a secret and only divulged it when he was publicly accused of something even more shameful: being cuckolded. The breakdown of their ill-fated marriage became the subject of several pamphlets, notably the very detailed account by George Abott, Lord Archbishop of Canterbury, in 1715, that drew on evidence given at court and rumours reported by members of the aristocracy and the king himself. Frances' case rested on the fact that Robert was incapable, despite many attempts, of having sex. Whether or not it was Frances that was the origin of the rumours, it remained that tales of Robert's sexual non-performance spread far and wide.

The couple married in 1606, when Robert was fifteen and Frances sixteen. By the time Robert had returned from a two-year grand tour to begin married life, the match had soured, and Frances was rumoured to be having an affair

40 *Athenian Mercury* 9, no. 28 (18 March 1693).

41 Elkanah Settle, *The New Athenian Comedy* (London: 1693), 16–17. For further discussion, see: Helen Berry, *Gender, Society and Print Culture in Late-Stuart England: The Cultural World of the* Athenian Mercury, Women and Gender in the Early Modern World (Aldershot: Ashgate, 2003), 144.

with the Earl of Somerset. Once they were eighteen, the couple began cohabiting. Frances told the commissioners that she hoped they would begin having sex 'after the fashion of other married Couples' leading to 'lawful Issue' and making her a mother, but when they were 'naked and alone in the same Bed', she 'offer'd her self, and her Body' to no avail.[42] Robert 'labour[ed] a quarter of an Hour carnally to know' Frances before accepting defeat and bidding her goodnight. He told commissioners that he had been unable to get aroused because she had insulted him calling him a 'Cow, and Coward, and Beast'.[43] Some speculated that he had been bewitched, whilst the archbishop diagnosed the problem as 'Want of Love, which restraineth all Motions of carnal Concupiscence, and not any Impotency'. He opposed the annulment of the match, assuming that if the couple could rekindle their romance, all would be well.[44]

The King himself reported that it was not just Frances he was not attracted to but all women. Robert's friends had 'put a Woman to him' to cure his impotence but 'he would not touch her'. He had also reportedly travelled to Poland to be 'unwitched' of his impediment.[45] Another source, a 'good friend' of the Earl, recalled how one Sunday morning, surrounded by five or six captains and 'Gentlemen of Worth' in his chamber, he had responded to talk of his impotence by rising out of bed, pulling his shirt up and showing all how 'able, and extraordinarily sufficient' his erection was. The men supposedly 'cry'd out Shame of his Lady, and said That if the Ladies of the Court knew as much as they knew, they would tread her [Frances] to Death' in jealousy.[46] Importantly, Frances claimed that the only reason she had shared details of their intimate sexual activities, or lack of, was because there were 'false Rumours of her Disobedience'.[47] The Earl, in contrast, was described by Abott as refraining from 'ill Speech of his Lady' altogether, 'for which we all much commended him', something Abott's account clearly shows was not the case, but served to represent Frances as failing in her duties as a wife and potential mother.[48] A mere three months after the annulment was granted, Frances married Robert Carr, first Earl of Somerset, the man she was supposedly having an affair with all along. They were both imprisoned in the Tower of London for poisoning Sir Thomas Overbury, and their daughter, Anne, was born in custody in 1615. Essex returned to his seat in Warwickshire and there 'lived a private Life' in embarrassment.[49]

[42] George Abott, *The Case of Impotency As Debated in England, In that Remarkable Tryal An. 1613. Between Robert, Earl of Essex, and the Lady Frances Howard, who, after Eight Years Marriage, commenc'd a Suit against him for Impotency* (London: 1715), 137.
[43] *Ibid.*, 35. [44] *Ibid.*, 117. [45] *Ibid.*, 24. [46] *Ibid.*, 42. [47] *Ibid.*, 139.
[48] *Ibid.*, 8. [49] *Ibid.*, 165.

Gossiping about one's husband's lack of sexual prowess was a frequent feature of satirical print that mocked men that were cuckolded by their wives. In *Fumblers-Hall*, for example, Alice All-Cock initially sought to remedy her husband's impotence and lack of desire by dosing him with anchovies, caviar and muscadine, well-known aphrodisiacs, but when this did not work, she asked a gaggle of women for their assistance and advice.[50] In A. Marsh's *Ten Pleasures of Marriage* (1682), an unflattering picture of the expectations of a middling newlywed couple in the seventeenth century, the 'good woman' sought the help of her neighbours to conceive (Figure 1.1). A mere three months after the wedding she asked her neighbours 'what caresses' they received from their husbands. In turn, she 'most shamlesly relates what hath passed between her and her husband, twixt the curtains, or under the Rose', hoping to ascertain 'whether her husband understands his work well, and whether he doth it well, and oft enough'.[51] The so-termed 'Councel of women' overwhelm her with stories of their own amorous activities whilst criticising the husband. The imagined reader was clearly male; the author intrudes into the narrative to joke that the silver lining of having one's failings shared publicly was that wives would then encourage their husbands to spend their days in the coffee house drinking chocolate and then 'embraceth you as if you were an Angel' in the evening. The wife was advised to discreetly supplement her husband's diet secretly with chocolate, spices, eggs, sweatbread, lambs' testicles and caviar. When her attempts to seduce him and this invigorating diet do not work, the wife turns to insulting him, calling him 'Fumbler', 'dry-boots' and 'good man Dolittle'. Quite bluntly, 'This makes him look as if he had beshit himself.'[52] The husband is represented as thoroughly disgraced by the public knowledge of his infertility.

Such texts were humorous, but they exposed a real anxiety for men about the homosocial company that their wives kept, the kinds of conversations they would have, and the dire consequences of not having children.[53] The suggestion that wives might be able to dose their husbands' meals with things that would encourage conception was something that some medical texts also catered to. Sarah Jinner's 1659 almanac included a 'Confection' that caused 'fruitfulness in Man or Woman' that could be secretly sprinkled 'upon the parties meat'. Almanacs were astrological books that encouraged readers to record daily happenings and provided lists of useful information including

[50] *Fumblers-Hall kept and holden in Feeble-Court, at the sign of the Labour-in-vain, in Dee-little-Lane* (London: 1675), 7.

[51] A. Marsh, *The Ten Pleasures of Marriage Relating all the Delights and Contentments that are Mask'd Under the Bands of Matriomony* (London: 1682), 76–77.

[52] *Ibid.*, 79

[53] Mark Breitenberg, *Anxious Masculinity in Early Modern England*, Cambridge Studies in Renaissance Literature and Culture (Cambridge: Cambridge University Press, 1996).

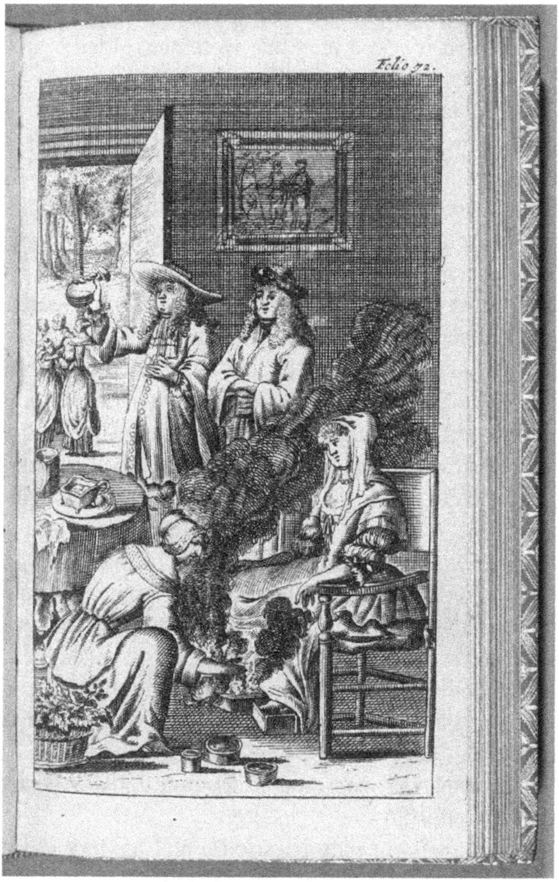

Figure 1.1 A. Marsh, *The Ten Pleasures of Marriage* (London: 1682), 72. RB102841, Huntington Library, San Marino, CA.

agricultural fairs, medical advice and advertisements. Jinner's was unusually focused on matters of sexual health. With the information she provided, she hoped people would be able to treat 'pain in the bottom of their bellies', a clear gesture to venereal disease, which as we know hampered fertility, without 'acquainting Physitians' with their indiscretions. Physicians, she noted, would not know the 'true cause of the Distemper' and therefore be incapable of treating it anyway.[54]

[54] Sarah Jinner, *An Almanack and Prognostication for the Year of Our Lord 1659* (London, 1659), sig. B1r.

Women's knowledge perceived intuition and expertise about generation was an ambivalent experience for men. At times it could be threatening and at others advantageous both as a source of expertise and because it allowed them to distance themselves from the responsibility for childlessness. In 1664, the diarist and naval administrator Samuel Pepys took advantage of being in the company of women after a gossips' feast – the celebration after a birth – to ask for advice on how to conceive. The women enthusiastically gave him ten pieces of advice that he numbered and duly recorded in his diary.

> 1) Do not hug my wife too hard nor too much: (2) eat no late suppers; (3) drink juyce of sage; (4) tent and toast; (5) wear cool holland drawers; (6) keep stomach warm and back cool; (7) upon query whether it was best to do at night or morn, they answered me neither one nor other, but when we had most mind to it; (8) wife not to go too strait laced; (9) myself to drink mum[55] and sugar; (10) Mrs. Ward did give me, to change my place.[56]

The couple should also lie with their 'heads where our heels do, or at least to make the bed high at feet and low at head'. Samuel noted that 'ne'r a man but I' had risen from the table at a gossips' feast and joined the women instead of the men, but his intrusion into the homosocial world of the gossiping feast provided him with otherwise hidden discreet knowledge about fertility. Despite Pepys' various efforts, the couple remained childless. Such was the perceived procreative agency of women that in some circumstances they were thought to be able to decide whether or not they got pregnant and whether it would be a boy or a girl. In 1627, John Holles, second Earl of Clare, wrote to his brother-in-law Sir Thomas Wentworth lamenting that both their wives had 'of late' been bearing 'wenches', or girls, instead of boys. He was petitioning his own wife to have some boys and hoped when Wentworth's wife saw this 'she will take faire warning, & doe as she should doe'.[57] Holles and his wife Elizabeth Vere actually had seven daughters and only one surviving son, the other died in infancy.

These ideas about women possessing troubling and even dangerous knowledge about generation owes much to the medieval tradition of terming this body of knowledge 'women's secrets'. Cheap print and correspondence were simply recapitulating a view that women could manipulate and control conception when it pleased them. By parsing out this field of knowledge from other kinds of medical and general knowledge, men also were able to claim

55 A kind of ale brewed from wheat malt and flavoured with herbs originally made at Brunswick, Germany (OED).

56 Samuel Pepys, 26 July 1664, *The Diary of Samuel Pepys: A New and Complete Transcription*, ed. Robert Latham (New York: Harper Collins, 1983), vol. 5 (1664), 222.

57 Sir John Holles to Sir Thomas Wentworth, 9 August 1627, Sheffield Archives, Sheffield, Volume 22 b, fol. 61.

that not being 'fruitful' was not their fault. They merely 'got' women pregnant, and their job was done. This, as men's letters and diaries indicate, was a fiction that even early modern people knew was inaccurate. Nor was getting pregnant only of interest to women. Elite families wrote about the generative lives of their neighbours, acquaintances and far-off relatives. Men like Nicolls or Paget might have liked people to think conception was as easy as having two 'bouts' or 'handling' a woman, but the anxiety present in such exchanges and the fixation with other people's fruitfulness point to the ways that this was often merely a narrative. It is noteworthy that when the Earl of Orrery, Roger Boyle's father, wrote that he knew the couple would 'imitate' their 'Ancestors' in being 'fruitful', a quick glance of the family tree reveals that Mary and Roger's 'ancestors' had not been particularly fertile. Mary's grandfather, Edward, who only had one heir, inherited the title of Earl of Dorset from his brother Richard Sackville, when he did not have any heirs. The Boyles had a similarly chequered past with procreation. Lord Orrery had only two sons. The new couple would go on to have only three children. Examining these narratives about success and pedigree makes painfully clear how much making babies was a family affair, and not merely confined to the world of women, however much men might have wanted to represent it as such.

Understanding the Causes of Childlessness

To understand how men could absent themselves from physiological and emotional responsibility for fertility, one only has to consider the ways in which medical authors wrote about the causes of childlessness. Although childbearing guides suggested that there were multiple causes of childlessness in women and in men, authors were far more interested in the ways wives might be able to moderate their bodies in order to conceive than in their husbands following suit. The 1595 text *Problemes of Aristotle* explained that a couple might struggle to conceive if the husband was too cold and his seed made 'vnfit for generation' or because his seed was too 'waterish' and would not stick in the womb. Sometimes the seed of husband and wife were not compatible – if the man were choleric, for example, and the woman sanguine. Fat women would struggle to bring a child to term because they had 'slipperie wombe[s], out of which the seede slippeth, and is not holden in'. Similarly, men and women that were too thin would also face problems.[58] And women

[58] Sarah Toulalan, '"Unfit for Generation": Body Size and Reproduction'. In *The Secrets of Generation: Reproduction in the Long Eighteenth Century*, ed. Raymond Stephanson and Darren Wagner (Toronto: University of Toronto Press, 2013), 299–318; Sarah Toulalan, 'To [o] much eating stifles the child': Fat Bodies and Reproduction in Early Modern England', *Historical Research* 87, no. 235 (2014): 65–93.

that were too hot would extinguish any seed cast into the womb. This was why women who were lustful rarely conceived. Having sex too frequently would 'corrupt and spill' the 'instruments of conception'. Notably, even though the answer gestured to the ways in which men's bodies might prevent conception as well as women, the question was framed in terms of why 'some women' were 'barren and can not conceaue'.[59] Similarly, the *Mercury*, asked 'Why are Common Women seldom or never with Child?' in 1691, rather than 'Why are some couples without issue?'. The response also centred on women's bodies and suggested that too much sex was deleterious to fertility:[60] 'Why does not the *Grass* grow in the *path way*?'[61] Although the frequency with which couples had sex was dependent on male as well as female activity, it was women who were held responsible, whose bodies underwent treatment and were often involved in diagnosis, as we shall see in the next section.

Other authors explained how if women did not menstruate sufficiently or regularly enough, they could 'neither conceive, nor ingender', and that this was the most frequent cause of childlessness. It was comparable to men possessing a 'defect or corruption', or whose seed was exhausted and wasted by 'his over-moist and cold conception'.[62] Culpeper told readers that in order to have healthy children, both spouses had to 'keep the *Instruments of Generation* pure and clean, and their Blood pure, that so their Seed being pure'.[63] This was accomplished through a moderate diet and 'Exercise of Body'. The womb might be too hot, too cold, too moist or too dry. All would hinder conception and could be remedied through a dietary regimen. The womb might be 'shut up' by humoral imbalance, or as Robert Barret explained, by some 'Tumor or Callosity'.[64] Moderate regimens connected the practice of piety to positive health and procreative outcomes.

The seed of spouses could also simply be incompatible rather than there being any defect. Sharp described how an 'impediment not fully seen' could mysteriously render a couple childless but with another spouse they would be very fertile. This was analogous to a broken watch that when thrown against the wall, in this case through remarriage, was jolted back into perfect working

[59] *Problemes of Aristotle with other Philosophers and Phisitions. Wherein are Contained Diuers Questions, with Their Answers, Touching the estate of Mans Bodie* (London: 1595), sig. E6r.
[60] *Aristotle's Master-piece; Or, The Secrets of Generation Display'd in all the Parts thereof* (London: 1690), 10.
[61] *Athenian Mercury*, 1, no. 18 (May 1691). Original emphasis.
[62] Jakob Rüff, *The Expert Midwife, or An excellent and most necessary treatise of the generation and birth of man* (London: 1637), 11.
[63] Nicholas Culpeper, *A Directory for Midwives, or, A Guide for Women* (London: 1675), 32.
[64] Robert Barret, *A Companion for Midwives, Child-bearing Women, and Nurses Directing them how to Perform their Respective Offices: Together with an Essay, Endeavouring to Shew the Influence of Moral Abuses upon the Health of Children* (London: 1699), 61.

order.[65] If spouses did not love each other, they would never be procreative, as many family correspondents feared. Culpeper explained that 'Want of Love between man and wife' would lead to barrenness because 'if their hearts be not united in love, how should their seed unite to cause conception?'[66] This was in part due to the dominance of the passions of the soul, or emotions, to understanding bodily health. Barret explained that only women who were of 'good Temperament, of a regular Life and Conversation' would conceive.[67] Grief or distress in women, in particular, could prevent conception or damage the health of an unborn child, as is discussed in more depth in Chapter 2. Culpeper instructed couples to 'avoid passions, anger, sadness, fear' and 'Let love be invited, and if it burn, there wil many Spirits flie to the womb and privities.'[68] Happiness begot lusty infants, but as we shall see in later chapters, the emotional tenor of the relationship was also dependant on women's efforts.

Childlessness could also come from a weak or non-existent erection in men, which as we have seen from family paperwork, was often represented as the most shameful and embarrassing cause. Like the Earl of Essex, this was often thought to be caused by bewitchment. Sharp noted that men in France commonly urinated through their wife's wedding ring to cure curses and enchantments that rendered them unable to have sex.[69] This kind of superstitious practice was normally discouraged in England but may very well have been practised in some households. Childlessness could also be no one specific party's fault and simply be divine will. Religious and medical explanations sat comfortably side-by-side in printed literature.[70] Eucharius Roeslin's *Byrth of Mankynde* celebrated conception as the most manifest and plain sign of 'the magnificent myghtynesse of that omnipote[n]t lyving god'.[71] Sharp explained that sometimes women were unable to conceive despite no obvious impediment because God reserved 'to himself a prerogative of furthering and hindering Conception where he pleaseth' so that spouses might 'more earnestly pray' and 'be thankful' when he granted conception.[72] Infertility then was something that might be caused by imbalance or imperfection in female, male or both bodies together or by the will of God.

While medical texts saw it likely that men as well as women could be in need of treatment for infertility, the number of pages devoted to the actions men could take are dwarfed by the chapters on what women could and should do to get pregnant. Roeslin notes, for example, that childlessness 'may be

65 Sharp, *The Midwives Book Or the Whole Art of Midwifry Discovered*, 79.
66 Culpeper, *Directory for Midwives* (1675), 70 67 Barret, *A Companion for Midwives,* 60.
68 Nicholas Culpeper, *A Directory for Midwives, or, A Guide for Women* (London: 1662), 139.
69 Sharp, *The Midwives Book Or the Whole Art of Midwifry Discovered*, 81.
70 Oren-Magidor, *Infertility in Early Modern England*, 51.
71 Eucharius Roeslin, *Byrth of Mankynde*, Richard Jonas (ed.) (London: 1545), fol. LXXX.
72 Sharp, *The Midwives Book Or the Whole Art of Midwifry Discovered*, 78.

defect and lacke in the mother receavynge the seade' but equally there might be 'faulte and defecte in the sower & in the seade it self'.[73] And yet, despite paying lip service to the possibility that men could suffer from bodily imperfections that made conception impossible, he fails to elaborate on these faults and instead devotes two pages to outlining the ways in which the womb might be too hot, cold, humid or dry. There may be a 'defecte and lacke' in the sower of the seed, if it was too hot, too cold or too thin, something he hoped the wife might be able to feel within her. There were 'dyvers' other reasons but he found them unnecessary to rehearse. A test to discover whether husband or wife was provided (a standard test that involved urinating on a plant and observing growth) but this was only necessary 'If ye be desyrous to know'. Another test involved placing a strong perfume beneath a woman's legs. If she smelt the perfume, she was fertile. If not, she was barren.[74]

In this way, women's bodies were regularly implicated in diagnosing childlessness as well as remedying it: yet another secret they had to keep and another way in which managing fertility sat within expectations of gendered labour within the household. This was in keeping with expectations of domestic labour. Culpeper's *A Directory for Midwives* included a similar urine test to discover which party was responsible for 'Accidental Barrenness', but noted that although it was 'sometimes caused on the mans part', it was 'most commonly on the Womans'. This 'accidental' barrenness was 'either common too both man and wife . . . or else tis proper to the woman only'. If a man's diet and exercise were governed 'according to the rules', Culpeper saw no 'accidental cause of Barrenness in him'.[75] It was not worth the space, Culpeper suggested, to outline the ways men could combat barrenness because it was so rare, in contrast to the multitude of ways the womb, and women, could obstruct conception.

Barret too suggests at times that fertility could be a joint enterprise in which wives and husbands might both need medical treatment, and yet in others seems wholly uninterested in detailing what the remedies might be for men. His *Companion for Midwives* provides an extensive explanation of how the womb might hamper conception and how these blockages and imbalances might be cured through diet and conduct, and fails to elaborate further on the point that 'No conception can be without the entrance of the Yard, and the consequent emission of Seed.'[76] As we have seen, this was not always inevitable or easy for men. The conclusion of his chapter on 'the Causes of Barrennness and the means to prevent it' encouraged couples to find out whether the cause was in the 'Instruments of Generation', in seed or problems

[73] Raynalde, *Byrth of Mankynde*, fol. 71. [74] *Ibid.*, fols 83v–84r.
[75] Culpeper, *A Directory for Midwives* (1656), 73–74.
[76] Barret, *A Companion for Midwives*, 61.

in the womb, again suggesting that men as well as women would be worthy of medical treatment for infertility.[77] François Mauriceau did not even deign to discuss male impediments, for, as he explained, 'Barrenness proceeds oftner from Women than Men' and that for every impotent man, there were more than thirty barren women.[78] Hypocritically, Mauriceau's chapter on 'Conception, and the conditions necessary for it' argued that when the seed in either party did not have the 'requisit qualities', was scarce or not 'well enough conditioned', the resulting infant 'may be the less & weaker for it', undermining his previous argument that male health was of marginal importance in healthy conception.[79] John Pechey in his 1698 *The Compleat Midwife's Practice Enlarged* hinted at male responsibility by suggesting that barrenness came from a 'defect either of the Genitals, or of the blood' as well as menstrual blood, but later only acknowledged disproportion of seed (a condition that was about the compatibility of spouses rather than male health) and bewitching (something that was not strictly the fault of the man and could only be lifted through external means, rather than management of diet and conduct).[80] The preceding fifty-four pages of his guide addressed difficulties and diseases of the womb that compromised fertility.[81]

The ways medical authors side-stepped the specific details of male sexual dysfunction parallel the avoidance of family members of similar topics in correspondence. Childbearing guides were increasingly, at least in title, directed towards midwives and female readers, so one might explain the lack of interest in treatments directed towards men to the fact that they were not the chief audience. This alone, however, is not sufficient as an explanation for the selective coverage of treatment for childlessness. In many ways, the take-away from this literature is that it may have been perceived as largely unnecessary to discuss what men might be able to do, because even if their bodies were disordered, it was women who were meant to diagnose and secretly treat them anyway. There was a significant schism between the explanations and expectations of medical practice in these childbearing guides.

This relative silence is possibly one of the key reasons that historians have assumed early modern people always blamed women for infertility. Even though men could suffer from 'brewer's droop' or impotence, Olwen Hufton has observed that 'under most conditions' childlessness was seen as

[77] *Ibid.*, 63.
[78] François Mauriceau, *The Diseases of Women with Child, and in Child-bed: as also, the Best Directions How to Help Them in Natural and Unnatural Labours* (London: 1672), 2.
[79] *Ibid.*, 14.
[80] John Pechey, *The Compleat Midwife's Practice Enlarged in the Most Weighty and High Concernments of the Birth of Man* (London: 1698), 243.
[81] *Ibid.*, 188–242.

punishment for female sin or a consequence of her misconduct.[82] Likewise, Randolph Trumbach has characterized the 'legal and social assumptions' of the period as so geared towards female incapacity that early modern people would have failed to consider the possibility of male impediment.[83] Helen Berry and Elizabeth Foyster have provided an important corrective to this view, suggesting that historians' own 'deeply gendered ideas' have shaped their representation of the past.[84] They criticize Lawrence Stone, for example, who notably calls Elizabeth Pepys 'childless and lonely', and assumes the physical impediment to be hers alone, rather than her husband's, Samuel.[85] The explanation of childlessness and treatments that medical authors recommended may also have been a product of the increasingly intensive interest in the womb as a source of female malady over the seventeenth century.[86] Combined with an intellectual preoccupation with understanding the 'secrets' of generation, this meant that although medical practitioners and authors clearly understood men to be theoretically possible of suffering from a host of conditions that made it difficult to conceive or led to weak and unhealthy babies, including simply poor health, the details of these impediments sat uncomfortably alongside the prevailing model of gendered domestic labour in early modern England. A close reading of records of medical practice elucidates the ways in which treating childlessness and encouraging fertility was embedded within daily routines of care and therefore easily hidden or minimised within the written record.

Treating Barrenness

The explanations for the causes of barrenness therefore mean we need to look more critically at sources documenting medical practice, bearing in mind the considerable pressure on couples to conceive and the push to represent childlessness as more often originating in women's bodily and emotional faults. Added to this, the advice given in medical texts for fostering fertility was often similar to advice on living healthily and preventing disease, making evidence

[82] Olwen Hufton, *The Prospect before Her: A History of Women in Western Europe, 1500–1800*, vol. 1 (London: Fontana Press, 1997), 174.

[83] Randolph Trumbach, *The Rise of the Egalitarian Family: Aristocratic Kinship and Domestic Relations in Eighteenth-Century England*, Studies in Social Discontinuity (London: Academic Press Inc., 1978), 167.

[84] Helen Berry and Elizabeth Foyster, 'Childless Men in Early Modern England', in *The Family in Early Modern England*, ed. Helen Berry and Elizabeth Foyster (Cambridge: Cambridge University Press, 2007), 159.

[85] Lawrence Stone, *The Family, Sex and Marriage in England 1500–1800* (London: Weidenfeld & Nicolson, 1977), 552–559.

[86] Mary E. Fissell, 'The Womb Goes Bad', in *Vernacular Bodies: The Politics of Reproduction in Early Modern England* (Oxford: Oxford University Press, 2004), 53–89.

of families treating men for infertility potentially everywhere. Eating sparingly, exercising moderately and taking care to quash excessive anger or sadness were all standard pieces of advice in many early modern regimens, but also central to promoting fruitfulness in women *and* men. In this sense, although some people sought the help of medical practitioners or purchased proprietary medicines from those who touted them, most of the time, treating infertility was a domestic exercise and embedded within the quotidian tasks of domestic management. One of the reasons for this was because yet again this kind of work was often subsumed within the labour women took on in households to feed and heal members and made discretion easier. This often included seeking out the answers to the medical problems that women themselves or other members of the household were suffering from.

Many elite families kept manuscript volumes containing, most prominently, culinary and medical recipes but also a miscellanea of household accounts, lists and useful information.[87] Remedies to increase fertility and aid childbearing make up a substantial amount of these volumes, and these recipes sat side-by-side to recipes for pickling walnuts or salves for sore eyes. These receipt books were often compiled by multiple family members, sometimes across generations, combining recipes taken from printed texts with those acquired through friends, family and medical practitioners. Authorship and attribution of recipes was often fluid and complex.[88] Women had a particularly important role in compiling and maintaining these collections, but this was not an exclusively female domain.

A substantial proportion of remedies to increase fertility were directed towards women only. Frances Springatt's recipe book contained a remedy 'To help conseption and strengthen Nature' of red sage, king's roots and comfrey roots mixed with nutmeg and the yolk of a newly laid egg, taken morning and night.[89] A remedy in Johanna St John's book, for example, cleansed the 'Mother' (womb) and caused 'Conception', attributed to Dr Row.[90] The Boyle family book contained 'A Course of Physick much tried and approued to purge the Womb of superfluous humours and to promote Conception in Barren Women' as well as one to 'cause conception' and

87 Leong, 'Collecting Knowledge for the Family'; Elaine Leong, 'Making Medicines in the Early Modern Household', *Bulletin of the History of Medicine* 82, no. 1 (2008): 145–168.

88 Michelle DiMeo, 'Authorship and Medical Networks: Reading Attributions in Early Modern Manuscript Recipe Books', in *Reading and Writing Recipe Books, 1550–1800*, ed. Michelle DiMeo and Sara Pennell (Manchester: Manchester University Press, 2013), 25–46. She notes that 'A recipe may have originated with someone, but it could also be that the compiler received it from an unnamed intermediary or copied it from a friend's manuscript', 27.

89 Frances Springatt & others, 1686–1824, WL, MS 4683, fol. 92r.

90 Johanna St John, WL, MS 4338/82 (1680), fol. 209v.

another to 'Remedy Barrenness and promote the faculty of Generation'.[91] The latter included 'salt of mugworth', which would open the womb when 'shutt up, cleanseth the Same, Cheriseth the Seminal Vessells, Comforteth and Enliveneth the Womb & maketh it fit for Conception'.[92] Rebeckah Winche's recipe book included a four-part regimen to purge the 'wombe from all hurtfull or superfulus humers w[hi]ch hinder conception', including a potion, pills, an electuary and a wine to drink.[93] The papers of the Scottish Cunninghame Graham family contained a similar four-part regimen that a woman should take before she 'accompany her husband'.[94] Jane Jackson's book contained a remedy 'For the stone stomacke and backe and to make a woman conceaue with child',[95] and another to 'To keepe her conceauing' that promised that 'she shall not lose the seede'.[96] A further remedy to 'make a woman conceaue' served both to increase the likelihood of conception and as a test for pregnancy. Soaking hemlock in water and giving it to the woman in the morning 'and the same day she shalbe able to conceaue'. If she was pregnant, she would 'brooke that drincke soone after', meaning concoct or digest.[97] All these remedies were specifically for women, and more often than not concerned with cleansing the womb, a priority entirely in keeping with the increasing interest of medical writers.

The sex of the intended patient for these domestic remedies, however, was often left unspecified or vague, suggesting that it was perhaps simply that men were not being explicitly addressed in recipes in the same way women were. Two remedies in the Jerningham family recipe book, one to 'stir up' lust and another to 'causeth conception', did not specify whether they were for men, women or both.[98] Other recipes were specifically made to be useful for both husbands and wives. Springatt's aforementioned remedy to help conception, for example, included the instructions that 'man should take of it as well as the

[91] 'Boyle family recipe book, 1675–c.1710', WL, MS 1340, recipe 114, fol. 35v; recipe 127, fol. 39r; recipe 312 fol. 86r. Michelle DiMeo has suggested that instead of being compiled by Katherine Jones, Lady Ranelagh (1615–1691), there are roughly fifty individual authors named in the manuscript, most of which are members of the Howard or Orrery families, connecting the manuscript to Lady Ranelagh's sister-in-law, Margaret Howard, Countess of Orrery (1623–1683). See: Michelle DiMeo, 'Lady Katherine Ranelagh or Lady Margaret Orrery?: Reattributing Authorship for the Boyle Family Receipt Book. 2010 Prize for a Graduate Student Conference Presentation', *Early Modern Women: An Interdisciplinary Journal* 6 (2011): 269–270.

[92] 'Boyle family recipe book', MS 1340, recipe 312, fol. 86r.

[93] Rebeckah Winche, Receipt book c. 1666, FSL, V.b.366, pp. 67–69.

[94] 'Medical recipe for inducing conception', Papers of the Cunninghame Graham family of Ardoch, Dunbartonshire, National Records of Scotland, Edinburgh, GD22/3/817.

[95] Jane Jackson 'Recipe book, 1642', WL, MS 373, fol. 47r. [96] *Ibid.*, 83r. [97] *Ibid.*, 82v.

[98] Jerningham family recipe book, Staffordshire Record Office, Stafford, D641/3/H/3/1, 63 and 67.

woman'.[99] Occasionally, domestic recipe books also included instructions to reveal whether the husband or wife was primarily responsible for childlessness. Jackson's book contained a common test, reiterated in both Roeslin and Culpeper and many other books about generation, in which spouses urinated on kernels of barley in separate vessels and observed the growth.[100]

These remedies were so closely tied to everyday domestic routine that several of them were to be administered through sex. Remedies 'to help conception' in Thomas Brugis' medical notes stated that a concoction of darnell weed, grass, barley meal, 'mirth and franconise' ought to be taken 'before ye goe to bed'. An additional recipe to promote getting pregnant with a boy instructed the woman to 'eate mercurie an hearb common befor you lye to gather'.[101] In Jackson's book, one remedy instructed the user to anoint the man's 'yard' with a concoction before sex in order to further chances of conceiving. Another suggests that both the yard and the 'womans privitie alsoe' should be anointed. Then, the husband should simply 'deale with her; and shee shall conceaue'. Unlike other entries in Jackson's book, this series of recipes addresses men specifically. One recipe that involved mixing the brain of a crane with 'gramders greac' and 'fox greac' [grease], kept in a silver or gold vessel, included the instructions 'at what time thou wold haue knowledge [sex] annoynt therewith *thy* yard and shee shall conceaue'.[102] Perhaps such language cajoled men into imagining themselves as rectifying female fragility through their own virility – he saw himself as administering the treatment even if he was covertly the intended recipient. Or perhaps women could secrete these concoctions inside her prior to sex without ever having to make it explicit that a treatment was being used. Richard Napier recommended that Anne Throckmorton use a pessary that was to be 'to be put up wit[h] y[o]u' (or her husband's penis) when she and Sir Peter Temple were struggling to conceive in 1614. Whether Peter was suffering from problems that might also be assisted or solved by the pessary is left unsaid.[103] The consultations continued over the ensuing weeks, and indeed the following years.[104] Lady Hester, Anne's mother-in-law also visited on a further two occasions, asking whether Anne would 'live to have issue'.[105] These multiple medical encounters that involved family members always centred Anne's body as the cause of

99 Springatt & others, WL, MS 4683, fol. 92r.

100 Jackson, WL, MS 373, 121r. Uroscopy was an important medical tool in diagnosis more broadly during the period and physicians often consulted urine when diagnosing whether a woman was pregnant. Michael Stolberg argues that uroscopy was 'one of the most important practices in the history of Western medicine', Michael Stolberg, *Uroscopy in Early Modern Europe* (Farnham: Ashgate, 2015), 1.

101 Thomas Brugis, Medical treatise describing illnesses and remedies, formerly laid into 'Vade Mecum or a companion for a Chirurgion', HEH, HM 59539, fol. 2r [labelled as p. 231].

102 Jackson, WL, MS 373, fols 82v–83r. My emphasis.

103 CASE23669, CB.

104 CASE23700, CB.

105 CASE23708 and CASE23711, CB.

their sexual and generative difficulties as a couple. Not once was the potential of Peter being responsible for their difficulties explicitly mentioned. Presumably this was unnecessarily shameful when cures might be prescribed that cured husband and wife at the same time.

Indeed, male sexual health was often written about in ways that entirely disambiguated it from considerations of fertility. St John's book, for example, included a remedy from a 'Mr Freeman' that purported to 'strengthen a weak member', containing many of the same ingredients that were common in recipes to cleanse the womb and promote conception: red sage, comfry and fennel to be taken morning and night, hot, as a bath.[106] James Shrowl's recipe book contained a remedy 'To heale any Lame Member' in which the 'member' was bathed for half an hour, 'chaft' with an ointment of ruse, rosemary and salad oil and then wrapped in lambskin before bed.[107] Dame Mary Lister's household book contained 'An Excellente receite for the running of the reines & all paines and Consumptions of the back.'[108] Jackson similarly included several remedies for injured or afflicted yards. One for 'sweling of a man's yard' involved heating a piece of cotton in 'new butter' and laying 'it to the place as hott as the patient can suffer it[.] this will helpe him within 3 or 4 dressings'. Another more curious entry sought to assist 'one that is burnt with a harlott', which included putting powder on the sores. Others remedied a 'burnt yard', 'a sore yard', 'For ones yard scalded', 'For any member that is scald or burnt' and six others just titled 'Another'. The Jerningham family recipe book contained a recipe for the 'Excoriation of the yard'.[109] The results of such treatments were listed as to 'help' or to 'heale'. Conception, or even the strength of erection, is never mentioned, despite the fact it must obviously have been a concern. Undoubtedly, many of these treatments were primarily concerned with getting rid of the painful, and sometimes fatal, symptoms of venereal disease. The silence on the greater ramifications and the stakes for generation involved in a sore, swollen, burnt, excoriated yard is notable.

When medical practitioners were asked about childlessness, they were also inclined to believe it was women that needed medical treatment. Forman and Napier often told the women who asked them about childlessness that that their wombs were insufficiently cleansed, they suffered from emotional distress or they did not love their husbands enough to be fruitful. Antonia Yersley, who asked Forman whether she would have any more children, was told that she was already pregnant, but because she was excessively fretful 'the child will

[106] Johanna St John, WL, MS4338, fol. 179r.
[107] James Shrowl, 1625–c.1750, WL, MS 749, unfoliated.
[108] Dame Mary Lister, 'Household Book, 1623–1635', Brotherton Library, University of Leeds, MS 621, 65.
[109] Jerningham family, Staffordshire Record Office, D641/3/H/3/1, fol. 76r.

hardly prove'.[110] Forman recorded that Susan van Hulste, thirty-three, who had asked about disease and whether she would have any children, had not had her periods 'in order', had 'moch pain in the head, reins, side, shoulders, heart', blood in her 'water' and 'sweas [sways] often tymes in her body'.[111] Lady Luce Oliver sent her urine. She had been married before, without issue, and her new husband, Napier noted, had had two children before. The problem was melancholy and windy humours in her womb.[112]

It was not completely unprecedented, however, for wives to be told it was their husbands who suffered from a physiological impediment that was stopping them from conceiving or having sufficient healthy children in the casebooks. When Margery Gudging, forty-four, asked 'whe[the]r she shall have Any child or noe', the judgement was that she would not have any children that survived but would become pregnant again at Michaelmas. The fault, Forman recorded, 'is in the man'.[113] Mary Goddard, married two years, asked the same question, but added that she wanted to know the cause of her childlessness. Again, the fault was primarily her husband's. Her womb was dry and her courses not 'well', but importantly her husband was also dry.[114] Ann Timbock, thirty-one, was told that although she would conceive twice in the future, it would not be by her husband because 'her husband & nature doth not Agree with her'. The 'greatest faulte', Forman recorded, 'is in the man' and she would have a child by someone else.[115] Men could be responsible not just for hampering conception but also poor procreative outcomes more broadly. When someone asked whether Jean Wintch had ever been pregnant in the past and how many children she would have, Forman judged that she would conceive four times but none of them 'will hardly live or come to good' and would have 'much strife' because of their father. They 'shall be gentle and mild in word but much embred of base people and evil in body'.[116] Medical practitioners took the possibility of male physiological infertility seriously, and although this was often not mentioned explicitly, they were often involved directly or indirectly in the cures administered, in a way that indicates they were catering to families at the stories they wanted to be able to tell about themselves and their fruitfulness at a later time.

In the same way as the remedies in recipe books for weak, sore or burnt yards evaded discussing fertility directly, so too did casebooks in discussing male genital problems. In January 1600, Napier noted that Richard Foster suffered from the sensation of something running like blood 'up into his joints

[110] CASE3399, CB. [111] CASE1862, CB. [112] CASE41562, CB.
[113] CASE3449, CB. [114] CASE6280, CB.
[115] CASE6494. Another shorter case is recorded for the same date and time for Ann Tymcok, CASE6490, CB.
[116] CASE5493, CB.

into his arms and belly with a pricking and into his head and then his eyes run and in the reins of his back and out of his yard matter white runneth', likely suffering from 'running of the reanes'.[117] Mr Ketteridge of Newport was 'troubled with the gonorrhea (sic) whose stones are exceeding hard for 3 weeks in great pain'.[118] Edward Plummer, forty- or fifty-years-old, had much pain in his member 'at the end of making water it prickes & throbs with extream payne'. His face and hands had swelled and he could barely keep anything down. He feared it was an ulcer 'for it is as matter that commeth from him & maketh it often', four times an hour to be precise, and was hindering his sleep.[119] In the casebook of the Derbyshire surgeon Joseph Binns, Mr Richardas, suffering from 'much payne in his yarde betwixte glans & prapulis', was diagnosed with gangrene.[120] Another case involved 'The Gardners man' who had a 'great tumor in all his yarde harde w[i]th Inflamation'.[121]

In all of these cases, practitioners and patients appeared comfortable discussing problems with penises, but shied away from discussing impotence and weak seed. Not a single case in Napier and Forman's casbeooks in which men between the ages of fifteen and fifty suffered from problems with their genitalia mentions fertility explicitly (an age group where one would imagine fertility was a concern). There are a mere four cases in the whole corpus that explicitly address failure to achieve or maintain an erection. Mr Gregory was impotent 'sine erectione',[122] Mr Piland's erections were not strong enough,[123] and Napier noted that Mr Paulin did not experience strong erections.[124] Mr Cooke asked on behalf of Richard Powell for 'some thing to thicken his seed' because he was troubled with gonorrhoea, a generic term for genital discharge and urinary problems. He also could not sleep and 'wanteth virility & erection'.[125] Aside from the brief mention of seed, these cases do not expand to discuss the ramifications of these difficulties for conception. This is surprising when we consider the frequency with which fertility is mentioned in any consultations with women.

Added to this, in all of Forman and Napier's cases that have been tagged in the database as being about fertility, there are only two men who approached the practitioners themselves to ask about their own bodies. Napier's cousin, George Kimpton, could 'beget no child' and was noted to have a 'very cold complexion', and very unusually his wife was not mentioned.[126] Lawrence Manlye asked whether he could have children, but in this particular case,

[117] CASE12962, CB. [118] CASE23538, CB. [119] CASE5092, CB.
[120] Joseph Binns, 'Medical Casebook, 1633–63', BL, Sloane MS 153, 20 July [unknown year], fol. 170v.
[121] *Ibid.*, 8 April [unknown year], fol. 171r. [122] CASE62699, CB. [123] CASE62793, CB.
[124] CASE62793, CB. [125] CASE55490, CB. [126] CASE41297, CB.

Napier did not include a judgement, and it is unclear whether he was even married.[127] In one instance, a married couple consulted the astrologers together. Dr Shephard of London and Sarah his wife visited Napier but were specifically requesting 'physick' for *Sarah* to 'cause fruitfulness'.[128] Goodman Barro[w] asked 'to take some thing for to become fruitfull' for his wife, Charity. They had been married for seven years and still not had a baby. He was turned away and advised to come back a few months later.[129] What we learn from this is not that fertility was not a shared enterprise, but rather the available scripts were so skewed towards talking about women's bodily impediments that even consultations involving both husbands and wives were written about in a way that stressed maternal responsibility.

Lisa W. Smith has suggested that examples of treating male sexual problems are scarce less because early modern people assumed women were always responsible for childlessness and more because of a prevailing view that male generative problems were irreparable. She notes that male fertility was dependent on healthy seed, which required abstinence from nocturnal pollutions, excessive or extra-marital sex, which was difficult to identify and tough to control.[130] Indeed, this goes some way to explaining the absences in these sources, although as we have seen, women's fertility was also dependent on their conduct and living healthily, and yet they received a litany of advice. Furthermore, both recipes in domestic books and case notes about male genital problems suggest at least a willingness to consider curing adjacent conditions that would affect male sexual performance. Edward Plummer, for example, was prescribed a clyster and then a 'dry dyet' for swelling in his face and hands and for pain and discharge from his penis in 1620.[131] He had had recurrent problems since 1601 when Napier noted he had gonorrhoea.[132] In surgical treatises, practitioners proudly recalled their patients' ability to have children after surgery as proof of their skill – more evidence that it was not necessarily that these problems were thought to be incurable.[133] This points to the ways in which although early modern people fully understood that conception required women *and* men to be attentive to their own health, there were very different ways of writing about this bodily experience.

Given fertility was interwoven into preventative healthcare and the work of feeding, healing and caring for family members, evidence for men taking treatment might be hidden behind generic medicines that strengthened, enlivened, warmed, cooled or increased appetite. It is important to remember

[127] CASE28583, CB. [128] CASE50159, CB. [129] CASE21729.
[130] Lisa W. Smith, 'Imagining Women's Fertility before Technology', *Journal of Medical Humanities* 31 (2010): 77.
[131] CASE50292. [132] See CASE18771.
[133] Jennifer Evans, '"They Are Called Imperfect Men": Male Infertility and Sexual Health in Early Modern England', *Social History of Medicine* 29, no. 1 (2016): 331.

that patients and practitioners co-created records of medical practice, and therefore we cannot be sure whether it was a practitioner, patient or both who were uncomfortable about writing about male infertility in blatant terms. Did thirty-two-year-old Roger Jeorge of Croydon, who was recorded as having 'Diz', or disease and was judged to be 'full of collor [choler] in the stomacke & belly & head syde', actually come because he was concerned about childlessness?[134] Other generic remedies like one in Lister's book 'ffor to make a man haue an appetite for his meate', might have been used for multiple reasons – sometimes for increasing appetite and strength, and at other times to increase libido and strength of erection.[135] A remedy that purported to kill 'heate within a man' when 'hee goeth to bedd' might have served multiple purposes.[136] It could be to facilitate recovery from disease caused by excessive heat, or to rectify a humoral imbalance between spouses. Could a corollary of a 'Cooling Purge' or a remedy to 'comfort the stomack & expel urine' used to promote health be the ability to produce lusty infants?[137]

When commercial drugs became available towards the end of the seventeenth century, they were often marketed as generically increasing bodily health but the proof of their efficacy was often that the patient went on to have children.[138] This again meant that people could take a medicine intended to increase fertility without advertising the fact. By having a broad use, such drugs not only increased their potential market but further entrenched the idea that living well led to fruitfulness.[139] Folded into Blanch Hooker's personal recipe book was a printed advertisement for a 'Prolifick Elixir' that promised to be the 'highest, richest and most powerful Cordial in Nature' and the 'only true and infallible Cure for Barrenness in Women and Impotency in Men in the

[134] CASE14, CB.

[135] Dame Mary Lister, Household Book 1623-1635, Brotherton Library Leeds, MS 621, p. 130. For the connections between food and lust see: Jennifer Evans, 'Provoking lust and promoting conception', in 'Provoking lust and promoting conception', *Aphrodisiacs, Fertility and Medicine in Early Modern Engalnd* (2014), pp. 87–130; Laura Giannetti, 'Of Eels and Pears: A Sixteenth-Century Debate on Taste, Temperance, and the Pleasures of the Senses', in *Religion and the Senses in Early Modern Europe*, 26 (Leiden, 2012), pp. 289–305.

[136] WL, MS 373, fol. 54r.

[137] Recipe book c. 1651-1700, once in the possession of Gertrude Holcroft, Brotherton Library, Leeds, MS 687, fol. 40r and fol. 40v. See also: Leah Astbury, 'Eat, Sleep, Lust, Repeat: Bedtime Routine, Health and Herbals in Early Modern England', *Cultural & Social History* 21, 2 (2024): 141-162.

[138] Mark S. R. Jenner and Patrick Wallis, 'The Medical Marketplace', in *Medicine and the Market in England and Its Colonies, c. 1450-c.1850*, ed. Mark S. R. Jenner and Patrick Wallis (Basingstoke and New York: Palgrave Macmillan, 2007), 1-23.; D. B. Haycock and Patrick Wallis, eds., 'Quackery and Commerce in Seventeenth-Century London: The Proprietary Medicine Business of Anthony Daffy', *Medical History* Supplement 25 (2005): 1-36.

[139] Jennifer Evans observes that medical handbills similarly advertised themselves as useful for barrenness in men and women. See: Evans, '"They Are Called Imperfect Men"', 13.

Universe', recommended by 'Thousands'.[140] Lady Ann Fanshawe's recipe book similarly contained an advertisement for 'Dr Anderon's, or, The Famous Scots Pills' that treated 'migrains, pains in the head, stomach or bellies of men, deafnes, weak or Blear'd Eyes' and barrenness. The pills could assist 'all Ages, Seasons and Hours' by men, women, children and even women who were pregnant.[141] One of the most popular and famous of such medicines was Daffy's Elixir, described as a 'most excellent preservative of Man-kind', which reduced all 'Extreams unto an equal Temper'.[142] Helping to balance humours, the medicine promised to remove all plethora of ills. Daffy's pamphlet told readers the medicine could cure stone and gravel in the reins; languishing and melancholy; and surfeits and the fits of the mother and spleen – all, as we have seen, linked to conception for men and women. It promised to cure green sickness, improve the colour of the face and smell of one's breath and make the body generally 'lusty'. It was further useful for '*Wet Nurses*, cleansing their *bloud,* and rendering their *Milk* wholsom[e] and *nutritive* to the sucking Babe'. '*Finally*', the medicine 'exalts the *Genderative virtue,* and restores *Radical Moisture,* cleansing and strengthening the Seminal vessels in both Sexes'. Daffy's Elixir was one of several proprietary medicines that made the transition from medical advertising and print into manuscript culture. Notably, Anne de Lisle and Letitia Mytton's collections contain the remedy.[143] These drugs suggest that efforts to conceive and increase fertility sat easily within other daily practices of procuring humoral balance, and the methodological difficulties of finding evidence of treatment when families were so keen not to mention it or actively conceal traces of these practices.

Looking at records of medical practice reveals that managing fertility was something that families sought not to broadcast far and wide, owing to the deep embarrassment that childlessness brought. Family correspondence was littered with gossip about who had conceived and when, we find that mothers went to medical appointments with their children, and families also collectively systematised knowledge about fertility in their recipe books. Despite this, there are notable silences in this record. Infertility was uncomfortable for families in a multitude of ways. It raised the possibility that, like Mary Rich later thought, God would prevent the perpetuation of the family and its name.

140 Blanch Hooker, 'Recipe book, 1690', Bedfordshire and Luton Archives and Record Service, Bedford, GY7/2, inside cover.

141 Lady Ann Fanshawe, 'Recipe book, 1625–1680', WL, MS 7113, fol. 213v.

142 Anthony Daffy, *Elixir Salutis: The Choise Drink of Health* (London, 1674), transcribed in D. B. Haycock and Patrick Wallis, eds., 'Daffy's Elixir Pamphlet', *Medical History* Supplement 25 (2005): 38–42.

143 Elaine Leong and Sara Pennell, 'Recipe Collections and the Currency of Medical Knowledge in the Early Modern "Medical Marketplace"', in *Medicine and the Market in England and Its Colonies, c. 1450–c. 1850*, ed. Mark S. R. Jenner and Patrick Wallis (Basingstoke: Palgrave, 2007), 147. See Wellcome MS 3295, fol. 46r and MS 3731, fol. 41.

Another explanation was the couple was a bad match. Even more damning and troubling was that the husband had weak seed or suffered from impotence. All of these separate explanations brought with them the threat of domestic disorder and public shame for the family. It is no surprise then that early modern people sought to represent women and their wombs as the reason for slow conception before any other explanation and the reason why they were keen to employ treatments that did not make male frailty too obvious.

Conclusion

Conception was meant to be quick and easy. When getting pregnant took a long time, did not happen or couples had sickly infants, it was not just spouses that were disappointed but the family and community around them lamented too. When the fifth Earl of Dorset's wife, Frances, was pregnant in 1655, the Earl of Northampton praised her 'vertuous qualitie of Multiplying the world'.[144] For elite families, this is exactly what generation promised: the perpetuation of their world and privilege. Making babies was inimical to personal and familial reputation, to the practice of piety, a source of gossip, and the mechanism of inheritance and lineage and thus sat at the apex of the concerns of individuals, communities, families, the state and Church.

A historian examining the paperwork that families kept alongside printed conduct and medical literature and casebooks might be inclined to agree with the chorus of medical authors that *all* early modern men and women wanted to have lots of children. The lifecycle of meeting, courting, marrying and conceiving that Marsh's *Ten Pleasures* claimed was universal left no space for those who were equivocal getting pregnant. Getting pregnant out of wedlock could lead to complete isolation from community, family and employment as well as prosecution for women.[145] In the same way as godliness was thought to beget further blessings, sin was thought to lead to more sin. Unmarried mothers were common characters in sensationalist pamphlets such as the 1614 *Deeds Against Nature*, which relayed the attempts of a young woman, Martha Scambler, to make 'away with the fru[i]t of her own womb', first through an unsuccessful abortion and then by delivering the baby into the privy, or toilet, and neglecting it.[146] A law in 1624 made unmarried mothers automatically guilty and likely to be hanged if the body of an infant was found and they had not acknowledged the pregnancy, even if they claimed to have

144 Earl of Northampton to Earl of Dorset, 12 January 1656, KHLC, U269/C86/3.
145 Gowing, 'Secret Births and Infanticide in Seventeenth-Century England'.
146 *Deeds Against Nature, and Monsters By Kinde Tried at the Goale Deliuerie of Newgate, at the Sessions of the Old Bailey, the 18. And 19. Of July last, 1614* (London: 1614).

suffered from a miscarriage or the child had been stillborn.[147] As a result, we know much more about these women than we do about married and wealthier women who sought to terminate pregnancies. Some historians have suggested that remedies in printed and manuscript recipe books that provoked the 'resumption' of menstruation may have been used covertly as abortifacients.[148] But while this information would no doubt have been available to women, it is impossible to estimate the frequency with which people made and took these cures, let alone the intended use. Menstruating regularly was central to women's health in the period,[149] and thus, resuming one's 'flowers' may have been simply a way to increase overall health.[150] As we have seen with fertility, the boundaries between regimen, health and fruitfulness were hazy in the period, often deliberately so.

Glimpses of married couples not welcoming conception are very difficult to find because expressing regret for God's doing was liturgically and socially condemned, and therefore not likely to have been written about. Alice Thornton reflected after the birth of her eighth child, Joyce, in 1665, that the joy of being pregnant was 'accompanied with thorny Caires & troubles, &

147 For a discussion of infanticide and illegitimate motherhood, see: Catherine Damme, 'Infanticide: The Worth of an Infant under Law', *Medical History* 22 (1978): 1–24; Gowing, 'Secret Births and Infanticide in Seventeenth-Century England'; Laura Gowing, *Common Bodies: Women, Touch and Power in Seventeenth-Century England* (New Haven, CT: Yale University Press, 2003); Peter Charles Hoffer and N. E. H. Hull, *Murdering Mothers: Infanticide in England and New England 1550–1800* (New York, 1984); Keith Wrightson, 'Infanticide in Earlier Seventeenth-Century England', *Local Population Studies* 15 (1975): 10–22.

148 Peter Biller, 'Birth-Control in the West in the Thirteenth and Early Fourteenth Centuries', *Past & Present* 94, no. 1 (1982): 3–26; Tim Hitchcock, *English Sexualities, 1700–1800*, Social History in Perspective (New York: Macmillan Education, 1997); Angus McLaren, '"Barrenness against Nature": Recourse to Abortion in Pre-Industrial England', *The Journal of Sex Research* 17, no. 3 (1981): 224–237; Angus McLaren, *Reproductive Rituals: The Perception of Fertility in England from the Sixteeth Century to the Nineteenth Century* (New York, 1984); Roy Porter, *Health for Sale* (Manchester: Manchester University Press, 1989), 148; John M. Riddle, 'Oral Contraceptives and Early Term Abortifacients during Classical Antiquity and the Middle Ages', *Past & Present* 132, no. 1 (1991): 4–32.

149 Wendy D. Churchill, *Female Patients in Early Modern Britain: Gender, Diagnosis, and Treatment* (Farnham: Ashgate, 2012); Patricia Crawford, 'Attitudes to Menstruation in Seventeenth-Century England', *Past & Present* 91, no. 1 (1981): 47–73; Jennifer Evans, '"Gentle Purges Corrected with Hot Spices, Whether They Work or Not, Do Vehemently Provoke Venery": Menstrual Provocation and Procreation in Early Modern England', *Social History of Medicine* 25, no. 1 (2012): 2–19; Cathy McClive, *Menstruation and Procreation in Early Modern France* (London: Routledge, 2015); Gianna Pomata, 'Menstruating Men: Similarity and Difference of the Sexes in Early Modern Medicine', in *Generation and Degeneration: Tropes of Reproduction in Literature and History from Antiquity to Early Modern Europe*, ed. Valeria Finucci and Kevin Brownlee (Durham, NC: Duke University Press, 2001), 109–152.

150 Jennifer Evans makes the argument that these remedies were designed to increase fertility rather than inhibit: Evans, '"Gentle Purges Corrected with Hot Spices, Whether They Work or Not, Do Vehemently Provoke Venery"'.

more to me then others' because she was worried she would not survive the delivery.[151] Mary Rich, the Countess of Warwick, bore two children, a boy and a girl, in the two years after getting married to Charles Rich but decided not to have any more children. Their daughter Elizabeth died when she was fifteen months old and their son, Charles died when she was thirty-eight in 1647, ushering an intensification of her puritan faith.[152] Mary thought that the death of her children and lack of an heir was 'justice' for their ungratefulness in not wanting any more children.[153] She explained her reticence to have more children as being provoked by 'great vanety' and a 'proude opinion'. Her husband was worried they would be unable to afford to care for a big brood.

The normative model in which a man and woman got married, immediately got pregnant and had a household of healthy, beautiful children that continued the family name, religion and inheritance rarely fit with the reality of the ambiguity and difficulty of fertility. In their paperwork, family members were keen to represent themselves as perpetually fruitful in all manner of ways that served political, spiritual and social hierarchies and to cement their own place as a 'branch' on the 'vine', as Hooke termed it. Making the perpetuation of the family line seem stable and continuous despite missteps and absences relied not only narrativising to flatten these embarrassing procreative lulls but also husbands and wives taking on substantial medical work. Whilst women consulting practitioners, self-diagnosing, seeking advice, moderating their conduct and taking medicines sat comfortably alongside a model of sacrificial motherhood, it jarred with prevailing ideals of masculinity. Virility ought not to be forced, cajoled or manufactured.

151 Alice Thornton, BL, Add MS 88897/2, 208.
152 Mary Rich [née Boyle], Countess of Warwick (1648–1678), Sara H. Mendelson, https://doi.org/10.1093/ref:odnb/23487, 23 September 2004, ODNB, last accessed 5/10/2018.
153 Rich, 'Some Specialities', BL, Add MS 27357, fols 33v–34v.

2 Pregnancy, Record-Keeping and Respectability

The wife in A. Marsh's parody of the emerging middling sort in *The Ten Pleasures of Marriage* (1682) conceives only months after their wedding. After she has shamefully prattled to her neighbours, a number of medical practitioners and others about her 'barrenness', she insists on buying a host of expensive treatments. It is only a matter of days before she proudly tells her husband that she is pregnant. He joyfully wrote 'the first day of her reckoning', or due date, in his almanac, a form of pre-printed astrological diary popular in the period,[1] 'as if it were printed with a red Letter!' The husband believes himself to be a 'noble Champion' who has behaved himself 'so gallantly' by impregnating her that he would 'continne now to reap the further conquests of your [his] honour'. His almanac publicly proclaims his virility and mastery over his domestic dominion.[2] In this example, the tension between cultural expectations of honourable and suitable conduct in sharing parts of pregnancy beyond the immediate household unit, and what a family might prefer to keep out of almanacs and other paperwork is rendered visible and is even mocked.

As Chapter 1 has shown, women were encouraged to keep the details of their husband's sexual performance and fertility treatment secret – the wife here shamefully tells all and sundry. The husband's desire to inscribe his wife's conception and reckoning so prominently in his almanac (and his suggestion that this victory would beget further fruitfulness) point to the parts of generation people were keen to show off and the desirability of being able to make specific predictions. A pious and chaste woman would be so attentive to any subtle bodily signs as to know she was pregnant quickly. Like fertility, this also rested on women maintaining a heightened awareness of their body and health throughout pregnancy in ways that were seen to reflect domestic piety

[1] See: Bernard Capp, *Astrology and the Popular Press: English Almanacs 1500–1800* (London: Faber and Faber, 1979); Louise Hill Curth, *English Almanacs, Astrology and Popular Medicine, 1550–1700* (Manchester: Manchester University Press, 2007); Lauren Kassell, 'Almanacs and Prognostications', in *The Oxford History of Popular Print Culture: Cheap Print in Britain and Ireland to 1660*, vol. 1 (Oxford: Oxford University Press, 2011), 431–442.

[2] A. Marsh, *The Ten Pleasures of Marriage Relating all the Delights and Contentments that are Mask'd Under the Bands of Matrimony* (London, 1682), 85–86.

and order more widely. Records of conception and reckoning in family paperwork, unlike the hidden evidence of treatment for infertility, fulfilled a wider self-examining imperative that reformers thought that families ought to practice individually and collectively. They also provided tangible evidence of marital fidelity and helped to imagine the unborn baby as part of the family.

Ten years earlier, Jane Sharp chastised young mothers-to-be in her midwifery guide, especially those carrying their first baby, because not one out of twenty kept a 'just account' of their bodies, including potential pregnancy and their menstrual cycle. This lack of attention and lax record-keeping caused them to be 'so ignorant commonly, that they cannot tell whether they have conceived or not'.[3] Nicholas Culpeper too criticised 'Some women' who 'do not know when they are conceived with Child'.[4] William Sermon fretted about the 'many women' who were 'foolishly perswaded that they were not with child' and their infants perished 'through indirect means', presumably poor diet and improper conduct, and when delivered were only 'five or six moneths old' (or at a gestational age of five or six months).[5] Knowing one was pregnant early and reliably was represented by medical authors as important in ensuring one's baby was born healthy. In the popular family conduct manual *Of Domesticall Duties* (1622), William Gouge thought that as soon as a woman 'perceiveth a childe to be conceived in her wombe', she 'ought to have an especiall care therof, that (so much as in her lieth) the childe may be safely brought forth'. The first part of the 'childs infancie' was in the womb. To neglect caring for it during this early period was just as morally corrupt as disregarding its welfare once it was born.[6] Writing about conception and pregnancy within households and families facilitated the performance of the preventative healthcare that medical authors expected: pregnant women would be able to promptly moderate their diet and avoid aggressive medicines so as to avoid miscarriage or other poor procreative outcomes, and were therefore represented as a kind of medical tool in their own right. Record-keeping, however, was, as the *The Ten Pleasures of Marriage* suggests, just a way that families sought to impose order and control on a largely unknowable and unpredictable process.

Historians have emphasised that uncertainty was an important feature of being pregnant prior to modern diagnostic testing.[7] The plethora of records

[3] Jane Sharp, *The Midwives Book Or the Whole Art of Midwifry Discovered*, ed. Elaine Hobby, Women Writers in English 1350–1850 (Oxford: Oxford University Press, 1999), 81, 82.

[4] Nicholas Culpeper, *A Directory for Midwives, or, A Guide for Women* (London, 1675), 100.

[5] William Sermon, *The Ladies Companion, or, The English Midwife* (London, 1671), 17.

[6] William Gouge, *Of Domesticall Duties Eight Treatises* (London: 1622), 505.

[7] Barbara Duden, *The Woman beneath the Skin: A Doctor's Patients in Eighteenth-Century Germany*, trans. Thomas Dunlap (Cambridge, MA: Harvard University Press, 1991); Laura Gowing, 'Secret Births and Infanticide in Seventeenth-Century England', *Past & Present*, no. 156 (1997): 87–115; Mark Jackson, *New-Born Child Murder: Women, Illegitimacy and the Courts in Eighteenth-Century England* (Manchester: Manchester University Press, 1996).

revealed in this chapter and the emphasis on smoothing out moments in which there was debate or confusion about whether a woman was pregnant or when she would deliver support this finding. Cathy McClive, for example, has described how even medical experts in eighteenth-century courts in France were unable to ascertain whether women who 'plead the belly' in order to avoid execution were genuinely pregnant. She notes that ambiguity about whether or not a woman was pregnant was not just a 'socially-constructed guise employed by unmarried women' but a 'medical and physical reality experienced by early modern women'.[8] Laura Gowing has noted that although quickening, the first movement of the child, might be a decisive sign of pregnancy for some women, others felt unsure until they went into labour. Uncertainty, Suzanne Bell and Mary E. Fissell have suggested, was not unique to childbearing in the early modern period but has persisted and continues to persist in different communities and situations when it is productive for gestating people.[9] This ambiguity, like the vagueness with which individuals wrote about fertility treatments, could be advantageous. The ambiguity of pregnancy could be useful for some women – if conceiving was undesirable or if they needed more time to make the pregnancy appear legitimate – and anxiety-provoking for others, who wanted to impose order and coherence on the experience. By subjecting the body to the same rigour that early modern people were increasingly turning to their lives, faith, household expenditure and financial bookkeeping, the 'accounts' that middling and elite families kept of pregnant or potentially pregnant bodies sought to inscribe legitimacy in a way that could not be scrubbed out by time or forgetfulness.

This chapter takes instruction from scholarship on family history and the nature of memory. Families created and continue to create archives that grant legitimacy and authenticity to certain individuals and invisibility to others.[10] Maurice Halbwachs, a sociologist, thus notes that memories are deemed important and hang together as a narrative less because they are events that happened in succession but more because they serve a function in furthering a certain idea or framework.[11] This is what Katie Barclay and Nina Javette Koefoed have called 'familial memory work'.[12] Keeping records of births, deaths and experiences with a view of constructing family history was work that women were

[8] Laura Gowing, *Common Bodies: Women, Touch and Power in Seventeenth-Century England* (New Haven, CT: Yale University Press, 2003), 113.

[9] Suzanne O. Bell and Mary E. Fissell, 'A Little Bit Pregnant? Productive Ambiguity and Fertility Research', *Population and Development Review* 47, no. 2 (2021): 505–526.

[10] Anna Woodham et al., 'We Are What We Keep: The "Family Archive", Identity and Public/Private Heritage', *Heritage & Society* 10, no. 3 (2017): 203–220.

[11] Maurice Halbwachs, *On Collective Memory*, trans. L Coser (Chicago: University of Chicago Press, 1992), 52.

[12] Katie Barclay and Nina Javette Koefoed, 'Family, Memory, and Identity: An Introduction', *Journal of Family History* 46, no. 1 (2021): 8.

particularly involved in, although as we shall see, men were avid compilers of this information too.[13] These interests intersect with the historiography of paper technology and the history of knowledge. Practices of collecting and systematising knowledge was closely linked to scientific endeavours in this period, and thus by collecting what might seem like everyday prosaic information about bodies and routine, early modern individuals were participating in a wider intellectual culture of record-keeping.[14] The records families kept, the pieces of paper they preserved and which memories made it into longer prose accounts of the family's life was not mere coincidence but because families put effort into making these pieces part of a longer trajectory and story. By being pregnant and creating matching accounts, couples and families were literally and figuratively making the family. This chapter follows in the same historiographic impulse to understand the imperatives that lead families to keep certain kinds of records and discard or ignore others.[15] Childbearing thus sat at the heart of the creation of familial identity as well as the daily routine of the household.

Announcing Pregnancy

The same ambiguity around the signs of pregnancy that allowed impoverished and unmarried women to tell courts that their bodies swelled fruitlessly, drove elite women to interpret non-specific symptoms into evidence that they were pregnant within months of conception. This process might be characterised as less one of discovery and more of wilfully deciding to read certain bodily signs as indicative of conception. Thus, in 1608 Anne, countess of Arundel, wrote to her daughter-in-law, Mary Talbot, the countess of Shrewsbury, reporting that Mary's daughter, Althea, was pregnant and in eager expectation of her quickening 'which I think will be about three weeks or a month'.[16] Anna Busbridge of a prominent Sussex family told her daughter, Mary, that she was feeling better in her pregnancy 'since my quicking' in 1651 (the first moment that a foetus moved).[17] The writer John Evelyn noted in his diary in early

13 Katharine Hodgkin, 'Women, Memory and Family History in Seventeenth-Century England', in *Memory before Modernity: Practices of Memory in Early Modern Europe*, ed. Ericka Kuijpers et al. (Leiden: Brill, 2013), 297–313.

14 Lorraine Daston, 'The Sciences of the Archive', *Osiris* 27, no. 1 (2012): 156–187; Elaine Leong, 'Writing the Family Archive: Recipes and the Paperwork of Kinship', in *Recipes and Everyday Knowledge: Medicine, Science, and the Household in Early Modern England* (Chicago: University of Chicago Press, 2018), 124–146.

15 Alexandra Walsham, 'The Social History of the Archive: Record-Keeping in Early Modern Europe', *Past & Present* 230, no. 11 (2016): 9–48.

16 Anne, countess of Arundel, to Countess of Shrewsbury, 3 March 1608, Lambeth Palace Library, London, MS 3205, fol. 141.

17 Anna Busbridge to Mary Busbridge, 18 August 1651, East Sussex Record Office, Brighton, Correspondence of the Roberts family, the Temple family, the Busbridge family, the Farnden family and other correspondence, DUN 51/62.

May 1652 that he had received word his wife, Mary, was pregnant and then several days later that she was 'quick'.[18] She gave birth on 24 August. Assuming she carried her pregnancy to term, she discovered and shared her discovery approximately six months after conception. With their second child, she was even swifter. Evelyn recorded she was 'quick' with child on 18 May 1653, when she was around four months pregnant.[19] Alice Thornton noted in her spiritual meditations that she had a particularly challenging first 'quarter' of her pregnancy, before she mentioned feeling the child move.[20] During her second pregnancy, she wrote that she could feel the infant move eleven weeks after conception, but she already knew herself to be pregnant prior to this point.[21] Margaret, Countess of Wemyss, wrote to her daughter, asking her to describe 'how you feell little devil stur', months after her pregnancy had been announced, indicating she knew and shared her suspicions with family members before quickening.[22] It is no wonder, given the intensity of correspondence asking women if they were pregnant discussed in Chapter 1, that women would have been keen to put fears and anxieties to rest by announcing they were pregnant.

In doing so, these women were framing their accounts in relation to the dominant ideal model of pious maternity set out in childbearing guides and other material that assumed married women who were relatively chaste would experience such a transformation in their physical selves that it would be obvious they were pregnant. Women's bodies were meant to feel, sound and look different after conception. This made it even more doubtful that unmarried women who said they had been unaware they were with child were telling the truth in courts. Thomas Chamberlayne described in *The Complete Midwife's Practice Enlarged* (1680) how immediately after 'she hath had the company of her Husband' she would start to experience 'signs of Conception' that were 'certain and apparent', or at least they should be. If 'hath received more content' or pleasure 'than ordinary', this was indicative.[23] Sharp described how after the man had 'cast his seed' into the womb, if she had conceived, the woman would feel 'the womb shut close, and a shivering or trembling to run through every part of her body'.[24] James Wolveridge similarly described the sensation of the womb shutting 'up the seed for

[18] John Evelyn, 7 May 1652, *Diary of John Evelyn: Vol 3: Kalendarium, 1650–1672*, ed. E. S. de Beer (Oxford: Oxford University Press, 1955), 65.

[19] *Ibid.*, 11 October 1653, 89.

[20] Alice Thornton, BL, Add MS 88897/1, 127.

[21] *Ibid.*, 133–135.

[22] Margaret, countess of Wemyss, to Anne, countess of Leven, 23 November 1695, GD26/13/401/23, National Records of Scotland, Edinburgh.

[23] Thomas Chamberlayne, *The Complete Midwife's Practice Enlarged, In the most weighty and high concernments of the Birth of Man Containing a perfect Directory, or Rules for Midwives and Nurses* (London: 1680), 72.

[24] Sharp, *The Midwives Book Or the Whole Art of Midwifry Discovered*, 82.

generation'.[25] William Sermon suggested that a woman might feel and hear her belly 'rumbling' as the womb 'suck'd' or drew in the man's seed and began to transform this matter. He similarly thought that a midwife could test to see if a woman was pregnant by inserting a finger or a needle 'into the womb' to see if it was shut.[26]

In the days after a couple had had sex, medical authors provided a list of other symptoms of conception. Chamberlayne described how a woman who had recently conceived might get headaches, vertigo, lose her sight and her eyes would appear sunken. The veins in her tongue would turn green, her neck would get hot and her back cold, her breasts would become cold, her appetite would wane, she would vomit and her belly would swell. Sharp supposed that the belly would initially grow flat, she would get a sharp pain above the navel, lose her appetite, her periods would stop, she would have difficulty defecating, 'sometimes she will be merry, or sad suddenly upon no manifest cause' and she might have 'a preternatural desire to something not fit to eat nor drink, as some women with child have longed to bite off a piece of their Husbands Buttocks'.[27] Robert Barret thought that ten days after conception a woman would have her 'Terms' or period, but this could be white or red, but these would soon cease. He also told readers that her breasts would become 'big and hard with pain, and the Nipples grown red'.[28] Her urine, according to Barret, would be white, and in Chamberlayne's terms, there would be 'certain live things, to creep up and down'.[29] Sharp thought that a pregnant woman's urine would produce worms if left for three days.[30] These symptoms could be seen, heard or felt by others too; 'Signs' could be 'collected', Sermon suggested, from the husband, the unborn child and from the midwife. Chamberlayne described how a midwife might feel the womb close shut.[31] The husband too might know immediately if he took 'extraordinary delight' in sex and felt a 'kind of sucking or drawing at the end of his yard'.[32] Simon Forman recorded in his casebooks that while having sex (or what he termed 'halk') with his mistress Elizabeth, he felt her womb suck his staff ('virgam virilem') and knew she was pregnant.[33] Later in pregnancy women could be sure they had

[25] James Wolveridge, *Speculum Matricis Hybernicum, or, The Irish Midwives Handmaid* (London: 1670), 1.

[26] Sermon, *The Ladies Companion*, 23.

[27] Sharp, *The Midwives Book Or the Whole Art of Midwifry Discovered*, 82.

[28] Robert Barret, *A Companion for Midwives, Child-bearing Women, and Nurses Directing them how to Perform their Respective Offices: Together with an Essay, Endeavouring to Shew the Influence of Moral Abuses upon the Health of Children* (London: 1699), 64–65.

[29] *Ibid.*, 64; Chamberlayne, *Complete Midwife's Practice Enlarged*, 73.

[30] Sharp, *The Midwives Book Or the Whole Art of Midwifry Discovered*, 83.

[31] Chamberlayne, *Complete Midwife's Practice Enlarged*, 72; Wolveridge, *Speculum Matricis Hybernicum*, 1.

[32] Sermon, *The Ladies Companion*, 23.

[33] NOTE112, CB.

conceived when they felt it move like 'the stirring of a flie when he flieth', called quickening.[34]

The complete bodily transformation that sexually continent women would experience when pregnant was a common theme in ballads of the period too. Stories of pre-marital sex and illegitimate conception were apt currency for both entertaining and educating. These narratives were at once instructive – warning younger readers of the dangers of promised marriage and pre-marital sex – and titillating.[35] Some, like *A Lamentable Ballad of the Lady's Fall*, were more sympathetic to the temptations of youth than others. It relayed how a 'gallant Lady' was persuaded to 'lead a wedded life' by a dishonest man.[36] '[E]spousals, bethrothings, assurings, contractings, affirmings (for they are all one)' to marry were in the clergyman Daniel Rogers's words, 'very solemn matters'.[37] For Gouge, this exchange of promise was 'the beginning of marriage' and breaking this contract was sinful.[38] But as there was no standard format for these promises, the formality that reformers imagined transforming couples into spouses was in the eyes of the beholders. If promising to marry was almost or quite literally getting married, then consummation could follow immediately. Ballads often explored this ambiguity between what women might assume was a formal promise but was, in reality, difficult to enforce owing to the often intimate and private nature of these arrangements. Up to 20 per cent of brides were supposedly already pregnant when they got married – the gallant lady's predicament was an all too common one.[39] Her wrongdoing in the ballad is represented as giving the 'consent' to sex 'too soon' upon the promise to get married. Not long after what she perceived as the consummation of the marriage, 'She felt her body alter'd quite':

> Her bright hue waxed pale;
> Her fair red cheeks turn'd colour white,
> Her strength began to fail:
> So that with many a sorrowful sigh,
> This beauteous maiden mild,
> With grievous heart perceiv'd herself
> To be conceiv'd with-child

[34] Sermon, *The Ladies Companion*, 23.

[35] For the instructive and entertaining purposes of ballads, see: Angela McShane, 'Ballads and Broadsides', in *The Oxford History of Popular Print Culture: Cheap Print in Britain and Ireland to 1660*, vol. 1 (Oxford: Oxford University Press, 2011), 341.

[36] *A Lamentable Ballad of the Lady's Fall (c. 1720)*, BL, Roxburghe Ballads, EBBA 31270.

[37] D. R., *Matrimoniall Honovr, or, The Mutuall Crowne and Comfort of Godly, Loyall, and Chaste Marriage* (London: 1642), 104–105.

[38] Gouge, *Of Domesticall Duties*, 198.

[39] David Cressy, *Birth, Marriage, and Death: Ritual, Religion, and the Life-Cycle in Tudor and Stuart England* (Oxford: Oxford University Press, 1997), 374.

With the marriage yet to be solemnised, the young woman endeavoured to hide her 'swelling' from her parents. Confronting her perceived husband-to-be, she told him: 'I go with child by thee', and pleads with him to marry her. The baby, she told him, springs in her womb 'To hear the father's voice.' If he refused to get married, she told him she would rather die than raise a bastard and that he should end her life 'with thy rapier'.

To an early modern audience accustomed to bawdy comparisons between swords and men's yards, the message was clear: his 'rapier' had already ended her chance at a normal life through illegitimate pregnancy. Importantly, the lady in this story was the protagonist and the reader is encouraged to view her mistake as a minor misdemeanour with tragic consequences. Several aspects of the story reinforce how close her experience was to the ideal model of married motherhood. She noticed her pregnancy immediately. She was not confused about whether she is ill or simply putting on weight. Nor does she struggle to identify the father, and tells him early that she is carrying his child. The baby also is described as moving vigorously within her, something which, as Chapter 3 suggests, was the kind of thing that elite and respectable women were meant to notice and record during their pregnancy. There was an implicit link between her (relative) chastity and innocence and the immediate and undeniable effects of sex and conception on her body. Such a cautionary tale would no doubt have warned readers how a slight deviation from godly familial life might bring a life of misery; sin begot sin. As Gowing notes, because painless birth was connected to promiscuity and moral disrepute of the mother, an easy pregnancy was also seen as suspicious.[40] Arduous pregnancy was linked to piety and penance. Pamphlets explored this cultural dichotomy and the ways in which women's bodies displayed and embodied their own and their family's piety (or lack of).

In *A Copy of Verses of a Baker and a Mealman*, two men conspire to convince women to have sex with them.[41] The mealman told a 'pretty Maid that in his house did dwell' that he will teach her to dance 'Which some People do report to be Alamode de France'. He deceived her into having sex. Shortly after their tryst, she suddenly experienced a 'Metamorphose' in her body. She thought she was poisioned but she was of course pregnant. Her 'Belly's like a Tun', or a cask of wine, and she is worried that her 'Guts will tumble out' with 'this plaguy Bout'. Here, her ignorance of sex goes someway to exonerate her from her sins. But once again the ballad links unequivocal bodily signs of pregnancy – a 'metamorphose' even – with relative chastity and inexperience.

[40] Gowing, 'Secret Births and Infanticide in Seventeenth-Century England'.
[41] *A Copy of Verses of a Baker and a Mealman: Giving an Account of their subtle Intreagues with their Mistresses, and how the Mealman got his Maid with Child*, EBBA 217071 (London, 1690–1700).

While she was unsure of the cause of her malaise initially, it is only too clear to the reader that the dishonest mealman has made her an unmarried mother-to-be against her will.

The Amorous Lady's Garland played on this pervasive fear that young unmarried women would be persuaded into having sex with men who promised to marry them and get pregnant almost legitimately.[42] A young lady met a butcher in St James's market, fell in love and got married. They kept their nuptials secret for twenty weeks until 'My lovely creature did begin/to thicken in the waist'. Her mother began to suspect she was pregnant, and given she assumed her daughter was still unmarried, she fretted to her husband 'alas! she is with child,/my jewel I do fear'. When confronted, the young woman pretends ignorance and says that her parents bid her to 'buy the best of meat' and she liked the offerings of the butcher so much 'Of it I made a hearty meal,/ which made my belly swell', before revealing they wed four months ago.

Other ballads representing the duplicitous and devious nature of women told of those who used their pregnancies or ability to get pregnant for gain and to trap men. Moggy in *Scotch Moggy's Misfortune* set her sights on the newly widowed Robin (Figure 2.1). She flirts with him and even visits a well to increase the likelihood of conception. Getting pregnant secures him as her new husband. She tells Robin 'gard my Belly swell' and loudly proclaims 'Robin he chash me about the stack,/Robin laid me on my Back,/Robin he made my Rump to crack,/Kind Robin loves me.' Such ballads expected readers would understand the tension between the assiduous bodily knowledge that married godly women laid claim to, which aided infant and maternal wellbeing, and the ways in which this same knowledge might be used for insidious and sinful purposes. Going to the well and noting how her belly swelled were not troubling in and of themselves but they transformed these normative parts of the experience of pregnancy into acts of feminine subversion.[43] Notably although her belly gets bigger, Moggy is not troubled with the dramatic transformation in response to getting pregnant in the same way that the more innocent women who were deceived into having what they hoped and expected would be marital sex were in ballads.

This helps to reveal the contours of an early modern cultural association between being certain one was pregnant and being morally and bodily continent. It is no wonder then that elite women announced their pregnancies quickly and assertively in diaries and letters. Added to this as well as gesturing to their

[42] *The Amorous Lady's Garland, Shewing how a young Lady going with her maid to St James's Market fell in Love with a young butcher, who desir'd him to walk with her into St James's Park, after some discourse they both agreed to be married the next morning* (London, c. 1740), EBBA 34197.

[43] *Scotch Moggy's Misfortune: Together With her cheerful Hops, that Shakum Guie will bury his Wife, and then make Moggy a happy Mother* (London: 1683–1696), EBBA 33786.

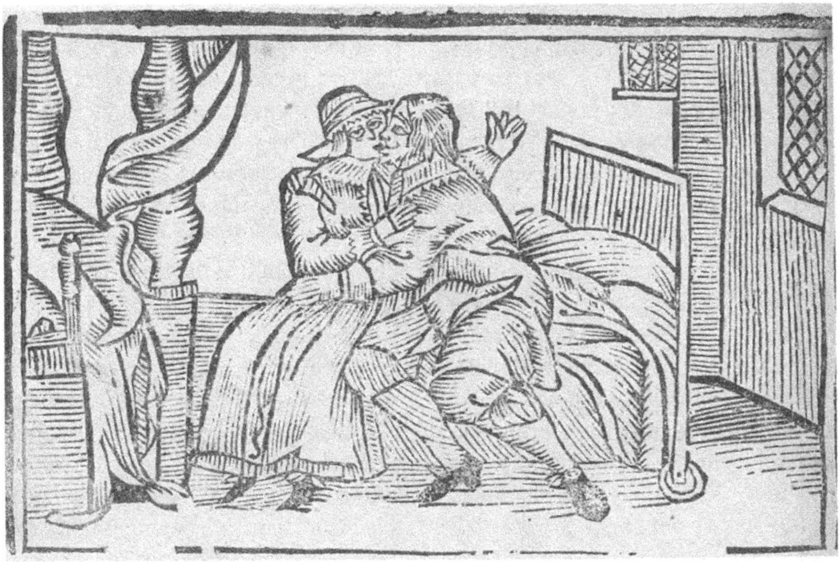

Figure 2.1 *Scotch Moggy's Misfortune: Together with her cheerful Hops, that Shakum Guie will bury his Wife, and then make Moggy a happy Mother* (London: 1683–1696). EBBA 33786, EBB6SH, Houghton Library, Harvard University.

relative chastity and bodily attentiveness, knowing one was pregnant early and certainly facilitated their engagement with preventative healthcare. First, if they knew they were pregnant as soon as they had conceived, women could eat appropriately, avoid certain activities and medicines, and be attentive to the medical needs of the baby within them and was therefore intertwined in the domestic labour of being a wife, mother and healer. Second, writing about pregnancy was part of a broader, particularly protestant, trend to keep 'good' accounts, financial and otherwise, creating and fostering a familial identity. Finally, these records proved and displayed the legitimacy of the conception.

Keeping Accounts, Health and Spirituality

When Jane Sharp encouraged women to take 'just accounts' and warned of the dangers of not doing so, she was not simply referring to noticing one's menstrual cycle, but a more extensive attentiveness to the body of the kind medical writers assumed in descriptions of the symptoms of early pregnancy.[44]

[44] Gowing, *Common Bodies: Women, Touch and Power in Seventeenth-Century England*, 121.

In this way, being certain about pregnancy would be much easier if individuals and families were keeping appropriate and attentive track of their bodies and health in their paperwork anyway. This was first because the authors of child-bearing guides were adamant that the cessation of menstruation alone was not a reliable sign of conception. Women could menstruate well into pregnancy, and therefore relying on one's periods as an indicator of how long one had been pregnant would lead to inaccurate reckonings. The author of *The English Midwife Enlarged* (1682) explained that if women dated their pregnancy from their first missed period, they might be out by a month, if they had conceived when menstruating, or even longer if she continued to bleed for the first several months of gestation.[45] The cessation of menstruation was more commonly thought to be a symptom of disease from a blockage or imbalance rather than conception. Menstruation was fundamental to the maintenance of health generally for women, not just in fertility, as discussed Chapter 1.[46] 'False' conceptions also mimicked the signs of pregnancy, making it even more difficult to rely on periods.[47] Knowing when one ought to be menstruating and keeping a record, however, was important. For Jakob Rüff, this meant women could appropriately take medicines with an 'expulsive vertue' to bring their period on.[48]

Knowing one was pregnant early also meant women would not take other treatments that might threaten the pregnancy. When in May 1651 Mary Evelyn took 'physick' for what she thought was a sickness, her husband, John, noted in his diary they had not known she was pregnant and the medicines had caused a miscarriage.[49] Domestic recipe books contained remedies to help women carry infants to full term that again suggest it was deemed medically important to be certain one was pregnant as close to conception as possible. Joanna Suddell's book, for example, contained a recipe to 'preuent Abortion approued by all that made use of the same Directions', which ought to be taken 'When you apprehend your self with child'.[50] A receipt 'To preuent Miscarriage' in an anonymously penned seventeenth-century recipe book

[45] *The English Midwife Enlarged* (London: 1682), 24.

[46] Alexandra Lord, '"The Great Arcana of the Deity" Menstruation and Menstrual Disorders in Eighteenth-Century British Medical Thought', *Bulletin of the History of Medicine* 73, no. 1 (1999): 38–63; Cathy McClive, *Menstruation and Procreation in Early Modern France* (London: Routledge, 2015); Gianna Pomata, 'Menstruating Men: Similarity and Difference of the Sexes in Early Modern Medicine', in *Generation and Degeneration: Tropes of Reproduction in Literature and History from Antiquity to Early Modern Europe*, ed. Valeria Finucci and Kevin Brownlee (Durham, NC: Duke University Press, 2001), 109–152; Sara Read, *Menstruation and the Female Body in Early Modern England*, Genders and Sexualities in History (Basingstoke: Palgrave, 2013).

[47] Sharp, *The Midwives Book Or the Whole Art of Midwifry Discovered*, 84.

[48] Jakob Rüff, *The Expert Midwife, or An Excellent and Most Necessary Treatise of the Generation and Birth of Man* (London, 1637), 49.

[49] Evelyn, 2 May 1651, *Diary of John Evelyn*, 31.

[50] Joanna Suddell, 'Receipt book, 1688', Clark Library, UCLA, MS.1950.023.

instructed women to take a piece of leather, spread it with civet (a yellow, musky-smelling liquid from the perineal glands of civet cats) and place it on the stomach 'as soone as they think themselues with child and weare it till they are deliuered'.[51]

These accounts sat within a web of other kinds of notes and observations that early modern people were encouraged to make and keep for themselves and their families. Reformers encouraged believers to engage in a continual process of self-examination in which paper became an important tool. But this paperwork was not just a space in which people evaluated their conduct, but also one in which they could justify their own perceptions, uphold their reputation, dispute the account of others, settle scores, convey cultural information and invent desirable futures.[52] This was also attended by an intensified interest in financial bookkeeping (another kind of account). Paperwork that was supposedly transparent, honest and accurate was venerated but this 'reality' was one 'manipulated to create the appearance of fiscal probity'.[53] James Aho has argued that while in counter-Reformation Europe double-entry bookkeeping emulated penitential confession, in England, this paperwork was often materially and functionally indistinguishable from other kinds of records that were kept to manage home spending. It was nevertheless bound up with epistemological practices that produced and systematised knowledge.[54] Domestic paperwork like recipe books were, as other historians have shown, an important space in which knowledge about the natural world and health were produced. Early modern individuals turned to paper to document their symptoms, diagnoses and cures. Practitioners too kept records.[55] These records were, it is important to remember, also part of the material culture of the early modern home, or at least the literate one. Keeping financial accounts was a moral act that reflected the 'compiler's moral worth' and projected 'that quality to the wider public' and records materially displayed this.[56] The author of a 1683 guide described how account keeping allowed one 'in an Instant' to see

[51] Anonymous, 'Seventeenth century receipt book', Whitney Cookery Collection, New York Public Library, New York, v. 8, recipe no. 92, p. 12.

[52] Sidonie Smith and Julia Watson, *Reading Autobiography: A Guide for Interpreting Life Narratives* (Minneapolis: University of Minnesota Press, 2010), 10.

[53] Jason Scott-Warren, 'Early Modern Bookkeeping and Life-Writing Revisited: Accounting for Richard Stonley', *Past & Present* 230, no. supplement 11 (2016): 152.

[54] James Aho, *Confession and Bookkeeping: The Religious, Moral, and Rhetorical Roots of Modern Accounting* (Albany: State University of New York, 2005).

[55] Roy Porter, 'The Patient's View: Doing Medical History from Below', *Theory & Society* 14, no. 1 (1985): 175–198. See also: Lauren Kassell, 'Paper Technologies, Digital Technologies: Working with Early Modern Medical Records', in *The Edinburgh Companion to the Critical Medical Humanities*, ed. Anne Whitehead et al. (Edinburgh: Edinburgh University Press, 2016), 120–135.

[56] Adam Smyth, *Autobiography in Early Modern England* (Cambridge: Cambridge University Press, 2010), 69.

'(as he doeth his Person in a mirror) his whole estate and what posture it is in at the time'.[57] The accounts that Sharp and other medical writers expected women to keep were therefore part of this paperwork that materially, practically, spiritually and emotionally ordered and defined the household. These diaries, spiritual meditations and recipe books sat on shelves in people's homes. Perhaps they were on occasion retrieved, looked at and shared and were part of collective and embodied memory practices.

The ways in which keeping written accounts of pregnancy was intertwined with spiritual practice is deftly displayed in the diary of Sarah Savage, living near Nantwich in Cheshire, wife of John Savage and the daughter of the nonconformist minister Philip Henry. She paid attention to all manner of things in her life and kept a written account of them for posterity. In the early years of her marriage, she was particularly concerned with noticing and recording things that might indicate she was pregnant. Four months after she married John, she expressed in her diary that she was 'a litle desirious yt God w[oul]d please to make me a fruitfull vine if hee see good'. If not, she vowed to 'submit to him'.[58] For Savage, keeping track of her body was a way that she spoke directly to her maker and placed her within a wider community of Christians, as well as being a practical medical tool to direct her diet and routine. These two facets were inextricable. Savage could wish, but she could not long for a child. That would be covetous and err too close to being desirous for something that contravened divine will. This led to a tension in such records between apparent attentiveness to generation and a shyness about naming it explicitly. Thus, three months earlier, she wrote on 8 March 'Lord supply mee . . .' but left a blank space where her desire should have been written. She was also 'drowsie' and reassured herself that 'my God will supply all my needs' (and if we read between the lines the needs of her suspected unborn baby).[59] On 12 May, she noted she was 'somth[ing] tired w[i]th house busines, yet on my bed my meditations of God w[e]r[e] sweet' and she 'run over in my mind' sermons she had heard.[60] By June, she still had not conceived and was a 'little discomposed by a fear of a disappointm[en]t tho it came not upon consideracon I was willing to submit yn had wt I desired viz'. In July, she was in hope again that 'he w[oul]d fulfill ye desire of my soul in a Partic. Thing', but only 'if hee see it good for mee'. A Tuesday later in July she still 'had hopes' that God would grant her 'lawf[ul] desires of my soul as far as is good for mee yet I trust all concernm[en]ts w[i]th him'. She crossed the next two lines out completely obscuring their legibility. In October she became

[57] Robert Colinson, *Idea Rationaria, or The Perfect Accomptant* (1683), 2. Cited in: *ibid.*, 71.
[58] Sarah Savage, 'Diary, 1686–88', Cheshire Archives and Local Studies, Chester, ZD/Basten/8, unfoliated.
[59] *Ibid.* [60] *Ibid.*

much bolder about her wishes and wrote 'If God should see good to delay or totally deny the mercy of children to me still by his grace I will wait on him, and love him not one jot the less, tho' I sometimes can scarce quiet my spirit as I would.'

It is not accidental, as Chapter 1 suggested, that her husband and his fertility were left out of these reflections, which were as much an attempt to prove her piety and wifely submission as they were a genuine concern for her ongoing childlessness. Despite a difficult beginning, including two miscarriages between 1687 and 1688, Savage went on to have nine children. Savage's use of her diary displayed her commitment to God and to her role as wife and future mother. She did not necessarily do so as an act of self-fashioning but also to bolster the family name and godly respectability. Making records of pregnancy and her body was part of the work of creating and recreating the family.

We can see this collective use in the ways in which husbands also wrote about their wives' health and bodies. Sometimes this was focused on discovering or verifying pregnancy, but at other times, it similarly served this broader culture of attentiveness that was encouraged at home. When Elizabeth, Samuel Pepys's wife, did not have her period for seven weeks, he wrote in his diary that he had been 'in hopes of her being with child', which were dashed by its eventual arrival several weeks later in January 1660.[61] For four months in 1654 Helen, the wife of Sir Archibald Johnson, a Scottish judge and statesman who would be executed by Charles II in 1663 for having served under Cromwell, had been unwell. Archibald noted that his wife was suffering with a 'seaknesse' in January and he had instructed her that it was most likely 'correction for hir neglect of secret worship and wayring [wearing] her strength and health on uther business'.[62] Later that month, Archibald recorded that Lady Libertoun suspected that Helen was pregnant, rather than unwell. We know from later entries that her period had stopped. On the 30 January, she 'grew unweal at night', which she and her 'friend' interpreted as the God preparing her 'eyther for great doings or great sufferings for His nayme'.[63] On the 24 and 25 February, she got a 'sore brash' (a sudden onset of pain), 'rysing of the spleen and bairnebed', a Scots word for womb, and her physician, Doctor Hayes, fretted for her life.[64] Archibald banished himself to the back-chamber and prayed incessantly that the Lord would 'pitye, pardon, sanctifye, and saive me and my wyfe and children, and to compassionate our present condition in

[61] Samuel Pepys, *The Diary of Samuel Pepys: A New and Complete Transcription Vol. 1 1660*, ed. Robert Latham (New York: Harper Collins, 1983), 1.

[62] Archibald Johnston, 20 January 1654, *Diary of Sir Archibald Johnston of Wariston 1650–1654, Volume II*, ed. David Hay Fleming, Publications of the Scottish History Society (Edinburgh: University of Edinburgh Press, 1919), 196.

[63] *Ibid.*, 30 January 1654, 199. [64] *Ibid.*, 24 and 25 February 1654, 209.

soule, body, estate and nayme,' a clear indication of the stakes if she miscarried. Physic in the form of a clyster appeared to resolve many of the more concerning symptoms. In March, Archibald still thought she was pregnant. Friends urged her not to travel in case it endangered the baby's life. He prayed that the Lord 'preserve hir and the chyld she is thought to haive'.[65] On 22 April, Helen announced that she had her 'flouers' [flowers], her period, 'which shew that she is not with chyld'.[66] For the Johnstons, the absence of her periods created an ambiguous state, but their resumption was conclusive proof she was not. It was only then, when it was clear that it was not pregnancy that was causing her ill health, that Archibald meditated on the 'dangerousnesse of hir condition'.[67] Archibald's record-keeping, which in turn rested on his wife's attentiveness to her body, reveals the focus families had on deciding whether a woman was pregnant and the resulting need to alter routine and regimen and, finally, that this process of noticing and writing was not something women did alone. Husbands, friends and doctors were all eager to notice potentially pregnant bodies and interpret them, even when this involved disputing the convictions women had. Good wives and mothers would supposedly know certainly and intuitively they were pregnant but were not always trusted in this knowledge.

At other times, husbands made notes about women's menstrual cycles or when couples had sex not deliberately to discover pregnancy but because, as we have seen, women's bodies and providing records of them redounded to male domestic honour. John Dee, the mathematician, astrologer and antiquary, made a note when his wife menstruated in his almanac as well as when they had sex. He also kept a record of the births of their children and episodes of ill health of family members.[68] Ralph Josselin recollected in his diary in 1640 that he 'began to have some hopes of my wives breeding', which he noted 'proved so', although he left out the things that led to their certainty.[69] In the eighteenth century, the wig maker Edmund Harrold documented his and his wife Sarah's health in great detail as well as his conduct and its spiritual significance. He also took care to record when, where and how he had sex with, or 'did', his wife. On the 9 June 1712, for example, he recorded that at night he 'did wife 2 tymes, couch and bed, in an hour and ½ time'.[70] For Harrold, the way he assiduously recorded his and Sarah's sexual habits was not always motivated by an interest in fertility or potential pregnancy. He 'did' his wife on the 16, 17 and 18 November, less than a week before she delivered their fourth

[65] *Ibid.*, 7 March 1654, 213. [66] *Ibid.*, 22 April 1654, 238. [67] *Ibid.*, 22 April 1654, 238.
[68] Lauren Kassell, 'Exhibit 14: Jane Dee's Courses in John Dee's Diary', in *Reproduction: Antiquity to the Present Day* (Cambridge: Cambridge University Press, 2018).
[69] Ralph Josselin, July 1640, *Diary of Rev. Ralph Josselin 1616–1683*, ed. E. Hockliffe, vol. XV, Camden Third Series (London: Royal Historical Society, 1908), 12.
[70] Edmund Harrold, 'Diary, 1712–1716', 9 June 1712, Chetham's Library, Manchester, fol. 2v.

daughter, also called Sarah.[71] In Harrold's diary, having sex was an indicator of the tone of the relationship; on 17 November, he 'did w[i]f[e] fine' and recorded that 'Shes very good now we live lovingly and contetedly blessed be God'. Other times he 'did' her 'clean', 'oddly', 'tit[e]ly', 'avi[d]ly', in the 'new' and 'old' fashion and 'stand[ing at the] ba[c]k [of the] sh[op] titely'. All of these details helped Harrold in the examination of his own and his family's conduct and show that knowing intimate things about one's body and having the accounts as of substantial interest to middling and elite families in early modern England. Harrold's accounts were not explicitly part of monitoring fertility but they sat within a web of written records of the self and other family members that early modern people were encouraged to make. Writing out these observations of daily life helped to furnish longer narratives about family and its identity with specific verifiable details, but it also helps to explain why elite families were able to announce their pregnancy so early. This culture of bodily knowledge was related to embodied devotion in complex ways that intertwined marital fidelity with clear verifiable signs in women's bodies, that implicated men and their honour too.

The Difficulty of Being Unsure

Ambiguity or confusion about whether a woman was pregnant was something that many families put considerable effort into resolving. In the same way that medical texts simultaneously expected women to know they were immediately pregnant but then also directed that many women would continue to menstruate throughout pregnancy, the guidance that authors gave on ascertaining pregnancy within months of conception was similarly contradictory and complex. Authors continually referenced the fact that it was difficult to reliably ascertain whether a woman was pregnant for medical practitioners. William Sermon's 1671 *The Ladies Companion* noted that midwives should be 'very careful' in such interactions. There was nothing more 'ridiculous' than assuring a family they were expecting only for the woman's belly to fall 'flat again' and for her to start menstruating again. A medical practitioner that had previously been 'well esteemed of' would become 'slighted and undervalued'.[72] He described an altercation with two women, both over fifty, who were adamant that they were pregnant. When their imagined due dates came and went, Sermon offered purgatives that showed they were simply unwell and they returned to perfect health once their bodies were purged. This was a common narrative in childbearing manuals written by physicians and midwives that served to verify their own credibility and claim to medical expertise:

[71] *Ibid.*, fol. 22r–v. Sarah Harrold was born 23 November 1712 and died 1 April 1713.
[72] Sermon, *The Ladies Companion*, 16.

women falsely believing they were pregnant only for this to be disproved by the intuition and expertise of the author. Sermon was cautioning midwives not because it was impossible to know for sure whether a woman was pregnant but because he assumed they would not have the knowledge and instinct he did.

Percival Willughby, a Derby man-midwife, offered a tale that had a similar moral in the published account of his professional activities. Midwives should 'bee cautious of their promises, and circumspect in their sayings and undertakings' he noted.[73] A 'good woman', meaning one of relatively high status, living near Nottingham had been assured she was expecting a baby when she actually had a 'swel'd cancerous tumour in the womb'. The midwives tried to deliver the imagined baby injuring her womb in the process.[74] Chamberlayne reported that a 'young Lady' thought herself to be four months pregnant, but she had not felt the baby move in some time. He told the reader he decided to believe her testimony – that she was pregnant and the baby had died – but doubt lingered that perhaps it was a false conception. When her day of 'Reckoning' came and went he asked her 'Friends and Physitians' whether they believed her to be with child and they corroborated her account. She was, as she and her friends had said, eventually delivered of a dead child sometime after.[75] The eighteenth-century German physician Johann Storch was often asked to determine the cause of symptoms that could or could not be parsing through women's testimony, that of her friends and family, and his own judgements. A thirty-year-old 'artisan's wife' complained of a growth. She had not felt her baby quicken and she continued to menstruate. A midwife determined her to be pregnant with a 'live child' and she gave birth shortly after.[76] Conversely, a forty-seven-year-old noblewoman was sure she was pregnant. She had not menstruated in months and she claimed to feel the child move within her. Storch notes 'I deferred to her opinion until the calculated date of the birth had passed, even though I never entirely concealed from her my reservations about the matter' that she was, indeed, not pregnant.[77] Storch explicitly waited until 'the whole thing would come to light by itself' before providing an unequivocal judgement about pregnancy to avoid appearing ignorant.[78] The irony that many of these practitioners expected women to know they had conceived from the moment they stopped having sex but fully comprehended the ambiguity and complexity of how difficult this might be reveals the ways in which being pregnant necessitated navigating between order and disorder.

Perhaps because of this, women and their families frequently sought the help of medical practitioners in trying to work out if they were expecting. The

[73] Percivall Willughby, *Observations in Midwifery by Percival Willughby*, ed. Henry Blenkinsop (Warwick: H. T. Cooke, 1863), 9–10.
[74] *Ibid.*, 1. [75] *Ibid.*, 2–3. [76] Duden, *The Woman beneath the Skin*, 160. [77] *Ibid.*, 161.
[78] *Ibid.*, 160.

astrologer-physicians Simon Forman and Richard Napier were asked close to 1,500 times to verify whether a whether a woman was pregnant. Relying on the stars, as well as other signs, Forman and Napier rarely displayed the reticence that other practitioners did in telling women whether they were with child. Elizabeth Gyniver was determined to be pregnant in no uncertain terms by Napier on 11 October 1600 and her 'courses haue bene stop this 10 or 12 weeks'.[79] When Elizabeth Borase asked Forman whether she was pregnant in 1597, Forman noted beneath the astrological chart 'She supposes her self with child, but I think it was not so.' Forman returned to his entry at a later date to note 'She proued shortly after not to be w[i]th child.'[80] Mary Braunch was told her symptoms were the result of a 'falls conceptio' but she described having felt her child move for the past thirty weeks.[81] At other times, the astrologers were also uncertain. Luce Ashmore visited Forman early July 1601. She had not had her period and was 'paind in the stomacke', 'mother [womb]', and 'head & backe'. He determined that not only was she pregnant, but it would only be four weeks until she delivered.[82] She returned later that month asking again whether she was pregnant to be told that it was a false conception.[83] Forman, however, again changed his mind. On 2 November 1601, Luce came again offering the dates that she suspected she had conceived with her husband Richard March, curiously described as a 'gent that lai w[i]t[h] here [her] 23 March'. Now he noted that she was '32 wicks' (weeks') pregnant. He calculated that she would give birth 21 December 'at 2 in the morninge'. Forman returned to his notes after the consultation recording 'She was deliuered of a boi' the 3 December at 9.45 pm.[84] The astrologers also had to negotiate with family members seeking help on behalf of women or weighing in. Mrs Froick brought her daughter's urine to Richard Napier's nephew, desiring 'to know whether she be with child'.[85] Mr Knight came to Forman to find out whether his wife, Alice, was pregnant in August 1600 without her 'consent'.[86] Alice herself came to Forman two months later in October for the same question to be told 'yt will not proue,' or she would never carry her child to full term.[87]

The philosopher Anne Conway and her husband, Edward, consulted a number of different medical practitioners in 1658 to confirm whether or not she was expecting a child. Anne suffered from an illness that evaded diagnosis for most of her married life. In 1658, her condition had deteriorated and her husband, Edward, the politician wrote to his private secretary and brother-in-law, George Rawdon, that the couple had resigned themselves to her inevitable death. He told Rawdon that they had long considered the possibility that her

[79] CASE8281, CB. [80] CASE2294, CB. [81] CASE6282, CB. [82] CASE9478, CB.
[83] CASE9529, CB. [84] CASE9846, CB. [85] CASE79869, CB. [86] CASE7996, CB.
[87] CASE8291, CB.

condition was not disease but pregnancy, but the severity of her symptoms suggested otherwise and these hints 'served only to torment' the family. The Conways consulted the 'best doctors and midwives' so they could be 'resolved' in the diagnosis, but the variety of opinions plunged them into the 'greatest uncertainty' for they were unequivocal that she was not carrying a child and had few explanations for her malaise. Finally, his wife felt something move within her, a symptom Edward described as 'not compatible with any disease'. He described how he and 'others' had placed their hands on her stomach and felt this movement that he compared to a 'fitt of the ague'. With relief, he told Rawdon that 'the violent extremity' she was in 'tended not to the concluding of her own life, but to the giving life to another'; Anne was pregnant for sure he thought. Although Edward was greatly relieved and delighted with the news, he was also embarrassed about how long it had taken to arrive at a diagnosis. Edward ruminated on how he and his wife had been 'so perfectly ignorant of the truth' and asked that Rawdon keep these details 'private as it is possible, till we have more assurance'. He fretted that they could all too easily 'be made a town-talk' and that only Rawdon's wife, Dorothy, should be told the circumstances of Anne's condition. In the same letter, he asked Rawdon to get an eagle stone, which would ease her pain and difficulties. Eagle stones were walnut-sized hollow rocks that rattled when shaken that ancient sources thought were carried by eagles to their nests to facilitate egg-laying. By the seventeenth century, they were increasingly regarded as a superstitious practice.[88] Again, he wanted Rawdon to be discreet; it was Anne's 'wish' that 'few people be aware' of her request and Edward asked that, if possible, the seller should be kept in the dark about their identity.[89] She gave birth to a little boy, Heneage, four months later who died in 1660 of smallpox. As the avid epistolary culture of writing about fertility and pregnancy indicates, the Conways were not unjustified in their fear that they would be gossiped about, and that her uncertainty would be a central theme. It was troubling when families could not understand bodily symptoms and knit them into an appropriate narrative. The interaction between Rawdon and Conway is yet another hint of the ways that record-keeping was narrativised in ways that elevated family status.

[88] Sandra Cavallo, 'Exhibit 17: Pregnant Stones as Wonders of Nature', in *Reproduction: Antiquity to the Present Day* (Cambridge: Cambridge University Press, 2018), 180–181; Mary E. Fissell, *Vernacular Bodies: The Politics of Reproduction in Early Modern England* (Oxford: Oxford University Press, 2004), 50–52; Ann-Sophie Thwaite, 'Magic and the Material Culture of Healing in Early Modern England' (Cambridge, University of Cambridge, 2020), 11–12.

[89] Edward Conway to Major Rawdon, 12 October 1658, Marjorie Hope Nicolson and Sarah Hutton (eds.), *The Conway Letters: The Correspondence of Anne, Viscountess Conway, Henry More, and Their Friends 1642–1684* (Oxford: Oxford University Press, 1992), Letter 92.

Even once a couple had announced they had conceived to family members and others, doubt could arise when the pregnancy did not appear to have progressed in an imagined or predicted way. In 1689, Anne Syderfin, the sister of James Lawes-Wittewronge, believed herself to be pregnant. In March, her brother James wrote to his father, Sir James Wittewronge, expressing his sadness that she had 'miscarried and in so great danger' but hoped that the next letter would bring news that she had recovered.[90] The miscarriage was seemingly staved off and her symptoms abated. Two months later he wrote noting that 'dayly' he prayed for his sister's safe delivery 'being much concerned for her'.[91] In a following letter, he noted that he had been 'in great hopes' that there would be 'wellcom newes of my sisters safe deliuery' but no sooner had he opened the letter 'then I perceiue'd the things I have long feard is like to proue true'.[92] The fear was that she had been deceived in her account and was not actually pregnant. On 5 June, he wrote offering his sister hope that she was simply overdue, 'you may please to tell her that Mr Musgraves' lady her neighbour in the country is lately brought to bed of a brave boy, haveing gone ten weeks beyond her reckoning'.[93] Only three days later, however, the situation appears to have become desperate, for he prayed that 'God send my sister well ridd of her supposed great belly.'[94] Towards the end of June, James's letters simply expressed his joy that Anne was well again, and no baby was born. For these families, uncertainty begged to be resolved one way or another. Interactions with medical practitioners show considerable ambiguity and anxiety around interpreting women's bodies as either pregnant or not. Even their professional reputation was embroiled in the politics of uncovering the secrets of women's bodies in the same ways that households and families felt that uncertainty reflected poorly on their family name. The next section shows how the pressure placed on women to know and moderate their behaviour only intensified once a woman had announced her pregnancy.

Being Cheerful and Careful: Preventing Miscarriage

One reason women were encouraged to know they were pregnant soon after conception was so they could do everything in their power to prevent miscarriage. Pregnancy was represented as delicate and easily disrupted by medical authors, and necessitated constant vigilance and immediate responsive action to ill health. John Oliver reminded women to be 'very careful of their bodies

[90] James Lawes-Wittewronge to Sir James Wittewronge, 11 March 1689, Hertfordshire Record Office, Hertford, DE/Lw F29, unfoliated.
[91] *Ibid.*, 6 May 1689. [92] *Ibid.*, 16 May 1689. [93] *Ibid.*, 5 June 1689.
[94] *Ibid.*, 8 June 1689.

while they were with child'.[95] Authors were particularly concerned about the flimsiness of the fibres and sinews that held the baby in place. Sharp explained how babies were held by 'cups' that kept the infant nourished could be easily broken by 'strokes, sudden fears, much sneesing, coughing, violent motion, extream joy, sorrow or trouble of the mind; or by medicaments that corrode, or bitter drinks the infant loaths'.[96] A 'Corrupt diet' governed by 'Gluttony and surfeiting', eating too much meat or drinking too much wine could supposedly choke the infant.[97] The author of *Every Woman Her Own Midwife* described how 'vehement motions or exercise' could disrupt the 'internall membrane of the Womb' and 'abortment presently followeth'.[98] So too could raising her arms too high, carrying things or sitting on 'hard and uneasie seats'. Instead, she could have her body gently 'rubbed and stroked'. Some activities like spinning and carding wool could 'stretch the body' in beneficial ways. Eating immoderately or drinking wine that was too strong could similarly cause miscarriage.[99] She should avoid all extremes of emotion: 'fasting, thirst, watching, mourning, sadnesse, anger, and all other perturbations of the mind'.[100] The imperative to be calm and happy in order to be fertile and conceive described in Chapter 1 also applied in pregnancy, and was yet another way in which family members thrust themselves into the experience of childbearing.

Conduct and medical texts constantly fretted about women being unhappy or scared while pregnant. Barret described the 'Tragical Consequences' when women did not 'qualifie' and 'temperate' their 'Humour Upon every Surprize' in pregnancy. If they were afraid, they should get into bed 'and indeavour to forget what's past'. She should abstain from 'all Mourning, Sighing, and extraordinary Grief'. Being happy and content during pregnancy was not just advantageous for the infant and mother but for those around her; it was important to Barret that 'her Company be agreeable'.[101] Culpeper also espoused the benefits of women leading '*contented* lives, that so their conception may be well formed'. To 'fret and fume, and flight and throw, and murmure and repine, and fill their minds all full of distracting cares and fears' was, Culpeper suggested, like 'an Egg full of meat, making a tumult in their spirits, and bringing all their thoughts into such confusion, that they look more like beasts then women', and would destroy and 'murthers both Body and

[95] John Oliver, *A Present for Teeming Women. By Their Husbands or Friends; Containing Scripture-Directions for Women with-child, how to prepare for the hour of Travel* (London: 1663), sig. Aa2v.

[96] Sharp, *The Midwives Book Or the Whole Art of Midwifry Discovered*, 147. [97] *Ibid.*, 147.

[98] *Every Woman Her Own Midwife, or, A Compleat cabinet opened for child-bearing women furnished with directions to prevent miscarriages during the time of breeding* (London: 1675), 2.

[99] *Ibid.*, 2. [100] *Ibid.*, 2. [101] Barret, *A Companion for Midwives*, 66.

Mind'.[102] He recommended Mr Jeremiah Burrough's *Christian Contentment*, a conduct book reprinted a number of times over the seventeenth century that provided guidance on how to accept the hand of God joyfully.[103] By the mid seventeenth century, there were several conduct books that were explicitly for women, or at least contained chapters directed towards them. In these texts women were encouraged to be 'chaste, silent and obedient'.[104] Mary Rich, the Countess of Warwick, was praised for her 'peculiar delight' in rendering 'the lives of all easie and pleasant and free from discontent, that they might serve God with chearfulness'.[105] Hannah Woolley instructed readers of the very popular and oft-reprinted *The Gentlewomans Companion* that 'greater assistance' was required in 'the framing and fashioning of a Woman' because her 'behaviour should be such as to please in all good companies'.[106] The conduct author Richard Brathwaite proclaimed that 'A cheerefull modesty' was a woman's 'best *Complement*, which shee ever weares about her as her chiefest ornament'.[107] Implicit in such advice was the expectation that women would manage the feelings of other household members. Women were also thought to be more permeable to the effects of emotion. Their bodies were especially impressionable to grief, sadness and fear.[108]

A vision of maternity here emerges in which women were expected to intensively manage their own pregnancies in a way that was pleasant and not disruptive for others. Her domestic responsibilities may have morphed while pregnant, but they did not stop. She may have been excused from strenuous household tasks but breeding a baby did not mean she was to stop ministering to the spiritual and bodily welfare of her husband, servants, other children and other family members, quite the opposite. Pregnancy then appears not as a moment of social or domestic inversion, but instead one in which women quite

102 Culpeper, *Directory for Midwives* (1675), 93–94.

103 Jeremiah Burroughs, *The Rare Jewel of Christian Contentment. By Jeremiah Burroughs, preacher of the Gospel to two of the greatest congregations in England; viz. Stepney and Cripplegate, London* (London: 1648).

104 Suzanne W. Hull, *Chaste, Silent, and Obedient: English Books for Women, 1475–1640* (San Marino, CA: Huntington Library, 1982).

105 Anthony Walker, *Eureka, Eureka The Virtuous Woman found Her Loss Bewailed, and Character Exemplified in a Sermon Preached at Felsted in Essex, April, 30,* 1678 (London: 1678), 95.

106 Hannah Woolley, *The Gentlewomans Companion; or, A Guide to the Female Sex Containing Directions of Behaviour, in all Places, Companies, Relations, and Conditions, from their Childhood down to Old Age* (London, 1673), 33.

107 Richard Brathwaite, *The English Gentlewoman drawne out to the full Body: Expressing What Habilliments due best attire her, What Ornaments doe best adorne her, What Complements doe best adorne her, What Complements doe best accomplish her* (London, 1631), sig A5r.

108 Olivia Weisser, *Ill Composed: Sickness, Gender, and Belief in Early Modern England* (New Haven, CT: Yale University Press, 2015).

literally heaped labour upon labour by an almost obsessive attentiveness to theirs and others' bodies within the household.

Family members writing to pregnant women freely used the threat of miscarriage in admonitions to eat certain things, behave a certain way and to stay cheerful, in a way that must have done anything but relax women. Anna Temple, for example, told her pregnant daughter, Ann Busbridge, that she could 'haue the mayron of beefe at the Butchers upon the greene, & the marrow, or pith of the sheepe'. She told her she had 'had expereince [of] it' and it was 'very good and strengthening'.[109] Likewise, Barbara Compton wrote to Walter Bagot, both of the Staffordshire aristocratic Bagot family, requesting he send obtained venison, a term used to mean meat obtained via hunting in the period, for her pregnant daughter for 'many times, great-bellied women think of such novelities'. Barbara had extended a loan she had made Walter and jested that this would be his recompense.[110] In childbearing guides, unsatisfied cravings were related directly to the ability of the maternal imagination to imprint on the child. Craving strawberries might cause children to be born with a sympathetic birth mark. If a woman thought about another man or saw an image of him while having sex with her husband, her baby would look like him rather than her spouse.[111] In her *Observations*, Sarah Stone, a midwife that practised in Bristol and London, recalled how she had attended a heavily pregnant woman who had lost a 'gallon' of blood and was afflicted by constant pains that came in waves. Stone believed she was suffering from unsatisfied cravings. Confronting her, Stone recorded in her observations that the woman continued to deny her longings, 'till I told her that both she and the Child would lose their lives, unless she speedily had what she had an Inclination for'. The mother-to-be responded, 'What should poor people Long for?', before eventually confessing that she was preoccupied with a desire for fresh peas. Stone, playing the role of the good midwife, told her charge that she would get anything in her power 'let the price be what it would'. When the patient eventually ate the longed-for peas, her pains ceased instantly and her health returned. Stone delivered the baby, a healthy baby boy, a month later. In this example, it was the woman who was responsible for recognising and interpreting her cravings, but those around her who needed to supply this need. 'Discreet women' would manage their imagination by avoiding 'lamentable, fearfull tales or storyes' and avoid seeing 'pictures or persons which are uglie or deformed, least the imagination imprint on the child the similitude of the

[109] Anna Temple to Ann Busbridge, 10 November 1632, The Keep, East Sussex Record Office, 51/48.

[110] Barbara Compton to Walter Bagot, 6 July 1616, Folger Shakespeare Library, Washington, DC, L.a.145, fol. 1.

[111] For a discussion of the maternal imagination, see Fissell, *Vernacular Bodies*; Marie-Hélène Huet, *Monstrous Imagination* (Cambridge, MA: Harvard University Press, 1993).

said person or picture'.[112] Ulinka Rublack notes that German towns often ordered beggars to hide visual evidence of their disability for fear it could cause pregnant women to pass on these features to their offspring.[113]

Attentiveness and vigilance were seen as paramount to preventing miscarriage. In draft letters to 'Mrs Tulloch' by an unknown correspondent, the writer was adamant that if the pregnant woman had 'taken any pains ab[ou]t' her health she 'might haue been perfectly ... well before ys [this] time', almost two months after she had supposedly conceived on 1 May 1721. It was 'easier to preuent yn [than] cure' the writer chastised, the same sentiment that childbearing guides expressed when they demanded husbands, but especially wives, moderate their diet and behaviour while trying to conceive. The writer warned that if Tulloch continued to 'neglect, & disregard yt w[hi]ch is so very valuable to all your acq[uaintan]ces & that be so to your self, your disease may end in ane incurable Decay' and she would come to 'repent your Indiffer [en]cy'. Seemingly, Tulloch did little to change her poor habits for another note was penned 8 August 1721 that warned that if she wanted to preserve her own life and that of her infant, she should 'begin to use' the medicine an unnamed doctor had prescribed, snidely noting that 'the sight of a Rec[ei]t' alone would not cure, only the taking of it. Again, on 28 September, the author was desirous of an update on Tulloch's health stating,

> I'm well convinced yt if you take ye proper care of your self, your Disease will not prove so dangerous as you imagine. But if you be careless & indifferent, & your illness prove obstinate or mortal (wch God forbids) you'll have your self to blame.[114]

Anna Temple similarly used the threat of a previous miscarriage to try and cajole her pregnant daughter Ann to be 'chear full' and not take 'a conceit'.[115] Families commonly proferred emotional distress as the cause of miscarriage. Isaac Archer, for example, described how his wife miscarried twice in 1622, once in April and again in August. The first baby was lost 'upon no occasion' but the result of her ongoing 'griefe and ilnes'. He judged that the baby 'was corrupted', meaning dead and so 'twas well it came away'.[116] She became pregnant again quickly and miscarried again in August 'through a sodaine fright, upon an unhappy occasion' but thought it impertinent to record who had caused the fright 'because 'twas beyond the intention of him that occasioned

[112] Jacques Guillemeau, *Child-birth or, The Happy Deliverie of Women Wherein is set downe the government of Women* (London, 1612), 26.
[113] Ulinka Rublack, 'Pregnancy, Childbirth and the Female Body in Early Modern Germany', *Past & Present* 150, no. 1 (1996): 96.
[114] 'Note on Mrs Tulloch's pregnancy, and copy of a note sending her advice and shoes, 1721', National Records of Scotland, Edinburgh, CH12/12/795.
[115] Anna Temple to Anne Busbridge, 10 November 1632, DUN 51/48.
[116] Isaac Archer, 'Diary', 25 April 1676, University of Cambridge Library, Add 8499, 179.

it'. This is another subtle reminder that journals and diaries were composed with an audience in mind and as a record of events – including both pregnancy and miscarriage – for posterity, of which generation, birth and miscarriage were important.[117]

Margaret, the Countess of Wemyss, wrote to her daughter, Anne, that 'there is nothing so good for you & ye childe both as to be merry so I intret you let not anie thing yt falls out, disquiet & vex you'.[118] In another letter, Margaret wished that her daughter would 'be soe wise and kinde to the childe in y[ou]r belly as not to grieve much as you did last'. Anne was particularly worried that her husband would be unable to be at the birth. She warned that as she was further along in her pregnancy now than she had been when she had been plagued by fear in her previous pregnancy, she would do far more damage.[119] This was not always just about infant welfare, however, but the wellbeing of the whole family. Anne's distress 'troubles us' Margaret explained '& does much displeass & dishonours God'.[120] When Anna Temple wished her daughter would be 'chear full' in her pregnancy, she asked her to consider that her fate was in the hands of the Lord and both living and dying were outcomes worthy of celebration.[121] These pregnant women were constantly scrutinised and subjected to considerable pressure to eat and behave in a certain way by family members. They were simultaneously encouraged to do everything within their power to avoid miscarriage but told that all experiences and events, including or perhaps especially carrying children, were ultimately the expression of divine will and therefore to a degree, unchangeable. Poetry that explored miscarriage and stillbirth similarly focused on God's hand, rather than maternal wrongdoing.[122] Although elite and middling women have been represented as occupying a privileged position during pregnancy and in particular being able to resist patriarchal imperatives, in fact their bodies were examined and laid open to scrutiny in family correspondence that childbearing guides and religious texts encouraged.

117 *Ibid.*, 22 August 1697, 179.

118 Margaret, countess of Wemyss, to Anne, countess of Leven, 23 November 1695, National Records of Scotland, GD26/13/401/23.

119 Margaret, countess of Wemyss, to Anne, countess of Leven, 30 November 1695, GD26/13/401/24.

120 Margaret, countess of Wemyss, to Anne, countess of Leven, 23 November 1695, National Records of Scotland, GD26/13/401/23.

121 Anna Temple to Anne Busbridge, 10 November 1632, East Sussex Record Office, Brighton, DUN 51/48.

122 Jennifer Evans and Sara Read, '"Before Midnight She Had Miscarried": Women, Men, and Miscarriage in Early Modern England', *Journal of Family History* 40, no. 1 (2015): 2–23; Pamela Hammons, 'Despised Creatures: The Illusion of Maternal Self-effacement in Seventeenth-Century Child Loss Poetry', *English Literary History* 66, no. 1 (1999): 29–49.

In hoping that women would be cheerful, conduct authors sometimes noted that husbands might also have a responsibility in this. John Oliver in *A Present for Teeming Women* (1663) noted that 'many Husbands' needed reminding of 'their duty' towards their wives during pregnancy.[123] He asked them to forget 'all bitterness, wrath, anger, clamour, and evil speaking' and have a 'tenderness for her health, protection, quiet, and tranquillity, a bearing with her infirmities, procuring all possible helps and supplyes'. Husbands had to promote their wives' 'cheerfulness and content in all fit and lawful wayes'.[124] Men that failed to do so were 'Divels or Monsters'.[125] *Every Woman Her Own Midwife* (1675) thought that women's 'familiar friends' had a responsibility too in shielding her from 'unwholsome' things lest 'she should desire it, and not be able to get it'.[126] Many of these instructions focus on actionable tasks that those around the pregnant women could do: remove unsightly things and provide food, medicine and safety. Whereas women are often instructed to be cheerful, men were simply asked not to be bitter, wrathful, angry or speak evilly. Male family members were also, crucially, not the recipient of letters that threatened miscarriage or infant illness. When Lord Lanesborough wrote to his mother-in-law about his wife's pregnancy, he noted that he understood it was important that all 'care' be taken to 'satisfy all scruples and apply as early preventatives as is possible', even though she had had a good pregnancy so far.[127] Although Margaret, Countess of Wemyss, was quick to warn her daughter that if she did not cheer up she might miscarry, she heaped praise on her son-in-law, the Earl of Leven, for his perceived attentiveness. She told her daughter she was sure that he had taken 'care of having every thing done for' her that would 'contribut[e] for her beter health'. He was 'one of the most carefull kinde husbands I ever saw, & yt makes me the less anxious of coming home this winter since she is in so good hands'.[128] This was despite the fact he had spent most of the pregnancy away from home and could not give his wife the certain promise of his return for her impending birth.

While husbands and other family members often viewed pregnancy and childbirth as a joint venture, airing their views and offering advice, adjudicating what would lead to positive procreative outcomes, they did so in a way that reinforced generation was women's work, even if they were constantly weighing in. Men 'got' material goods and wives worked to bring this to fruition. Being a 'good' husband or father-to-be during pregnancy was tangible, observable and, simply put, easy. Being a 'good' wife and mother was intangible and was measured constantly and inconsistently. Writing about

[123] Oliver, *Present for Teeming Women,* sig. Aa2v. [124] *Ibid.*, sig. Aa3r.
[125] *Ibid.*, sig. Aa4v. [126] *Every Woman Her Own Midwife,* 3.
[127] George Lane to Lady Frances Cranfield, 1 August 1674, KHLC, U269/C21/1.
[128] Margaret, countess of Wemyss, to Anne, countess of Leven, 8 October 1695, GD26/13/401/8.

pregnancy often policed women and conditioned what they claimed to know about their own bodies, but it also imposed order on an otherwise unknowable and uncertain experience.

Reckoning and Fidelity

Beneath the need to be certain was the very real possibility that the child within might not be legitimate. In this way, making specific predictions, especially with regards to when the baby would be born, was related to verifying wives' sexual fidelity. This was yet another intensive focus for families that was displayed in obvious ways in their paperwork, but it was also a concern for women themselves who might seek the advice of medical practitioners to help them in making 'reckonings'. Thus, Elizabeth Underhill asked Napier whether her 'reckening is past' and Goody Phillips was 'according to her [rec]kning a fortnight past the tyme of her accounte'. This delay in being delivered had led her to be 'extreme sicke & looketh euery hour to be deliuered & yet is not'.[129] Goody Morgan told Forman that her daughter, Ann Gale of Goldington, 'looketh to be delivered about sonday', which was the 'last day of her reckning'.[130] It is no accident that the other common meaning of 'reckoning' was meeting one's maker. Birth forced women to confront their mortality but also labour painfully but redemptively.

Although Protestant reformers saw having sex as a marital debt that spouses owed one another and, crucially, an intrinsic part of the formation of godly families, there were delicate parameters to the amount of sex even spouses should be having. Too much sex, as we have heard, was thought to have deleterious consequences for health and prevent the conception of healthy infants. Although the Church of England was no longer as concerned with enforcing abstinence on days of the liturgical calendar such as Lent and Advent, as sermons and religious texts constantly reminded parishioners, marriage and the sexual license it provided was to avoid other kinds of fornication and for the perpetuation of the Church through procreation. Sex within marriage was therefore acceptable, even encouraged, but not carte blanche for indulgence. A woman who did not know she was pregnant quickly might not be keeping 'accounts' but she might also be having sex so often it was difficult to even work out when she could have conceived. Accounts and reckonings served as tangible and material records of the child's legitimacy. In making these predictions, couples helped to place themselves and their prospective issue within certain family narratives, albeit in ways that were often difficult for women.

[129] CASE20595, CB. [130] NOTE5484, CB.

As well as this role, establishing a reckoning helped families practically prepare for when delivery was going to happen. Goody Phillips asked when she would be delivered so as to know how long to keep her midwife with her 'for shee loketh every day for a happy delivery wch god granite her'.[131] Goody Bird, a midwife, came to Napier to ask when her patient, Goody Lane, would be delivered.[132] Ellen Selby used her sister's 'reckening' to calculate when she might be able to visit her. If Mary Arthington was able to 'hold out' until then, it would be possible and, in the meantime, wished her 'many prayers' as Mary's had brought her comfort when she was heavily pregnant.[133]

Yet again, however, the expectation that women could be accurate and specific in their reckonings was undermined by the fact that even medical authors could not agree on how long pregnancy was meant to last. Helkiah Crooke described how an infant could be born after seven, eight, nine, ten or eleven months of pregnancy, but those who gave birth after eleven months were probably 'deceiued in the time of her conception'. Babies born at eight months 'do neuer liue' and 'The birth at nine months is most legitimate and to Nature most familiar.'[134] Barret claimed he was drawing on Hippocrates, stating that a child would be formed in forty-five days, a woman would normally quicken ninety days after conception and give birth after 270 days or nine months. The rule was that the time from conception to quickening could be tripled to get the day of birth, although he admitted that girl babies were often born in the tenth month of pregnancy because they needed extra time for the 'increase and perfection of the infant'.[135] The distinction between full term and premature or undeveloped babies, however, was not always clear. In her meditations, Alice Thornton described giving birth to a daughter that lived an hour and a half as a 'miscarriage'. She was seven months pregnant.[136]

Despite this, the pressure to give specific and accurate due dates meant women were encouraged to overcome this potential confusion. Lady Frances Cobham wrote to Elizabeth St Loe, later the Countess of Shrewsbury and known as Bess of Hardwick, in October 1564, stating that she had travelled to Cobham in preparation for delivery 'wher I intend god wyllynge to be browght a bed i loke a weke before sente anderous day' [St Andrew's Day, 30 November].[137] Anne Meautys wrote to Jane Bacon in July 1630, telling her 'I am now with child; my time if God permit me life, will bee about

[131] CASE20595, CB. [132] CASE24397, CB.

[133] E[llen] S[elby] to Mary Arthington, undated and copied out into 'Letter book c. 1680–1700', Bodleian Library, Oxford, MS Add A 119, fol. 1r.

[134] Helkiah Crooke, *Mikrokosmographia a description of the body of man* (London: 1615), 269–270.

[135] Barret, *A Companion for Midwives*, 57 [136] Thornton, BL Add MS 88897/1, 129.

[137] Frances Brooke, baroness Cobham, to Lady Elizabeth St Loe, 21 October 1564?, Folger Shakespeare Library, Washington, DC, Cavendish-Talbot MS, X.d.428 (16).

Crismas.'[138] When Lucy Scrope wrote requesting updates from her pregnant sister, Abigail Newton, she noted that, 'I shall not be long after you for I recken at the beginning of July'.[139] Other women sought the assistance of astrologers to be able to profer a certain time when they would give birth. In 1609, Richard Napier's sister-in-law asked how many weeks it would be until she gave birth.[140] One woman who 'hath bene 21 weekes quick as she supposeth' could not 'tell whe[n] she shall be brought a bed but is desyrous to know it'.[141] Margaret Morley of Lumbard Street, twenty-five years old, asked 'Vtrum sit sit grauida *et quado ptriet* et vtru sit mascul aut femina' [Whether she is pregnant and *when she will give birth* and whether it will be male or female].[142] Elizabeth Russell, forty-five years old, asked 'Whether she is pregnant and when she will be delivered'. The judgement was that she would be delivered '23 days hence'.[143] At times, women were not necessarily told when they would deliver but when they had conceived so as they might come to their own reckonings; Margaret Bedall asked whether she was pregnant and told she was carrying 'a boy of ten dais', or was only ten days pregnant.[144] Like being able to announce pregnancy early, families also frequently turned to astrologers to calculate their reckonings. Julian Wilson, fifty years old, who asked Forman whether she was pregnant, reported to him that she only had '12 daies to goe' until delivery.[145] It is unclear from the notes whether he reified her calculations.

Perhaps the clearest indication that reckonings were intertwined in proving fidelity is found in the tensions that arose when babies were born before or after the time they were expected. What might otherwise seem a quirk – writing out reckonings – became part of husbands' interrogations to pinpoint marital indiscretion in their wives. *Aristotle's Master-piece* explained how 'Many bitter Quarrells happen between Men and their Wives, upon the Man's suspition that his Wife comes too soon; and by Consequent that he could not be the Father.' Instead, it was his want of 'Understanding the secrets of Nature that brought the man unto that Error'. One woman, the book narrated, a married woman of 'a noble family of unspotted Fame', delivered a baby a mere twenty-seven weeks after the calculated date of conception. Rather than simply assuming that the woman had been inaccurate in her prediction, the author of *Master-piece* suggested that instead the baby had been born early for the baby did not appear to look like others born at 'full 9

138 Anne Meautys to Jane Bacon, 2 March 1641, in Joanna Moody (ed.), *The Private Correspondence of Jane, Lady Cornwallis Bacon, 1613–1644* (London: Associated University Presses, 2003), 263–264.

139 Lucy Scrope to Abigail Newton, 11 May c. 1690, Lincolnshire Archives, Lincoln, MON 13/122.

140 CASE35256, CB. 141 CASE23810, CB. 142 CASE949, CB.

143 CASE7684, CB. 144 CASE7446, CB. 145 CASE1249, CB.

Months'.[146] Edward de Vere became estranged from his wife, Anne, countess of Oxford, when he suspected her of unfaithfulness because 'he lay not with his wife but at Hampton Court, and that the child could not be his because the child was born in July' and he was under the impression that it took twelve full months for a child to be gestated.[147] Once he was corrected and reassured his wife had been faithful, he accepted the child as his own and reunited with his wife. Consultations in the astrologers' casebooks also point to the importance of reckonings to working out whether a woman had been faithful. On 5 November 1618, Mr Cowley was 'wonderfully desyrous to know' from astrologer Gerence James when Vere Bouth would give birth.[148] This was in addition to the five consultations of her own.[149] William Bouth also asked when his wife would give birth in 1618. Napier notes that 'his wife is mistaken in her c[oun?]t', which he had taken 'impatiently & was troubled in his hed & could not rest well that night'. The dates his wife had given him were confusing and he sought external validation that she had been faithful.[150]

Ballads similarly explored the ways that men might be able to discover infidelity through interrogating the reckonings that women proffered. In the *Lass of Lynn's New Joy*, the protagonist has a tryst with an unnamed man only to find herself pregnant. Initially, she tries to hide her state by lacing her stays 'So hard all day' that they 'Pinch'd both her Back and Side'. With her mother, she conspires to find a husband to be a 'Cloak' for her 'Great Belly'. She convinces George the Tapster at the Bull to marry her, and on their wedding night, ensures the match is consummated. As they lay in bed, he placed his hand 'On a soft place' and 'found she'd a Rising Belly'. Although he suspects she is pregnant with another man's child, he is quickly satisfied by her assurances that she is simply 'fat and plump' from the wedding feast, and she quickly enlists the help of a midwife to fudge her reckoning so as to make the new baby appear legitimate. She flatters his ego by suggesting that it is because he is so virile that the baby has come surprisingly early and tells him that pregnancies last last 'Five Months by Days, and five by Nights', and so she has 'gone her full time to a day'. Here creating accounts and predictions about her reckoning is a crucial part of the lass and midwife's collusion.

This fear of misplaced reckonings opening families to accusations of infidelity is perhaps the reason that elite families, and particularly husbands, were eager to publicly correct reckonings retrospectively. Hugh Cholmely noted in

[146] *Aristotle's Master-piece; Or, The Secrets of Generation Display'd in all the Parts thereof* (London, 1690), 51.

[147] Johanna Rickman, *Love, Lust, and License in Early Modern England: Illicit Sex and the Nobility*, Women and Gender in the Early Modern World (Aldershot: Ashgate, 2008), 30.

[148] CASE47793, CB.

[149] CASE47609, CASE47608, CASE47607, CASE47606, CASE47583, CB.

[150] CASE47770, CB.

his memoirs written for his sons that when his wife gave birth to their first child, Richard, in 1624, earlier than expected, she was adamant that she 'went full forty weeks'.[151] The fact that families noted when women were mistaken in their calculations points to the importance of these dates in the narratives families told about their own generation. Judith Isham described in a letter to her husband how her sister had been 'deceived in her reckoning' and gave birth earlier than she had expected to.[152] Likewise, Isabella Wentworth wrote to her son c. 1712, telling him that although Lady Bathurst had 'reckoned a month after y[ou]r Lady', she had been wrong in her calculations and 'yesterday brought to bed of a very Little Girl'.[153] The astrologers sometimes returned to cases in which women had asked when they would deliver to add the day and time that the child was born. Goody Phillips was 'brought a bed the 29 of febr about 9 of the clocke' and Goody Lane 'the next morning about six'.[154] As with keeping accounts, accuracy was important to ways people tried to understand and fashion generation into ways that accorded them and their families honour, even if this accuracy was an invented one. Getting it wrong led to the kind of 'town talk' that Edward Conway fretted about when he asked his brother-in-law to keep the uncertainty of Anne's pregnancy to himself.

By sharing reckonings, women sought to declare the legitimacy of their pregnancy but in doing so they simultaneously laid their marriage open to scrutiny and interrogation. This also helped to define the boundaries of the family and involve others in the creation and recreation of this lineage. It also meant individuals could have their accounts doubted and corrected. Margaret, the countess of Wemyss, told her daughter that she doubted she would give birth at the end of January. Margaret told her that if she did give birth before February, 'it will be before your time', but promised if this was the case to 'haste over so soon as I can'.[155] In another letter, she reassured her daughter that even if she went beyond her reckoning, it would not necessarily endanger her or her child's life – 'wee have severall women in this place that has gone by there [sic] reckoning, one of them was delivered yesterday & had a very good Labour'. One woman had had very similar symptoms to Anne 'had pains these 9 weeks & is a Lean small woman' and had had a healthy child.[156]

[151] Hugh Cholmley, *The Memoirs of Sir Hugh Cholmley, Knt. and Bart. Addressed to His Two Sons* (London, 1787), 40.

[152] Judith Isham to Justinian Isham, 23 April 1666, Northampton Record Office, Northampton, MS IC 583.

[153] Isabella Wentworth to Thomas Wentworth, 24 February c. 1712, BL, Wentworth Correspondence, Add MS 22225, fol. 373.

[154] CASE20595, CASE24397, CB.

[155] Margaret to Anne, c. 1675, National Records of Scotland, GD26/13/401/14.

[156] *Ibid.*, GD26/13/401/13.

Prognosticating together served the dual purpose of starting to make preparations for the delivery and involving Margaret in the pregnancy and family that Anne and her husband were perpetuating. Isabella Wentworth similarly used correspondence to offer her own interpretation of when her daughter-in-law would give birth in 1712. '[I]t being my Ladys first', she figured 'she may come at 38 weeks which is the 16 of next month', which would be February but 'she may goe on to ye end of ffeb or ye first week in march,' because 'none can be exact' she admitted.[157] Sir Anthony Denton wrote to Sir John Isham in 1608, telling him that his sister 'is near a good tyme, God thanked'.[158] These kinds of letters were only written to close members of family. Sharing this knowledge enveloped them in the couple's marriage and procreative experiences in intimate but important ways.

Conclusion

Looking at the records that families, and particularly women, kept, domestic paperwork reveals that announcing pregnancy early and making accurate reckonings imposed order on what was otherwise a fluid and unpredictable experience. But these notes served a greater purpose in making certain respectable aspects of childbearing public, whilst downplaying others like efforts to increase fertility, and, as we shall see, pain and difficult recoveries. Authoritatively knowing when one had conceived was firmly linked to marital fidelity and (relative) chastity, and the resultant paperwork formally inscribed this commitment to the family project, as well as involving others within the fold of the new family. This involvement, however, often left women open to scrutiny and criticism. Family members were all too quick and willing to blame women for regrettable procreative outcomes. Writing about conception and pregnancy was a key part of the experience of having babies for middling and elite families. Although Sharp expected that women would keep 'just accounts', it is apparent that these accounts were both intellectually and practically connected to broader cultures of record-keeping and representing familial identity as well as spiritual practice.

157 Isabella Wentworth to Thomas Wentworth, 27 January 1713?, BL, Add MS 22225, fol. 353.
158 Sir Anthony Denton to Sir John Isham, 28 December 1608, Northamptonshire Record Office, Northampton, IC/137.

3 Big Bellies, Imagining Babies and Cultures of Display

After a new pregnancy was announced, families threw themselves into preparations for the birth and speculated about what the baby would be like; whether it would be a boy or girl, whether it would be large or small, and whether it would be good natured or 'dull'. In the same ways that elite married women wilfully interpreted certain bodily signs to mean they were pregnant and calculate when they were going to deliver, this same prognosticating impulse was turned to looking for outward signs that would reveal the unborn child's nature. Women's bodies, like the records that families kept of conception and pregnancy, and the material items they gathered for the birth and after-birth period, were part of an embodied culture of display in which swelling bellies and the imagined large lusty infants contained within them were thought to represent families' burgeoning prospects. Individuals engaged in a process of collective imagining, which defined the emotional and social boundaries of the family and household, and simultaneously policed women's conduct. To refuse gifted or lent items or fail to participate in the written practices of predicting threatened to open rifts within families. The things that households gathered and the written records that they created during this phase formed an important body of tangible things that defined the family in question as godly, reputable and fruitful, and placed childbirth right at the centre of domestic life. As with reckoning, male family members were very much active participants in this imaginative and material preparation for new life.

By placing written accounts alongside material culture – linens, expenditure on food and drink, infant clothes and birthing stools – which have featured prominently in histories of childbirth previously, we might better see them as part of a larger impulse to embed unborn children within familial contexts and narratives. For some historians, the objects that women were given or gathered prior to birth was a mechanism of temporary seclusion from the domestic unit. For Adrian Wilson and others, these items and the practices associated with them served to literally and figuratively sequester women away from the rest of the (male) household during birth and helped to create a relatively egalitarian space in which class, religious denomination and other markers mattered less than they normally would. The birthing woman occupied a room that had been specially designated for the birth and the month afterwards, called her lying-in. She was surrounded by other women she had invited and the ritualistic, and at times talismanic, items she had chosen for up to a month, and this period was far more of a social and community ritual than a familial one in this argument. Once this month, or lying-in, was up, she went to church to give thanks and was supposedly reabsorbed into the family and its priorities.[1] Thus, Patricia Crawford described the ceremony of childbirth as the 'female rite of passage *par excellance*'. For Linda Pollock, although women did not invariably support one another during pregnancy and labour, birth was a nonetheless wholly female event in which material culture played a central role in creating and solidifying female solidarity.[2] Things and the reorganisation and demarcation of space have been central to this argument that stresses childbirth and particularly this late stage of pregnancy was a unique and subversive time in the gender order of households. This chapter finds quite the opposite. The preparations in the later stages of childbirth did not sequester women away from family and the household. They served to make childbirth a family affair and in keeping with the argument of this book, although women took on the bulk of work in generation, they did so in ways that was set out and circumscribed by male priorities. Although husbands, brothers, fathers and uncles may not have been literally present in the room when birth occurred, the items that they had carefully selected and procured were, and they were only metres away in practical and culturally significant ways.

Growing Big

Early modern correspondence is awash with reflections on pregnant women's 'big bellies', and they were celebrated in the same way that announcements and reckonings were. This was chiefly because the bigger the belly, the more likely it seemed that the baby would be large, healthy and potentially male. In writing about pregnant stomachs, families collectively and vocally hoped for positive procreative outcomes, but also simultaneously made the birth of 'lusty' infants seem inevitable within narratives about how ascendant the family was. In October 1695, Margaret, Countess of Wemyss, wrote to her pregnant daughter asking if she had 'grown bige yit' and if she was nauseous – did she 'keep' her 'meat'. She hoped she would 'grow stronge' and 'be better & better' with every pregnancy until she had the twenty children

[1] Adrian Wilson, 'The Ceremony of Childbirth and Its Interpretation', in *Women as Mothers in Pre-Industrial England: Essays in Memory of Dorothy McLaren*, ed. Valerie Fildes (London: Routledge, 1990), 68–107, *The Making of Man-Midwifery: Childbirth in England, 1660–1770* (London: Routledge, 1995).

[2] Linda A. Pollock, 'Childbearing and Female Bonding in Early Modern England', *Social History* 22, no. 3 (1997): 286–306.

she 'usid to wish for' when she was a child.[3] A month later, she wanted to know again 'if you be grown bige'.[4] Lord Broghill gleefully told his father-in-law, Richard, in January 1667 that his wife, Mary, was 'verry bigg' despite the fact she was not due to deliver until the 'Latter end of Aprill'. These signs pointed to the impending birth of a 'Lusty Sonne'.[5] This was not the first mention of Mary's belly since getting married. In March 1666, Broghill's father expressed to Richard that he wanted nothing more than for her to have 'a great belly', which he invited Richard to now 'Come & see' it.[6] Frances Sackville's husband, George Lane, wrote to Lady Frances Cranfield, his mother-in-law, describing how her 'great Belly' was 'very pleaseing'.[7] Henry, Earl of Bath, passed on the well wishes of John Finch, chief justice, to his wife, Rachel, 'for you and particularly for your Belly', meaning her burgeoning bump.[8]

The interest in pregnant bellies at times appears to have been prurient and potentially erotic. Women's swelling bellies were a visually interesting representation of male virility and sexuality. They were looked at in ways that confuse relief with the healthy progression of pregnancy with desire. If we recall how the husband in *The Ten Pleasures of Marriage* gleefully recorded his wife's pregnancy in his almanac, he now focused his attentions on the sight of her apron, which 'day from day rose'. Now, 'all the World may plainly see you have behaved your self like a man, and every one acknowledge that you are both good for the sport'.[9] The wife in the parody suddenly becomes more affectionate, potentially even libidinous in response to the sight of her burgeoning stomach as a visual representation of her husband's virility. She 'imbraces and kisses' her husband because he had 'furnish'd her shop so well'. The author impresses upon the reader that 'the procreating of children, makes the band of wedlock much stronger, and increaseth the affections', but we see that there was a prevailing cultural idea in these jokes that women's pregnant bodies would display men's sexual skill and the couple's ascendancy.[10] This was a common metaphor in cheap print of the period: that the furnishing of women with their baby bumps was similar to the way husbands furnished wives with clothes, linens, food, medicine, shelter and

3 Margaret, countess of Wemyss, to Anne, countess of Leven, 21 October 1695, National Records of Scotland, Edinburgh, GD26/13/401/21.

4 Margaret, countess of Wemyss, to Anne, countess of Leven, 23 November 1695, GD26/13/401/23.

5 Lord Broghill to Richard, fifth earl of Dorset, 7 January 1667, KHLC, U269/C218/12.

6 Lord Orrery to Richard, fifth earl of Dorset, 2 March 1665/6, KHLC, U269/C219/3.

7 George Lane to Lady Frances Cranfield, 1 August 1674, KHLC, U26/C21/1.

8 Henry, earl of Bath, to Rachel, countess of Bath, c. 1639, KHLC, U269/C267/10.

9 A. Marsh, *The Ten Pleasures of Marriage Relating all the Delights and Contentments that are Mask'd Under the Bands of Matrimony* (London: 1682), 102.

10 *Ibid.*, 104.

other domestic items. Pregnant women were like ships, the anonymous author of *Fifteen Real Comforts of Matrimony* jested, and they 'never looks so handsome' as when they were 'completely rigg'd and trimm'd' with a pregnant stomach.[11] Conversely for some, the sight of a burgeoning belly in others could provoke shame and sadness. When Samuel Pepys saw his sister 'fat gone' in her pregnancy in May 1669, he noted in his diary that 'I know not whether it did more trouble or please me, having no great care for my friends to have children; though I love other peopl's.'[12] The joy he felt for his sister and her husband, John Jackson, was tempered by his own childlessness. Big bellies were potent social symbols for men and women, for they tangibly and visibly reflected what prior to this point families had only wished for or imagined in their correspondence.

Elite women often sought to display and highlight their changing parturient forms, so much so that Mary of Modena, wife of James II, was suspected to have fashioned a fake belly to pretend she was pregnant in 1688.[13] Mary Tudor wore a stomacher that emphasised her 'belly laid out, that all men might see she was with child'.[14] Some elite women bought new stomachers with matching sleeves, soft stays or had their existing stays altered to include side lace-up panels during pregnancy.[15] Honor Grenville, Viscountess Lisle, an aristocratic Cornish woman whose life in the sixteenth century is exceptionally well-recorded in the Lisle papers, was offered a stomacher cloth of gold by William Lock, a mercer, in 1536, when he found out she was pregnant. Jane Seymour, Henry VIII's third wife, was 'open-laced with stomacher' when she was pregnant.[16] Such garments did not hide parturient bodies but drew attention to them.[17] Pepys described Catherine of Braganza, then queen of England, wearing a 'white pinner and apern [apron], like a woman with child', a suggestion that wearing aprons and pinners (pinafores) had become a kind of maternity dress in themselves, albeit one potentially more often of convenience rather than fashion.[18]

For other women, buying new clothes to accommodate their changing shape was financially impossible. In the ballad *The Lass of Lyn's sorrowful Lamentation for the loss of her Maidenhead* c. 1657–1696, the young woman

[11] *Fifteen Real Comforts of Matrimony being in Requital of the Late Fifteen Sham Comforts, with Satirical Reflections on Whoring and Debauchery of this Age Written by a Person of Quality of the Female Sex* (London: 1683), 1.

[12] Samuel Pepys, 12 May 1669, *The Diary of Samuel Pepys, Vol. 9, 1668–1669*, ed. Robert Latham (New York: Harper Collins, 1983), 553.

[13] Cited in: Rachel J. Weil, 'The Politics of Legitimacy and the Warming-Pan Scandal', in *Political Passions: Gender, the Family and Political Argument in England* (Manchester: Manchester University Press, 1999), 67.

[14] Harriet Waterhouse, 'A Fashionable Confinement: Whaleboned Stays and the Pregnant Woman', *Costume* 41, no. 1 (2007): 58.

[15] *Ibid.* [16] *Ibid.*, 56. [17] *Ibid.*, 58. [18] Pepys, *The Diary of Samuel Pepys, Vol. 9*, 557.

who got pregnant out of wedlock fretted that 'My Petticoats which I wore,/and likewise my Aprons too,/Alas! they are all too short before,/I cannot tell what to do.'[19] It was not just the prohibitive expense of buying new clothes to accommodate her pregnant form but the fact that she had conceived out of wedlock that the lass of Lynn sought to conceal. Even wealthy women like Sarah Churchill, duchess of Marlborough (1660–1744), might make do by adapting existing clothing. She reflected in a letter to her granddaughter, Diana, that three months before her 'reckoning', she could not 'endure to wear any bodice at all, but wore a warm waistcoat wrapped about me like a man's and tied my petticoats on top of it. And from that time never went abroad but with a long black scarf to hide me, I was so prodigeous big.'[20] One might say even writing this was a form of displaying her pregnant form in lieu of clothes. It was not until the nineteenth century that specific pregnancy corsets and dresses were manufactured.[21] Bellies and the way they were noticed, written about, clothed and, as we shall see, depicted, were part of a system of signs of bodily, financial, religious and social fortune, which men were equally if not more invested in than women. Whilst this symbolism is not so obvious to us now, it was seemingly immediately apparent to early modern individuals, so much that it appears in a wealth of different kinds of printed and manuscript material.

Pregnant stomachs were also celebrated in portraits of aristocratic women in the sixteenth century. Catherine Carey's (Lady Knollys') large belly protrudes from beneath her dress in her picture (Figure 3.1). She carries a gold girdle chain and large oval tablet representing the god Mars, armed with a spear and shield, gesturing to the Greek proverb 'Be prepared'.[22] Her dog stares unflinchingly out of the portrait, a symbol of marital fidelity.[23] Karen Hearn has described how works like this and others by the Dutch painter, Marcus Gheeraerts the Younger, of English aristocratic women acted as a 'form of visual evidence of anticipated dynastic success'.[24] 'Pregnancy portraits' such as that of Lady Knollys (1562), *Portrait of an Unknown Lady*, c. 1595 (Tate T07699) and *Portrait of a Woman in Red*, 1620 (T03456), the latter, believed

[19] *An Answer to I Marry and thank ye too: Or, The Lass of Lyn's sorrowfull Lamentation for the Loss of her Maiden-head*, EBBA 22080 (London: 1657–1696).

[20] Cited in Phillis Cunnington and Catherine Lucas, *Costumes for Births, Marriages and Deaths* (New York: Barnes & Noble, 1972), 15.

[21] Emma O'Toole, 'Dressing the Expectant Mother: Maternity Fashion in Eighteenth- and Early-Nineteenth-Century Ireland', *Women's History. The Journal of the Women's History Network* 2, no. 5 (2016): 26–32.

[22] Karen Hearn, 'A Fatal Fertility? Elizabethan and Jacobean Pregnancy Portraits', *Costume* 34, no. 1 (2000): 40.

[23] Pauline Croft and Karen Hearn, '"Only Matrimony Maketh Children to Be Certain…": Two Elizabethan Pregnancy Portraits', *The British Art Journal* 3, no. 3 (2002): 19.

[24] Hearn, 'A Fatal Fertility?', 40.

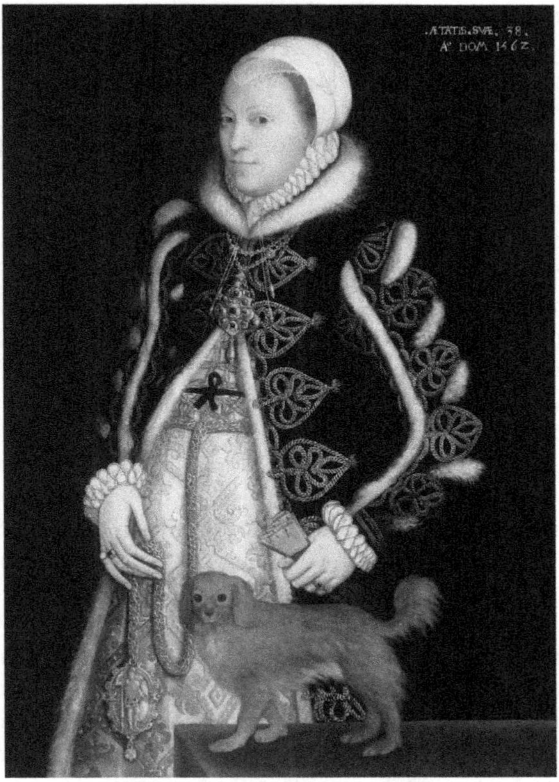

Figure 3.1 Portrait of Catherine Carey, Lady Knollys, by Steven van de Meulen, 1562. Oil on panel, 108.6 × 79.4 cm. Paul Mellon Collection, Yale Center for British Art released under CC-BY licence.

to be a member of the Constable family, repeated the bigness and fecundity of these women's 'bellies' in a similar way as correspondence.[25] The women painted in this way were in their late thirties, already having borne several children, and carrying their last or penultimate child. The portraits were not celebrations of youthful fertility but rather of continuity, obvious ascendancy and the permanence of these families. The portrait of Mildred Coke, Lady Burghley, painted in c. 1563, highlights rather than disguises her maturity. Hearn suggests that cultural anxieties about succession and the queen's waning fertility provoked families to commission these tangible reflections of maternal

[25] Tate Gallery Online Catalogue, 'Portrait of a Woman in Red 1620' and 'Portrait of an Unknown Lady c. 1595', www.tate.org.uk/art/artworks, last accessed 14/03/2025.

travail for the family and its title.[26] Although there was a little boom in these portraits in the late sixteenth century, generally it is very difficult to find obviously parturient bodies in European art of the period because this was supposedly deemed unseemly or vulgar.[27]

The medical and culinary recipe book of an anonymous early eighteenth-century English or Scottish family suggests that obviously pregnant bodies could also be a source of fascination and celebration in very domestic contexts too. The book contains numerous remedies relevant to generation such as 'A Very good Receipt against miscaringe', 'A present Remidie for a Woeman with childe, wch hath taken hurt by a fall or fright or any Mischanc to staye the Child and to Comfort it' and 'For the falling doune of the Matrix after Child birth'.[28] It includes a series of naïve images, perhaps the work of a child, drawing his or her family members. First there is what we might gather is a male figure carrying maybe a riding crop, spade or rod for disciplining children and servants (Figure 3.2a). Then there is what appears to be a female figure – she wearing a dress (Figure 3.2b). The next page possibly depicts a baby. The figure is substantially smaller than the others and its dress is distinctively cross-hatched, a possible representation of swaddling bands (Figure 3.2c). On the next page, the drawer has made another figure with a big, distended, possibly pregnant, belly (Figure 3.d). On the following page, using the bleed-through, this belly becomes breasts, with a bigger, rounder belly drawn in below (Figure 3.2e). The identity of the drawer and their intentions are irrecoverable, and yet the prominence of big bellies within a book that is primarily concerned with domestic wellbeing and order points to the ways these concerns overlapped within households. Perhaps more than their composition, it is that they have been kept and not erased or removed that reveal the meaning behind visibly pregnant bodies in the construction of family identity in the period.

In court settings, calling a woman 'big' and drawing attention to the size of their pregnant stomach was often used to signify how close a woman was to delivery, as well as their performance of godly maternity. It was used to stress pregnant women's vulnerability and their need for social and legal protection. Crimes committed against pregnant women were deemed more barbaric and ungodly, especially so at this later stage of parturiency. Describing women as 'big' emphasised not only their bodily infirmity but also the maturity of the babies they carried; these infants were just on the cusp of outside life and therefore to rid them of the possibility of it was more morally reprehensible.

[26] Hearn, 'A Fatal Fertility?'.

[27] Croft and Hearn, '"Only Matrimony Maketh Children to Be Certain…"'; Hearn, 'A Fatal Fertility?'; Michael de Winkel, 'The Interpretation of Dress in Vermeer's Paintings'. *Vermeer Studies*. Edited by Ivan Gaskell and Michiel Jonker. Symposium Papers, 55, no. 33 (1998).

[28] 'Recipe book', University of Glasgow Special Collections, Glasgow, MS Gen 831, 46–47.

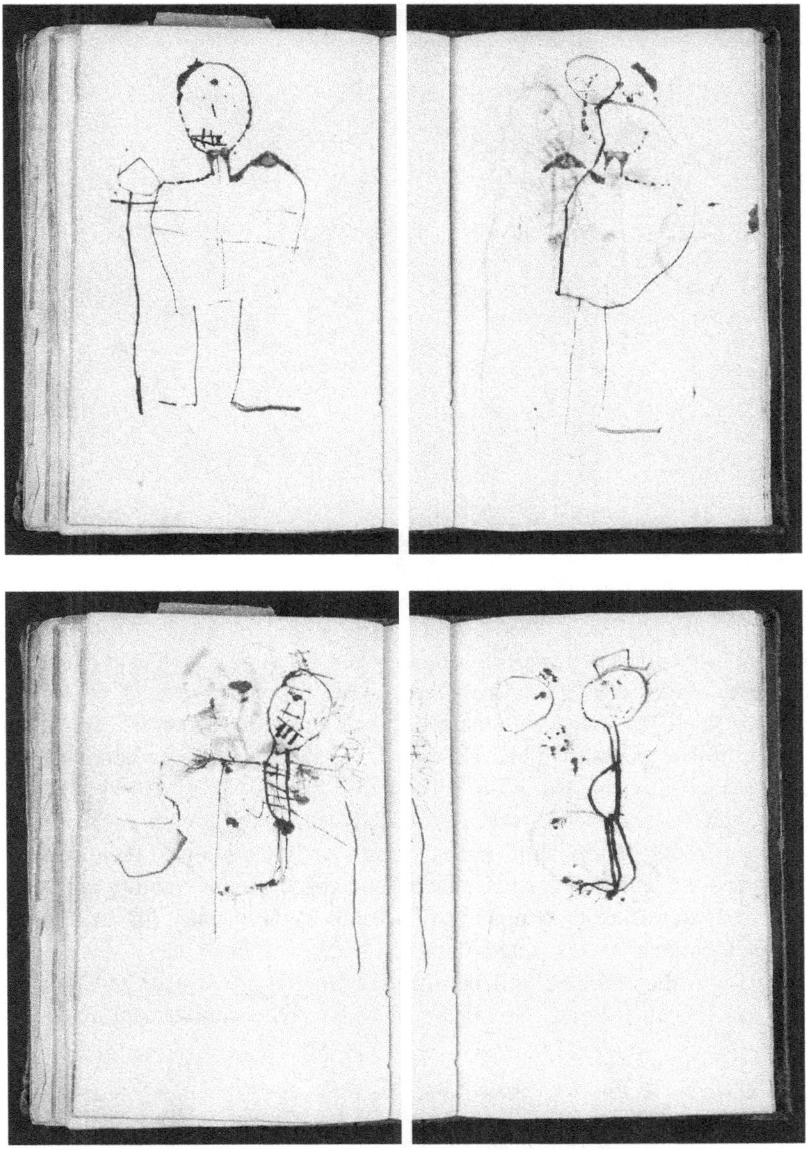

Figure 3.2 (a–e) 'Medical recipes, seventeenth to eighteenth century', MS Gen 831, 76–80. By permission of the University of Glasgow Archives and Special Collections.

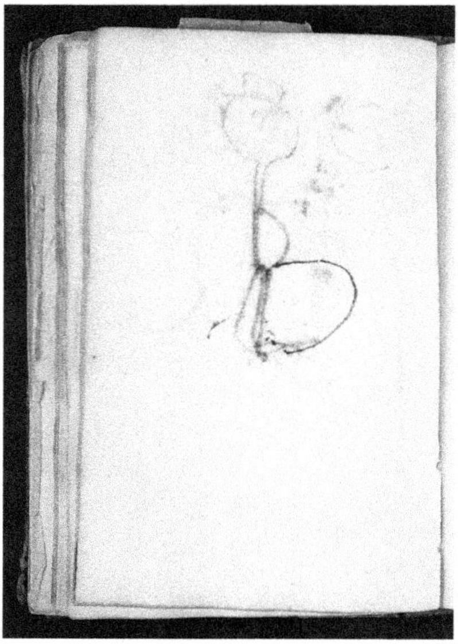

Figure 3.2 (*cont.*)

Big bellies recurred as a trope in sensationalist murder pamphlets to emphasise the depravity of criminals. In *A True and Perfect Relation of A Horrible Murther* (c. 1678–1680), an unnamed man brutally murdered his 'neighbour' who is 'full bigg with Child'. The child was delivered after its mother died and lived on to avenge the death.[29] The wife of David Williams was 'most big with child to bee' when she was cruelly murdered by three soldiers.[30] In assault cases, Jenine Hurl argues victims drew attention to their pregnant states where relevant to 'increase their appearance of vulnerability before the court and command its sympathy'.[31] In France, the penalty for assaulting a pregnant woman was adapted in accordance with how close she was to delivery – if the child had quickened, the perpetrator was executed, if not, a fine was levied.[32] Being pregnant excused women from execution across

[29] *A True and Perfect Relation of A Horrible Murther, Committed by a woman in Golden-lane, on her Neighbour big with-Child, who had borrowed Thirty shillings of her, who is since fled*, EBBA 20741 (London: 1678–1680).

[30] *A Warning for all Murderers. A most rare, strange, and wonderfull accident, which by Gods just judgement was brought to passe, from Rithin in Wales*, EBBA 30323 (London: 1601–1640).

[31] Jenine Hurl, '"She Being Bigg with Child Is Likely to Miscarry": Pregnant Victims Prosecuting Assault in Westminster, 1685–1720', *The London Journal* 24, no. 2 (1999): 30.

[32] François Mauriceau, *The Diseases of Women with Child, and in Child-bed: as also, the Best Directions How to Help Them in Natural and Unnatural Labours* (London, 1672), 64–65, cited in: Hurl, '"She Being Bigg with Child Is Likely to Miscarry"', 29.

Europe in this period. Women who 'plead the belly' were interrogated and inspected by a jury of matrons to attest to whether they were telling the truth.[33] Pamphlets similarly played on the idea that seeing a pregnant belly elicited sympathy and the desire to protect. The sight of a 'bigge belly' of a 'handsome, and decently apparelled' 'wandring yong woman' in one ballad provoked such pity in Mother Watts that she offered her a room for the night, 'sucker [succour], helpe and furtherance … at the painefull hower of her deliuerie'. The woman delivered a monstrous and misshapen child that night, but her vulnerable appearance had convinced Mother Watts to take her in despite her better judgement.[34]

Although being big was often celebrated, for pregnant women themselves, particularly unmarried ones, the word could also be used to signify a stage of pregnancy that was cumbersome and difficult. Female writers, therefore, often used the term to describe the moment when their pregnant state made life uncomfortable, when delivery was imminent and their child had reached a certain level of maturity. Frances Hutton, in a letter to her husband Christopher, relayed how 'Mrs Allen', possibly a midwife or nurse, thought she was carrying a 'very great child' because of her size. Hutton wondered whether she night be carrying twins, 'I am so exceeding big'. Her size and recurring pains meant she could no longer walk.[35] In this exchange, being 'big' conveyed how much the infant had grown, how imminent delivery would be and how taxing bearing children could be. The next day, Francis was still struggling; she was in 'Every hour in expectation of my labour' and her condition tied her to her bed and 'chamber above this three weeks. Mrs Allen will not let me stir out of it I am so extreme big.'[36] Alice Thornton similarly gestured to her size to emphasise that she was ready to give birth. In her second pregnancy, a month before she assumed she would give birth, she grew 'bigge' and 'was in a wearish condition'. When pregnant with her third child, 'a week before my full time', she was 'in much paine through the heavinesse of my Childe; haveing the midwife in constant expectation each houre', exacerbated by her mother's absence. Again, in her fourth pregnancy, she was 'heavy, bigge, & weary' and 'Full of paine; & the labour each day'.[37] At other times, bigness was used by others to gesture to how imminent delivery was. Thomas Busbridge in a 1682 letter to his sister, Anna Farnden, described his wife's struggles to get home to give birth – she was 'big with

33 Cathy McClive, 'The Hidden Truths of the Belly: The Uncertainties of Pregnancy in Early Modern Europe', *Social History of Medicine* 15, no. 2 (2002): 209–227.

34 *Strange Newes out of Kent, of a Monstrous and Misshapen Childe, Borne in Olde Sandwich, upon the 10 of Julie Last* (London: 1609).

35 Frances Hutton to Christopher Hutton, 20 April 1678, BL, MS Add 29571, fol. 459.

36 Frances Hutton to Christopher Hutton, 21 April 1678, BL, MS Add 29571, fol. 463.

37 Alice Thornton, BL, Add MS 88897/1, 134.

child', the roads tricky and 'not well in a coach'.[38] In 1645, Isabella Twysden recorded in her almanac that she had ridden on horseback to Peckham 'great with child' and was grateful to 'land no hurt'.[39] Lady L'Estrange was 'very well & is as bigg as if she were near Lying downe' or going into labour, '& so I suppose she is'.[40] Penelope Mordaunt appealed to her husband to return home from Walton and Bedford because she 'begin to groe big', 'biger and heavear' than with any of her previous children.[41]

Although being big was something that was celebrated when women conceived within wedlock, for unmarried women, this was often the moment when their bodies began to betray their indiscretions. Single women were surveyed by neighbours, and when they were suspected of having pre-marital sex and being pregnant, their stomachs and breasts were watched for signs of conception.[42] The neighbours of Gertrude Law of Rotherham thought she might be pregnant in 1671 when she got big and then 'suddenly grown less in her body'. A man said 'thou was with child but thou art swampe [flat] now'.[43] Five months later, the body of a baby was discovered in a well on her street, cementing their suspicions that she had had a child out of wedlock. When women were accused of having illegitimate children and committing infanticide, they often claimed that their big stomachs were caused by something other than being pregnant. Showing they were unaware of their pregnancies, or that their stomachs were swelling because they were unwell or had eaten too much, could save them from being hanged. These claims might allow them to circumvent the part of the 1624 law that held them automatically responsible for the baby's death if they had not shared their pregnancy with anyone: how could they tell anyone they were pregnant if they did not know they were? Isabel Barton, who was suspected of infanticide in Yorkshire in 1663, told the court she had been 'ravished' by a man in June and that her body 'grew big' but she had no idea she was with child until she miscarried in December.[44] In these court cases, the size of women's bellies was used as evidence that either incriminated them or helped to exonerate them, and supports the suggestion by historians that the term being or growing 'big' had contemporary parlance as signifying a stage when pregnancy was visually

38 Thomas Busbridge to Anna Farnden, 6 September 1682, DUN 51/88.

39 Isabella Twysden, 8 February 1644/1645, BL, Add MS 34169, *Mercurius Coelicus: Sive Almanack, Et Prognostication, Vel Speculum Anni à Nativitate I. C. 1647*, fol. 2r.

40 John Mordaunt to Penelope Mordaunt, 27 October 1698, Warwickshire Record Office, Warwick, CR 1368/vol. 1, fol. 2.

41 Penelope Mordaunt to John Mordaunt, 9 September 1701, CR 1368/vol. 1/36.

42 Laura Gowing, 'Secret Births and Infanticide in Seventeenth-Century England', *Past & Present*, no. 156 (1997): 91.

43 *Ibid.*, 94. 44 *Ibid.*, 91.

verifiable.[45] For elite married women, however, this was an act of display more than a fraught process of visual verification. Big bellies helped families furnish accounts of what the unborn child would be like. Noticing, depicting and writing about big stomachs was part of this same attentive culture of record-keeping and sought to impose order and a sense of processual predictability to pregnancy. That bellies could swell for all kinds of other purposes was often left out of elite correspondence and instead celebrated as being a portent of positive procreative outcomes to come.

The 'Litle One Within'

Pregnant bellies were important to families primarily because they suggested that the child was alive and well within, and helped to imagine it as part of the household already. When William Chaytor sent a letter to his pregnant wife, Peregrina, in 1691, he offered well wishes to her as well as 'the litle one within'.[46] Interpreting the signs and symptoms of pregnancy to engage in these imaginative and speculative ventures was one of the ways families imposed certainty on the process of childbearing. It also made the unborn child part of the family before its birth. This kind of specificity was similar to the ways in which women and families proffered particular dates when they thought they might give birth or their reckoning that we have heard about in Chapter 2.

Family members were particularly interested to know whether the baby was a boy or girl. When Lord Broghill wrote to his father-in-law to announce that his wife had quickened, he noted 'they tell me by all signes yt will bee a Boy'.[47] When Grace Wallington gave birth, her husband, Nehemiah, recorded in his diary that when she had a 'man child', they were surprised because this was 'contrary to our expectation.[48] Jane, wife of Ralph Josselin, claimed that one of her births was 'very strange to her' because it was a daughter, 'contrary to all her former experience and thought'.[49] Isabella Wentworth wrote to her son, Thomas, to ask him to buy lace to make a 'cressning [christening] suit' fit

[45] Linda A. Pollock, 'Embarking on a Rough Passage: The Experience of Pregnancy in Early-Modern Society', in *Women as Mothers in Pre-Industrial England*, ed. Valerie Fildes (London: Routledge, 1990), 44. Kathryn M. Moncrief similarly suggests that the common parlance of such terms indicates that pregnancy was 'identified by what could be observed', '"Show Me a Child Begotten of Thy Body That I Am Father to": Pregnancy, Paternity and the Problem of Evidence in All's Well That Ends Well', in *Performing Maternity in Early Modern England*, ed. Kathryn M. Moncrief and Kathyrn R. McPherson (Aldershot: Ashgate, 2007), 30.

[46] William Chaytor to Peregrina Chaytor, 11 August 1691, North Yorkshire Record Office, Northallerton, ZQH 9/3/24.

[47] Lord Broghill to Richard, fifth earl of Dorset, 6 April 1666, KHLC, U269/C218/3.

[48] Nehemiah Wallington, 1 December 1628, *The Notebooks of Nehemiah Wallington, 1618–1654: A Selection*, ed. David Booy (Aldershot: Ashgate, 2007), 60.

[49] Ralph Josselin, 13 January 1658, *The Diary of Ralph Josselin, 1616–1683*, ed. Alan Macfarlane (Oxford: Oxford University Press, 1991), 415.

to dress a boy but expressed her suspicions that his wife was carrying a girl.[50] Thomas only agreed to pay an exorbitant fee for a man-midwife (100 guinneys) because he was convinced it would be a boy. He was ultimately disappointed when Isabella's hunch proved right. The astrologer-physicians, Richard Napier and Simon Forman, were often asked to determine whether women were carrying a boy or a girl. Mary Robinson asked Forman in 1599 whether she would have a boy or girl.[51] Likewise, Elizabeth Scarlet who was 'neere upon her tyme' asked when she would give birth and whether it would be male or female.[52] This was at times motivated by anxieties about procuring an heir. Vere Bouth asked whether she 'shall have an hayre', having previously had a little girl that died.[53] Sir Thomas Middleton asked whether he would have a son.[54] Lady Elizabeth Dacre also asked whether she would have a boy, suggesting she was concerned with primogeniture.[55]

It seems that parents were not making these guesses randomly, but they might have drawn on extensive guidance in childbearing guides about how to read bodily signs to discover the sex of unborn babies. Carrying a girl was described as much more taxing on maternal health than carrying a boy, and therefore women who felt weak and sick during their pregnancies were assumed to be having a 'wench'. Jane Sharp explained that 'If it be a boy she is better coloured' and she would be 'more cheerful and in better health, her pains are not so often nor so great'.[56] Jacques Guillemeau suggested that women who were pregnant with girls would be 'wayward, fretfull, and sad' due to the excess of moisture produced by female children.[57] Girls were bred on the left side of the womb, where it was colder and moister, and boys on the right, where it was hot and dry. This supposedly led to bodily asymmetry that could be read to discover the sex of unborn children. If movement was felt only on one side of the womb; if one breast 'rise and swell beyond' the other;[58] this would reveal the sex of the baby.[59] Thomas Chamberlayne and Jane Sharp recommended observing how a pregnant woman moved. If she put her right foot forwards, 'and in rising she eases all she can her right side sooner than her left', she was carrying a boy.[60] Even the milk that came into a woman's breasts in the latter months or weeks of pregnancy might reveal the sex. Sharp

[50] Isabella Wentworth to Thomas Strafford, 13 January c. 1713, BL, MS Add 22225, fol. 345.
[51] CASE4857, CB. [52] CASE23786, CB. [53] CASE47606, CB. [54] CASE25935, CB.
[55] CASE48073, CB.
[56] Jane Sharp, *The Midwives Book Or the Whole Art of Midwifry Discovered*, ed. Elaine Hobby, Women Writers in English 1350–1850 (Oxford: Oxford University Press, 1999), 83.
[57] Jacques Guillemeau, *Child-birth or, The happy deliuerie of vvomen* (London: 1612), 10.
[58] Thomas Chamberlayne, *The Complete Midwife's Practice Englarged, In the most Weighty and High Concernments of the Birth of Man Containing a perfect Directory, or Rules for Midwives and Nurses* (London: 1659), 80.
[59] Sharp, *The Midwives Book Or the Whole Art of Midwifry Discovered*, 83.
[60] Chamberlayne, *The Compleat Midvvife's Practice Enlarged*, 80.

suggested women expressed a drop into a basin of water – 'if it swim on the top it is a Boy, if it sink in round drops judge the contrary'.[61]

These findings challenge the prevailing idea that children remained largely ungendered until they reached a certain level of maturity. In particular, historians of medicine have noted that unlike the ways sex and gender conditioned the diagnosis and treatment of adult bodies, for children, sex made little difference in terms of diagnosis and treatment of disease.[62] Hannah Newton argues that sex was not 'as significant as other variables' in understanding children's bodies and their medical needs,[63] nor was it important in informing medical treatment.[64] It was only when children reached a certain age that gender was imposed upon them, chiefly through dress and the practice of breeching when boys were around six.[65] Yet, the interest in working out whether babies were boys or girls when it seemed they might not live long, and the ways in which people sought to assign sex to infants when this was not immediately apparent, points to a pressure to classify newborns as decidedly male or female within families, as well as a belief that male and female babies must be humorally distinct enough to have a different impact in gestation on the maternal body. Goody Marshall's child was 'Christnd for a wench' in 1624, despite being described by Richard Napier as a 'hermaphrodite' and living only a week.[66] Scientific, alchemical and philosophical works were keenly interested in intersex individuals or 'hermaphrodites'.[67] This interest was often as much prurient as it was intellectual and served to sustain sexual and gender boundaries.[68] In medical texts, physicians adjudicated whether their patients would live their lives as men or women, a decision that was enforced by authorities.[69] Family members, medical practitioners and pregnant women engaged in an important and symbolic cultural ritual in imagining infants in which their sex was central. Although treatment for infants may not

[61] Sharp, *The Midwives Book Or the Whole Art of Midwifry Discovered*, 84.

[62] Wendy D. Churchill, *Female Patients in Early Modern Britain: Gender, Diagnosis, and Treatment* (Farnham: Ashgate, 2012), 19.

[63] Hannah Newton, *The Sick Child in Early Modern England, 1580–1720* (Oxford: Oxford University Press, 2012), 40.

[64] *Ibid.*, 90.

[65] Anthony Fletcher, *Gender, Sex and Subordination in England, 1500–1800* (New Haven, CT: Yale University Press, 1995), 297.

[66] CASE57733, CB.

[67] Leah DeVun, 'The Jesus Hermaphrodite: Alchemy in The Late Middle Ages and Early Renaissance', in *The Shape of Sex: Nonbinary Gender from Genesis to the Renaissance* (New York: Columbia University Press, 2021), 163–200.

[68] Jenny C. Mann notes that the authors of sixteenth- and seventeenth-century medical texts represent the bodies of hermaphrodites as demanding 'visual exploration' that is complete and unfettered. Jenny C. Mann, 'How to Look at a Hermaphrodite in Early Modern England', *Studies in English Literature, 1500–1900* 46, no. 1 (2006): 86.

[69] *Ibid.*, 85.

have diverged significantly for boys and girls, their bodies were already thought to be humorally male or female, which would have different impacts on their mothers during pregnancy, in ways that confirm the work of other scholars who have suggested that gender and sex were important categories of difference over the medieval and early modern period.[70]

In addition to working out the sex of babies before they were born, some parents named their children prior to delivery. This practice perhaps more than any others strongly suggests the desire to knit infant lives into larger familial narratives. Robert Woodford, a Northamptonshire lawyer, relayed in his diary how on the day of his son's baptism, he forgot to instruct the chosen godparents that the 'name should be John'. Godparents were in charge of holding and naming infants at baptism ceremonies in early modern England, usually in consultation with parents.[71] This practice was common enough that Alice Kenyon's mother, Jane, joked with her that she should find 'convenient godmothers' who would promise to call her daughter 'Anne or Alice' and definitely not Jane.[72] One of baby Woodford's godparents, Mr Readinge, in a flash of divine inspiration. judged the child to be called John. This was not an uncommon narrative for godparents to name children from divine inspiration. Elias Ashmole was named because his godfather, Thomas Ottely, had an epiphany to cease the family tradition of naming boys after their fathers. However, where the Woodford narrative departs is that Robert noted that not only was John the name he had hoped for, but it was 'the name by which I and my wife used to call it before it was born'.[73] Another touching glimpse into this practice can be found in a letter from Eliza Cope, of the Dorset Sackville family, who told her sister that for the entire pregnancy and the two weeks since she had given birth she and her husband had been calling their son 'little Cakebread'. He would have a new more formal name at his christening.[74]

How the baby moved within the womb might also reveal things about its future character. Wemyss asked her daughter how her little 'devil sturred'.[75] Thornton compared the ways that her different children felt in the womb. Her

70 For a summary of these debates see: Helen King, *The One-Sex Body on Trial: The Classical and Early Modern Evidence* (Farnham: Ashgate, 2013).

71 This practice was changing over the seventeenth century so that parents eventually held and named their own infants. Ralph Josselin recorded in his diary on 17 August 1644, 'This day I baptized 3 children. John Read held his own child; the first I ever baptized so' in Josselin, *The Diary of Ralph Josselin*, 44.

72 Alice Kenyon [II] to Alice Kenyon, 29 May c. 1630, Lancashire Record Office, Preston, DDKe/9/93/11.

73 Robert Woodford, 20 August 1637, *The Diary of Robert Woodford, 1637–1641*, ed. John Fielding (Cambridge: Cambridge University Press, 2012), 96.

74 Eliza Cope to sister, 21 September 1651, KHLC, U269/C273/6.

75 Margaret, countess of Wemyss, to Anne, countess of Leven, 23 November 1695, GD26/13/401/23.

fourth child, Katherine, was 'more weighty & not so nimble as naly & betty'. Katherine was 'very liuely' in the womb, which made Alice 'uery feauorish & hot, causing much sicknesse'. Sometimes such sensations were used to direct medical care. Alice had her blood let and described how the baby 'sprange in my wombe'. She was healthier and stronger from this point onwards.[76] These efforts to understand and visualise the infant imbued the infant with an identity – a sex, personality and even name – in a collaborative process with other family members. Many of these exchanges insisted on the specificity of the experience of pregnancy to the mother and the child. When Althea Talbot, Countess of Arundel, was pregnant in 1608, her mother-in-law noted to her father, Gilbert, that 'all children were not bred alik[e]'.[77] It was comforting for families to imagine that their infant's personality was already fully formed and imagine the ways that it might resemble its ancestors.

In imagining their unborn babies, early modern English families had a long-standing visual code from which to borrow from – the representations of infants in the womb in printed medical texts. These were useful in two ways. They not only allowed people to understand the basic physiological process of pregnancy, but they depicted babies that would have been comforting to individuals anxiously waiting for the birth of a new family member: these babies all appeared large, lusty and very much cognisant of their surroundings. These sixteenth- and seventeenth-century images bore many similarities to the highly stylised older tradition of babies in Muscio's Latin treatise from the ninth century that appeared to be suspended in flasks or jars.[78] Unborn infants were almost always represented as male and they were often pudgy or muscular. This trend remained 'remarkably constant' from the medieval period to the eighteenth century.[79] In Sharp's *Midwives Book*, the infants swim in luxurious space, and appear in a variety of lively positions (Figure 3.3). They are large and lusty – they have hair on their heads, their eyes are open and they stare out at the viewer with various facial expressions. Whereas older images depicted the womb as a single membrane, by the seventeenth century, authors and artists were interested in the layers of the womb and in depicting the stones, or female testicles. In these pictures, the womb is represented in isolation as if cut out and separated from the maternal body. Karen Newman and Eve Keller have argued this absence was an act of artistic and intellectual exclusion of maternal effort.[80] Both suggest that

[76] Thornton, BL, Add MS 88897/1, 144.

[77] Anne, countess of Arundle, to Gilbert Talbot, earl of Shrewsbury, March (?) 1608, Lambeth Palace Library, London, MS 3205, fol. 139.

[78] Karen Newman, *Fetal Positions: Individualism, Science, Visuality*, Writing Science (Stanford, CA: Stanford University Press, 1996), 26.

[79] *Ibid.*, 26.

[80] *Ibid.*; Eve Keller, *Generating Bodies and Gendered Selves: The Rhetoric of Reproduction in Early Modern England* (Seattle: University of Washington Press, 2007), 125–155.

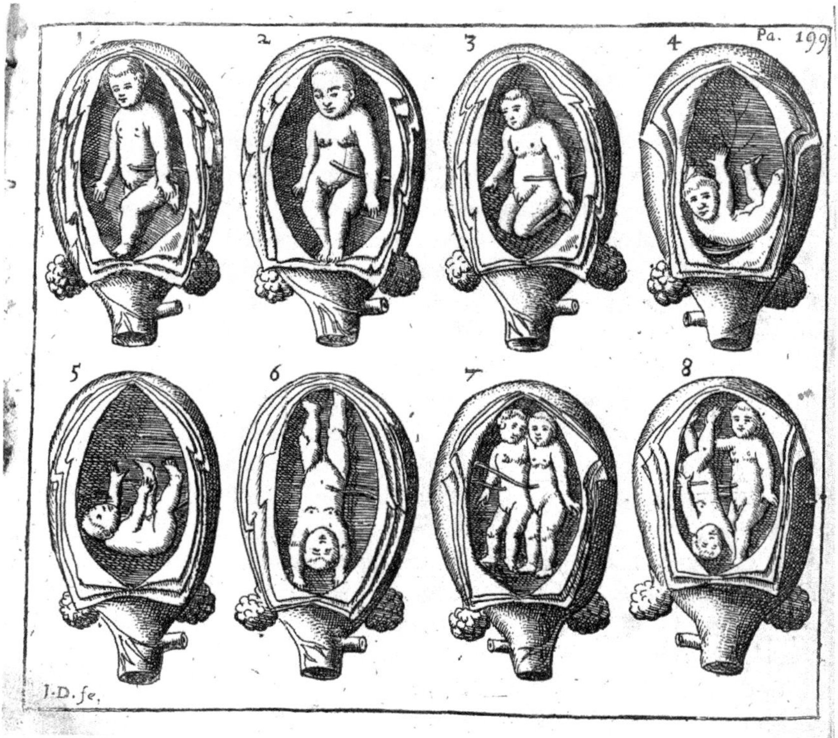

Figure 3.3 Jane Sharp, *The Midwives Book Or the Whole Art of Midwifry Discovered. Directing childbearing women how to behave themselves* (London: 1671), 199. Wellcome Collection.

this was part of a deliberate effort by early modern male obstetrical authors to deny, ignore and minimise the action of women's bodies in generation. These visual changes supposedly signified and enacted a transformation in ideas of personhood too – male authors and infants were imbued with agency, while female generative knowledge and work was undermined. These images made an unborn 'person … from the first moment of his conception'.[81]

Rebecca Whiteley has called for such obstetrical images to be redefined as 'birth figures', stressing their discursive purposes as tools of understanding birth positions. She proposes that such images could perform several simultaneous but diverse functions for different audiences. First, images of the unborn in childbearing manuals provided midwives with practical

[81] *Ibid.*, 155.

information about how to ensure infants were delivered safely. Secondly, learned readers were engaging in philosophical questions about the nature of creation and the universe. Finally, she suggests that for labouring women, their friends and family, images in midwifery manuals visualised the infant as large and lusty, not 'fragile, scrawny neonates' – and that this, rather than an effort to erase the maternal body, led to their highly stylised appearance.[82] Whiteley suggests that in the same way pregnant or labouring women might avoid troubling or disturbing images that could damage infant health and would instead gaze on pleasing objects and pictures to improve infant health, the babies in bottles in childbearing manuals were a tool in securing positive medical outcomes.[83] These images presented a hopeful and reassuring visualisation of pregnancy – they focused on the outcome: a baby, just as correspondents did in their letters imagining the size, sex, name and personality of the new family member.

These signs had meaning to early modern families perhaps because of the ways that authors equated the movement of foetuses with maturity and viability. James Wolveridge explained that forty-five days after conception, the infant was 'divinely infused' with a soul and therefore 'receiveth life' and was 'no longer called a young one, but an infant'. Robert Barret, borrowing from Hippocrates, similarly suggested an infant was 'formed' by day forty-five and this could be doubled to work out quickening and tripled to work out the day in which the infant 'will make haste to the Birth'.[84] Jakob Rüff described how after quickening the infant sought to widen his 'narrow little Cottage' by moving, and it was this that helped to swell pregnant stomachs. When they could no longer be contained they 'moved with great force and violence in the womb' to be born.[85] Sharp described the 'violent motion of the child' that forced the waters to break and that the infant 'can no longer stay there than a naked man in a heap of snow'.[86] Medical writers assumed that infants had a certain awareness and that from when they began to move, their character and bodies were largely formed.

[82] Rebecca Whiteley, *Birth Figures: Early Modern Prints and the Pregnant Body* (Chicago: Chicago University Press, 2023); Rebecca Whiteley, 'Figuring Pictures and Picturing Figures: Images of the Pregnant Body and the Unborn Child in England, 1540–c.1680', *Social History of Medicine* 32, no. 2 (2017): 241–266.

[83] Whiteley compares such images to Katharine Park's work on birthing trays in early modern Italy that mothers hoped would raise their chances of 'producing a well-formed son', Katharine Park, *Secrets of Women: Gender, Generation, and the Origins of Human Dissection* (New York: Zone Books, 2010), 145.

[84] Barret, *A Companion for Midwives,* 57.

[85] Jakob Rüff, *The Expert Midwife, or An Excellent and Most Necessary Treatise of the Generation and Birth of Man* (London, 1637), 61, 76.

[86] Sharp, *The Midwives Book Or the Whole Art of Midwifry Discovered,* 160.

In this context, it makes sense why family members were particularly interested in how unborn children moved and also why big babies were thought to be particularly healthy infants. We might say that this process of understanding the infant body through reading a patchwork of signs is similar to the one that Olivia Weisser describes early modern people doing for other kinds of illness including boils, pustules and wheals on bodies.[87] Richelle Munkhoff describes the ways plague searchers engaged in 'acts of interpretation' when they looked at dead and alive bodies for signs of the plague.[88] Family members interpreted a mess of bodily, religious and social signs to create an identity for the baby before it was born and were careful to write these predictions in a variety of different kinds of paperwork. This culture of investing in and imagining the future life of the babies from elite families intensified with the process of gifting, borrowing and gathering things for the new child. These items, like the accounts written about babies and their mother's big bellies, formed part of a familial ritual of display that was largely inaccessible to unmarried and vulnerable women.

Some Things to Be Had

As well as imagining what the baby would look like, these months of pregnancy, when families were sure a child was on its way, were dominated by the process of buying and gathering things for delivery such as bed linen, clouts, cloths for swaddling the newborn, cradles and sometimes birthing stools and negotiating these gifts, loans and purchases. Food and alcohol were needed to feed and entertain the women who attended the birth, the men sitting anxiously waiting downstairs and for both the baptism and churching ceremonies. Indeed, gifting women with things to prepare for birth was so ubiquitous it was inscribed in the title of John Oliver's 1688 popular text for childbearing women – *A present to be given to teeming women, by their husbands or friends Containing Scripture.* [89] In 1697, a heavily pregnant Peregrina Chaytor wrote to her husband requesting twenty pounds and 'to bring me down and buy som things which must be had' for her impending delivery.[90] Peregrina was in

87 Olivia Weisser, 'Boils, Pushes and Wheals: Reading Bumps on the Body in Early Modern England', *Social History of Medicine* 22, no. 2 (2009): 321–339.

88 Richelle Munkhoff, 'Searchers of the Dead: Authority, Marginality, and the Interpretation of Plague in England, 1574–1665', *Gender & History* 11, no. 1 (1999): 1–29.

89 John Oliver, *A Present To be given to Teeming Women, By their Husbands or Friends* (London: 1688).

90 Peregrina Chaytor to William Chaytor, 29 July 1697, North Yorkshire Record Office, Northallerton, ZQH 9/12/51.

temporary lodgings in London, while her husband was at their home in Croft, North Yorkshire. She asked for:

3 paire of good sheets
2 paire of such as the boyes lye in
5 pair of pillobear [pillowcase]
3 towells
the rest of the huggaback napkins to what are at London
the broad Diaper Napkins and table cloath
one duzen and half of the course huggaback napkins
2 table claoth of huggaback or linen
the [destroyed] huggaback table cloath
Holland in her trunk [destroyed] to make sleeues either here or be sent up
some more holland left their and any old linen of hers or mine for night close for the child
half a dozen of De mask napkins and table cloath
The dressing glasse and boxe
The silk mantles and quilt 4 silver spoons and forks
2 silver salts
1 silver podinger
the cup wth the cover or tankerd
bacon hams and tongue and cheses salt
butter a firkin of salt butter
[destroyed] bushels of wheat flour
Aile [ale]
3 litle pillows laced pillowbeers
one or two dimothy pillows w[hi]ch came from Richmond

Although most early modern family paperwork was not quite as detailed in their record-keeping of the materials gathered for birth, Peregrina's letters to her husband point to the variation of expensive, cheap, repurposed and borrowed items that were key to this practice. Peregrina sought to gather pricy items like the silver porringer (a shallow silver dish often given for christenings), some cheaper items (like flour) and others repurposed (like the holland linen in her trunk). Some things, which Peregrina hints at in her request for 'linnen of hers or mine for night close for the child', were borrowed or gifted by other family members. Perhaps most notably of all, Peregrina negotiated with her husband the gathering of these materials rather than approaching her female friends. Janelle Day Jenstadt explains that childbearing furnishings appear in account books less often than other domestic goods because they were often borrowed and returned rather than purchased. Added to this, childbearing items did not often appear in probate inventories because they had other uses and because constant use rendered the linen used for birth substantially less valuable.[91] This was not because aristocratic families could not afford a set of their own, although in the 1690s the Chaytors perceived themselves to be in dire financial stakes, but a careful and deliberate practice of exchange helped to solidify friendships and alliances between families.

Some of these exchanges and negotiations must have happened orally and so the extent of this material culture of exchange is irretrievable from family

[91] Janelle Day Jenstad, 'Lying-in Like a Countess: The Lisle Letters, the Cecil Family, and a Chaste Maid in Cheapside', *Journal of Medieval and Early Modern Studies* 34, no. 2 (2004): 374.

paperwork. When individuals did write to either request or offer items in the lead up to a birth, these written accounts served as yet another material stamp of investment and involvement of the family in its perpetuation by young and fertile members and sat alongside almanacs, letters and diaries that attested to women's godly conduct through pregnancy and occasionally portraits. Anne Holles wrote to her 'good friend' Mrs Marris, requesting the return of a 'mydwyves Chaire' in 1632. Presumably this was not enough to identify the object, for Anne continued, describing it as a 'dutch Chaire all of wood, and when it came downe was not sett together, but one side of it layd cloce [close] to the other, and soe packed up in Canvas'. With it, she asked for the return of two wooden boxes, possibly storage boxes for childbed linen.[92] This was possibly one of several chairs Marris had received or accumulated. Importantly, the chair and boxes were not Anne's originally but her 'daughter haughtons' or 'her mothers' – she could not remember which.[93] She needed them close because she expected that 'my daughter may have use of it ere long'.[94] Jane Cavendish kept 'A note of my childbed linen' in her commonplace book consisting of seven sheets, 120 double cloths, swaddling clothes for the newborn along with '26 pillowberes [pillowcases] course & fine, 1 torn for rags. These are in the childbed linen trunk.'[95] The fact that Cavendish used torn pillowcases to make 'rags' hints at the ways less wealthy women might have dealt with the mess of delivery, staunch bleeding after birth and fashion nappies.[96] Linen and bedsheets were, as Sasha Handley has shown, particularly emotive and affective objects within early modern households and often kept for their meaning across generations.[97] Sarah Fox notes that this culture of borrowing (which in the eighteenth century became institutionalised when poorer mothers could apply to charities to receive bundles of linens) was a flexible and adaptive practice that survived well into the eighteenth century.[98]

92 Anne Holles, countess of Clare to Mrs Marris, 11 December 1632, Strafford papers, Sheffield Archives, Volume 22 b, fol. 105.

93 Her daughter 'Haughton' was most likely Elizabeth Holles [née Vere] (d. 1683), the wife of her son, John, who styled himself as Lord Haughton. Her mother was Mary de Vere [née Tracy] (1581–1671).

94 This was most likely her daughter Eleanor who married Oliver FitzWilliam, first earl of Tyrconnell, around this time. Their marriage was childless.

95 Jane Cavendish, 'Commonplace book', HEH, Ellesmere MS EL 11143, unfoliated. For more on chairs and linen in childbearing and these exchanges, see: Pollock, 'Childbearing and Female Bonding in Early Modern England', 289.

96 Sara Read suggests that menstruation was often managed by the use of 'clouts' made by ripping up old fabric. See: Sara Read, 'Thy Righteousness Is but a Menstrual Clout: Sanitary Practices and Prejudice in Early Modern England', *Early Modern Women: An Interdisciplinary Journal* 3 (2008): 1–25.

97 Sasha Handley, 'Objects, Emotions and an Early Modern Bed-sheet', *History Workshop Journal* 65 (2018): 169–194.

98 Sarah Fox, 'Birth and the Household' in *Giving Birth in Eighteenth-Century England* (London: University of London Press, 2022), 51–77.

Lady Lisle obtained an extensive list of items of clothing and bedding for her and her unborn child between 1536 and 1537, all negotiated by her chief servant, John Husee.[99] These items were not always borrowed because the family were unable to afford to buy their own but the material letter detailing a loan and the objects themselves 'cemented social and political relationships'.[100] Sometimes, however, women wrote expressing real need for objects that they could not afford or find themselves. In 1590, Elizabeth Molyns was worried about her heavily pregnant daughter and wrote to Cicely, Lady Buckhurst, Countess of Dorset, hoping she would be 'allow & p[ro]vyde for her that ys mete for a woman in her case'. Molyns' son-in-law had commited 'wronges vexations & Inspeakable Inyuryes' through his 'crueltie & wyckednes' to her daughter, chiefly by denying her items needed for her impending delivery. Molyns asked Buckhurst to find her daughter some 'honest matrons' to accompany her in her delivery 'as may be for her saffetie'. It was 'evident', she wrote, that her husband 'hathe no car[e] for the p[r]-esvacion of her Lyffe'.[101] Thomas Peyton wrote telling Henry Oxinden that his daughter was 'towards lying in' and that her husband was so uncaring that he paid as much attention as if it was his cow that was calving, rather than his wife giving birth. 'Shee', he cautioned, 'is as unprouided as one that walks ye highwaies'. Peyton lamented that the beginning of the marriage was as 'unblessed' as its current 'incesant troubles'.[102] This was most likely Margaret Oxinden, who married the wayward John Hobart in August 1649, plunging Henry into lawsuits on his son-in-law's behalf.[103] Men were severely judged for not providing for their wives at other times too, but this was particularly reprehensible during pregnancy and birth.

Although these items took on an important emotional and social significance within households, women were very careful to ensure they were only requesting what was 'mete' or 'fitting' for their deliveries.[104] Bridget Willoughby, for example, reassured her pregnant daughter Elizabeth in 1611 that she would be 'readye to supplye you with any thinge that shall be *fittinge*, as yor occasions shall requueyre'.[105] Elizabeth Molyns stressed that her daughter only needed what was 'mete', nothing more. Obtaining only what was strictly necessary, and never excessive, tapped into a dominant religious cultural discourse in the

99 Catherine Mann, 'Clothing Bodies, Dressing Rooms: Fashioning Fecundity in the Lisle Letters', *Parergon* 22, no. 1 (2005): 137–157.
100 *Ibid*., 152.
101 Elizabeth Molyns to Lady Buckhurst, 1590, Bodleian Library, Oxford, Herrick MSS, English hist.c.474, col. 1, fol. 132.
102 Thomas Peyton to Henry Oxinden, 9 August 1653, BL Add MS 28003, fol. 163.
103 ODNB.
104 Pollock, 'Childbearing and Female Bonding in Early Modern England', 290–291.
105 Bridget Willoughby to Elizabeth Gell, 2 May 1611, Derbyshire Record Office, Matlock, Chandos-Pole-Gell MS D258/20/42. Author's emphasis.

early modern period of moderation. While this duty to consume food, drink, material goods, sex and company with care was configured in prescriptive texts as important for men *and* women, plays, satires and even some conduct manuals suggested that it was women alone who often spent too much in the lead up to delivery. The preacher Richard Adams, for example, noted that women should gather simple linens that were 'fine', 'clean' and 'white' and refrain from purchasing ornate, expensive or decorated objects. He chastised women who 'find you have conceiv'd, and grow pregnant, are highly concern'd to put on, and use these Ornaments', which they all too readily involved their 'mates' in.[106] This was a culture that local authorities were also keen to regulate. As early as 1540, the Chester Assembly Book expressed concern about the 'great excess' of food and drink at childbed gatherings, churchings and christenings.[107] The material culture of childbirth was consistently represented as being bequeathed to women by their husbands, the Church and state to ease and support their childbearing but it was conditional on their godly and moral conduct.

The stereotype that wives used parturition as an excuse to trick their hardworking husbands out of money to buy frivolities was regularly referenced and satirized in plays and cheap print of the period.[108] Thomas Middleton's *A Chaste Maid in Cheapside*, written in 1613 and published in 1630, parodied the pregnancies of middling sort women who sought to emulate the increasingly lavish lying-ins of elite women. Alan Brissenden has suggested that Middleton was directly mocking the lavish lying-in of the countess of Salisbury, wife of William Cecil, who John Chamberlin reported had her chamber hung with 'white satin, embroidered with gold (or silver) and perle' valued at £14,000.[109] In the play, Mrs Allwit is ridiculed for the excess of 'embossings,/Embroiderings, spanglings, and I know not what,/As if she lay with all the gaudy shops'.[110] Allwit equates the toll of spending that men

[106] Richard Adams, 'How may Child-bearing Women be most encouraged, and supported against, in, and under the hazard of their Travail?' in Samuel Annesley (ed.), *Continuation of morning-exercise questions and cases of conscience practically resolved by sundry Ministers in October, 1682* (London, 1683), 661.

[107] The First Assembly Book, 12 May 1540, Cheshire Archives and Local Studies, Chester, ZA/B/1/70v.

[108] Sara Read, '"Pregnant Women Gaze at the Precious Thing Their Souls Are Set On": Perceptions of the Pregnant Body in Early Modern Literature' in Jennifer Evans and Ciara Meehan (eds.), *Perceptions of Pregnancy from the Seventeenth to the Twentieth Century* (Basingstoke: Palgrave, 2017), 133–159.

[109] Jenstad, 'Lying-in Like a Countess', 373; Thomas Middleton, *A Chaste Maid in Cheapside*, ed. Alan Brissenden, New Mermaids (London: Bloomsbury, 2002), xiv. The National Archives Currency Convertor (www.nationalarchives.gov.uk/currency-converter, last accessed 25/7/2024) suggests that £14,000 in 1613 was the current equivalent of £1.7 million in 2017.

[110] Thomas Middleton, *A Chaste Maid in Cheapside*, Drama Classics Emma French (ed.) (Nick Hern Books, 2007: London), 1.2.30-38.

undertook with the emotional and bodily work of breeding a child for women: he tells the audience that it was more often husbands' backs that broke through their wives spending, rather than wives' through birthing.[111]

Ten Pleasures of Marriage mocked the first-time mother-to-be who acquired so much stuff that 'the Child-bed linnen alone, is a thing that would make ones head full of dizziness, it consists of so many sorts of knick knacks; I will not so much as name all the other jinkombobs that are dependances to it.'[112] Whilst the expectant mother was meant to devote herself to ensuring her body and soul were prepared for delivery, the woman parodied in *Ten Pleasures* instead turned herself to diligently measuring 'Beds, Bellibands, Navel clouts, shirts, and all other trincom, trancoms!' as if 'she had gone seven years to school to learn casting of an account'.[113] In such satirical texts, the work of pregnancy is equated with, even outstripped by, the labour and exhaustion husbands endured to buy things for their wives. Within this account, it is not just her excessive spending but also the fact that she does so without her husband's supervision or other family involvement that makes it reproachable. Husbands in *The Bachelers Banquet* saw their wives' bellies growing big although they had been cuckolded and the child was begot 'by the helpe of some other friend', but they were foolishly bothered about getting only the best things for their wives' lying-ins.[114] The husband had to 'trot up and down day and night, far and near, to get with great cost that his wife longs for'. When his wife gives birth, he must entertain her friends visiting for half the day, while 'the poor man' is 'handled behind his back' with salacious gossip.[115]

These pamphlets reveal the subtle but pervasive links between the material culture of childbirth and the legitimacy of conception and the ways in which men perceived themselves as giving their wives things in a way that was dependent on their good conduct. This in turn complemented and sat alongside manuscript accounts of the experience of bearing children in family archives. In the *Lass of Lynns*, it is only once the midwife has reassured the sceptical father-to-be that the child is his that he grants his wife and her gossips 'a Barrel of stout Ale,/and send for a Groaning Cake' to 'us Merry make'.[116] His purchasing and celebrating is only mocked by the gossips and audience who know full well that the child is not his. Moderate and abstemious pregnant women were idolised as the ideal. It was not necessarily that women like Peregrina, for example, were really surviving with the bare minimum, but it

111 *Ibid.*, Act III, Scene ii. 112 Marsh, *The Ten Pleasures of Marriage*, 105.
113 *Ibid.*, 106.
114 Thomas Dekker, *The Bachelers Banquet: or, A Banquet for Bachelers* (London: 1604), 13
115 *Ibid.*, 17.
116 *The Lass of Lynns New Joy For finding a Father for her Child. Being a Third Song of Marry and Thank ye too*, EBBA 21315 (London, 1682–1692).

was advantageous to the family's pious reputation to be seen to be doing so. Print culture's intensive focus on women being good mothers meant that some were discarded as 'lewd and vnnatural women, as leaue their new-borne children vnder stalls', and others perceived as selfish and ungodly for their immoderate gathering of baby things.[117]

Whereas Peregrina Chaytor might have considered her list a reduction of her normal and expected means, the vast majority of early modern women would not have owned, been able to borrow or purchase this plethora of expensive pieces. One family's definition of 'mete' or 'fitting' could be quite different from another's. Poorer early modern women might have borrowed heavily from family and friends to make up a full set of childbearing linen and would suffice with fewer, plainer and cheaper pieces.[118] Low-status women might use a straw bed instead of the increasingly fashionable pallet bed, a mattress or bed that was lower to the floor. The straw could be burned after delivery to save on the cost of linen.[119] Since providing proof of preparation for birth could be crucial evidence in exonerating women from infanticide,[120] one might expect details of a lower-status lending culture to feature prominently in the court cases of unmarried mothers, this appears to have been an uncommon defence. This may have been because this material culture of childbirth was so firmly bound up with male involvement and legitimate pregnancy to make it seem wholly unnecessary to single mothers proving to courts that they had intended to keep their children. Only two women out of a surviving seventy cases of neonatal infanticide tried at the Northern Circuit Assizes between 1642 and 1680 used this as a defence.[121] These pregnancies were normally concealed from family, friends, masters, mistresses and fellow servants. Unmarried mothers did not have the immediate support of a husband and family. They were additionally excluded from the emotional and practical support of fellow women. Aiding an unmarried pregnant woman could lead to legal ramifications: one woman was prosecuted for 'keeping of whores and lewd women in childbed and suffering of men to come in and lie with them before they be churched'.[122] Another woman tried at the Old Bailey for infanticide in

[117] William Gouge, *Of Domesticall Duties Eight Treatises* (London: 1622), 507.

[118] Ann Buck, *Clothes and the Child: A Handbook of Children's Dress in England 1500–1900* (Bedford: Ruth Bean Publishers, 1996); Alice Dolan, 'The Fabric of Life: Linen and Life Cycle in England, 1678–1810' (unpublished PhD thesis, University of Hertfordshire, 2015), 91.

[119] Sarah Fox, 'Reconceptualising the Birth Process in Eighteenth-Century England' (unpublished PhD thesis, University of Manchester, 2017), 53.

[120] Mark Jackson, *New-Born Child Murder: Women, Illegitimacy and the Courts in Eighteenth-Century England* (Manchester: Manchester University Press, 1996), 34.

[121] Gowing, 'Secret Births and Infanticide in Seventeenth-Century England', 99.

[122] Laura Gowing, *Common Bodies: Women, Touch and Power in Seventeenth-Century England* (New Haven, CT: Yale University Press, 2003), 157.

1691 asked a midwife in Stepney whether she could 'Lye In in private, which the Midwife promised she should' if she could provide for the child. Instead, the mother 'made away with the Child, throwing it into a Puddle of Water on the backside of the House'.[123] In this way, although many of the rituals and practices of delivery were female-only, they were culturally directed and bestowed upon them by men. The discussions of illegitimate motherhood displays how central the family project was in structuring the experience of bearing children.

Within elite families, the boundary between what was perceived as necessity and decadence was often debated. Isabella Wentworth, who served as lady of the bedchamber to Mary of Modena, for example, was particularly adamant that her daughter-in-law should have only the finest childbed accoutrement. This concern was not an aberration. She took an avid interest in her son's life, and particularly his marital prospects. Prior to his marriage to Anne Johnson in 1711, Isabella expressed what can only be described as desperation that her son wed and produce an heir. When Anne was pregnant with her first child in 1713, Isabella was similarly heavy-handed in her involvement. Isabella was dismayed that Anne was not interested in the 'new fation' for cradles and sumptuous birthing linens. Isabella took it upon herself to find and present Anne with new trends but Anne, Isabella wrote to her son in disappointment, liked 'her own fancy much better then any elc'. She told Thomas how she 'durst not' suggest anything else to Anne other than what she perceived as the bare necessities for birth – she protested 'thear is nothing of ffancy in them', and yet Anne still turned up her nose.[124] When Thomas sent his wife bedding and linen for the baby's arrival, Isabella told her son that Anne was insufficiently grateful. Isabella, in contrast, was delighted and gushed that he had sent 'enough for fower or five times Lying in'. She liked the 'clouts very well' and a quilt was 'very handsom'.[125] The tension between the two women is palpable, with Thomas as the mediator, and crucially the one who gave permission for purchases for both his wife and mother for the impending birth. Isabella told her son in one letter that she doubted Anne even loved her.[126] By rejecting Isabella's offers to procure and provide material things, Anne was also rejecting her involvement in the project of multiplying the family.

Indeed, men were often asked explicitly for their permission when women wanted things to prepare for birth. When in Barbados, William Swynsen wrote to his brother John requesting that he bring childbed linen with him for his

[123] Elizabeth Deal, 22 April 1691, The Proceedings of the Old Bailey, www.oldbaileyonline.org/record/t16910422-22?text=t16910422-22, last accessed 7/8/2018.
[124] Isabella Wentworth to Thomas Wentworth, 16 January 1713, BL Add MS 22225, fol. 347.
[125] *Ibid.*, 9 January 1713, fol. 341. [126] *Ibid.*, n.d. January 1712, fol. 348.

pregnant wife.[127] The chief servant of Lady Honor Lisle was responsible for negotiating the purchase and borrowing of items needed for Lady Lisle's pregnancy and delivery in 1537, and it was he that had to write to donors when the baby was stillborn and never 'occupiede' the swaddling clothes that had been obtained.[128] William Chaytor, if we recall, was in charge of gathering and purchasing 'some things to be had' for Peregrina's birth. Wives updated their husbands on the process of preparing for birth. Penelope Mordaunt wrote to her husband, Sir John Mordaunt, in October 1699 while heavily pregnant that she felt increasingly uneasy 'now a days as well as nights', which made her send to a 'Mrs Barnes for blankets and things for the Child, Lest I should be cate [caught]', with the suggestion being that he too might work to procure her some necessary items.[129] Lettice, the wife of Framlingham Gawdy of West Harling, Norfolk, wrote to her father, Sir Robert Knollys, c. 1617, asking him to negotiate with 'my lady', possibly her mother-in-law, Ann Framlingham, on his visit to her in Oxfordshire for 'some clouts' for her upcoming delivery.[130] 'Clouts', like the aforementioned 'rags', were pieces of fabric that were often used for hygiene purposes, explicitly for managing menstruation or for babies' nappies.[131] The woman in question had promised Lettice clouts during her first pregnancy but Lettice explained 'I was so well provided that I thought to reserve them till I had need of them, which is now.' Her eight children took a toll on her stash of linens. She told her father that she had had 'so many children that they have worn through all my things and therefore I must try my friends again'. She asked her father to search for 'some old shirts in a corner for me or some old things', which presumably she might be able to tear up as clouts, thanked him for his gift of two 'wrought stools', which her husband had collected from him. Her final request was for him to send a 'yellow taffeta quilt' that she perceived he no longer needed.[132] Lettice's exchange with her father shows that male family members were often intimately involved in the process of procuring materials for delivery – both her husband and father were key in acquiring and moving goods, but it also mattered that she would deliver her baby on a stool used by other family members. This also hints that there was a subtle etiquette to these material exchanges – a face-to-face request was politer, and possibly, one from a man was more authoritative.

In turn, men framed the things that women asked for and needed for birth as conditional on the performance of godly maternity and their sexual fidelity.

[127] Cited in Pollock, 'Childbearing and Female Bonding in Early Modern England', 290.
[128] Mann, 'Clothing Bodies, Dressing Rooms'.
[129] Penelope Mordaunt to Sir John Mordaunt, 12 October 1699, Warwickshire Record Office, Warwick, CR 1368, vol. 1, fol. 21.
[130] Lettice Gawdy to Sir R. Knollys, c. 1620–30, BL Add MS 27395, fol. 125.
[131] Dolan, 'The Fabric of Life', 73; Read, 'Thy Righteousness Is but a Menstrual Clout'.
[132] Gawdy to Knollys, BL Add MS 27395, fol. 125.

Men engaged with domestic material culture in ways that constituted family relationships,[133] and childbirth accoutrement and materials were no different. The linens and baby clothes, like other items of dress, mirrored the ways men as heads of household clothed their wives, children and servants to signal their own 'personal prestige and honour'.[134] Giving gifts was rarely entirely about need or altruism in early modern England but defined a relationship between the giver and the receiver that was symbolised in the material object.[135] These items alongside paperwork confirming assiduous and careful conduct of women during pregnancy formed part of a family archive. Men framed their contribution to successful procreative outcomes as procuring and paying for material things, making it difficult to see the period shortly before, during and after delivery as one in which women challenged patriarchal structures and separated themselves from the household and men. In fact, childbirth and the material culture surrounding it reinforced and re-enacted many of the tropes and cultural expectations of the early modern home.

Conclusion

During pregnancy, women and their families were interested in understanding and predicting what the unborn infant would be like. The size of women's stomachs and their symptoms throughout pregnancy promised to reveal whether the baby would be a boy or a girl, big or small, or lively or dull, and this all helped to impose order and certainty on generation. When women were 'big', they were undeniably pregnant, something that was celebrated and displayed when the woman in question was married, and particularly middling or elite. Correspondence, conduct manuals and popular print played on the idea that men furnished, trimmed or rigged their wives with their conceptions, big (pregnant) bellies and then the stuff to deliver safely. But for women themselves, this moment of growing big could be troublesome. For unmarried women, it might betray their condition and lose them their job and livelihood.

[133] Karen Harvey, *The Little Republic: Masculinity and Domestic Authority in Eighteenth-Century Britain* (Oxford: Oxford University Press, 2012), 128. For more on the myth of separate spheres, see: Hannah Barker, 'Soul, Purse and Family: Middling and Lower-Class Masculinity in Eighteenth-Century Manchester', *Social History* 33, no. 1 (2008): 12–35; Karen Harvey and Alexandra Shepard, 'What Have Historians Done with Masculinity?', *Journal of British Studies* 44, no. 2 (2005): 274–280; Amanda Vickery, 'Golden Age to Separate Spheres? A Review of the Categories and Chronology of Women's History', *The Historical Journal* 36, no. 2 (1993): 383–414.

[134] Mann, 'Clothing Bodies, Dressing Rooms', 137. See also, Ann Rosalind Jones and Peter Stallybrass, *Renaissance Clothing and the Materials of Memory* (Cambridge: Cambridge University Press, 2000).

[135] Felicity Heal, *The Power of Gifts: Gift-Exchange in Early Modern England* (Oxford: Oxford University Press, 2014), 9.

Even for married women, the later stage of pregnancy might be accompanied by pain and immobility. The material goods that women borrowed and purchased were not just essential but involved in a larger culture of the display of respectability. The stuff of childbearing was represented as being gifted to women but was conditional on the perceived legitimacy of the pregnancy and their good conduct. Paradoxically, although some men were criticised for failing to provide for their wives properly, the anxiety around women's conduct during pregnancy, what the child would look like and the dates women proffered matched up, reveal how men's domestic and fiscal honour was carefully intertwined with the performance of women's bodies, as well as how central childbirth was in defining and cementing familial relationships and identity.

4 Men, Midwives and a Place to Give Birth

w?>As families gathered linens, clothes and items for delivery, they also started to make practical arrangements for birth about where women would deliver, who would be there and who would be the midwife. These were decisions that, like other aspects of the experience of having babies, were driven by family interests and a desire to protect and enhance social standing. Midwives are dominant figures in histories of early modern childbirth, at least in part because of the dramatic rise in man-midwives that took place in the eighteenth century. Prior to this, it was highly unusual for men to be present in the room where women gave birth, and usually only when surgeons were called in when the mother or child had already died. From 1750 onwards, however, male practitioners, newly fashioned as 'doctor midwives' or 'accoucheurs', became the default practitioner to deliver babies for many elite families. By 1790, between a third and half of all deliveries in England had man-midwives in attendance.[1]

Historians have long speculated as to how and why this rapid shift in the sex of midwives changed in the period. For James Aveling, an obstetrician writing in the late nineteenth century, this shift was simply the direct result of medical, scientific and rational progress.[2] Man-midwives were supposedly handed 'the key to the lying-in room' because they offered women forceps and other instruments that made birth quicker, less painful and safer.[3] Their incursion (in his opinion) constituted the timely emergence of the discipline of obstetrics. Generation was supposedly wrestled away from the inexpert and untrained hands of midwives and anchored within the male and institutionalised world of medicine and science. This is a teleology that Adrian Wilson has echoed in much milder terms more recently when he noted that before belonging to

1 Irvine Loudon, 'Childbirth', in *Western Medicine: An Illustrated History*, ed. Irvine Loudon (Oxford: Oxford University Press, 1997), 209.
2 J. H. Aveling, *English Midwives; Their History and Prospects* (London: Churchill, 1872).
3 Walter Radcliffe, *Milestones in Midwifery with a Foreword by David Brown* (Bristol: Wright, 1967), 30.

'medicine', childbirth belonged to women.[4] When the majority of medicine took place at home in the period, including childbirth, it seems anachronistic to separate out these fields of knowledge and practice. Within these explanations there is an implicit assumption that before man-midwives, childbirth was more of a social affair and one that was confined to women. As early as 1919, Alice Clark noted that in many ways, this narrative mirrored a more general and longer story of women being shunted out of skilled and highly valued work.[5] Following in Clark's footsteps, feminist scholars tackled the men-equal-progress narrative head on in the 1970s, and afterwards, claiming that it was precisely because midwives were highly trained that they were perceived as a threat by male authority figures. Barbara Ehrenreich and Deirdre English suggested that female midwives were often accused of being witches in order to limit and control their power, a theory that was later undermined by David Harley.[6] Man-midwives, in fact, supplanted expert, relatively well-educated women.[7] For historians in the 1970s, this shift was the result of young surgeons and physicians trying to create a new career path in an increasingly competitive medical marketplace. Female midwives were simply collateral damage. Wilson similarly sees competition for clients as key to this story of the rise of the man-midwife but sees women themselves as driving the shift from female to male practitioners as they sought to demarcate themselves socially by securing high-profile, quasi-celebrity man-midwives that accelerated this trend.[8] This chapter finds that man-midwives' success was in a large part because making babies was already an affair that men were deeply involved in. This shift appears less dramatic when we find from family

[4] Adrian Wilson, 'The Ceremony of Childbirth and Its Interpretation', in *Women as Mothers in Pre-Industrial England: Essays in Memory of Dorothy McLaren*, ed. Valerie Fildes (London: Routledge, 1990), 70.

[5] Alice Clark, *Working Life of Women in the Seventeenth Century*, Studies in Economics and Political Science (London: George Routledge & Sons, Ltd, 1919), 265–285.

[6] Barbara Ehrenreich and Deirdre English, *Witches, Midwives, and Nurses: A History of Women Healers* (Oyster Bay, NY: Glass Mountain Pamphlets, 1971). David Harley combatted this argument: David Harley, 'Historians as Demonologists: The Myth of the Midwife-Witch', *Social History of Medicine* 3, no. 1 (1990): 1–26.

[7] Doreen Evenden, *The Midwives of Seventeenth-Century London*, Cambridge History of Medicine (Cambridge: Cambridge University Press, 2000); Hilary Marland, ed., *The Art of Midwifery: Early Modern Midwives in Europe* (London: Routledge, 1993).

[8] Loudon, 'Childbirth', 211; Adrian Wilson, 'Two Female Cultures', in *The Making of Man-Midwifery: Childbirth in England, 1660–1770* (Cambridge, MA: Harvard University Press, 1995), 185–196; Adrian Wilson, 'Midwifery in the "Medical Marketplace"', in *Medicine and the Market in Early Modern England*, ed. Mark Jenner and Patrick Wallis (Basingstoke: Palgrave, 2007), 153–174. Judith Leavitt argues that in the late eighteenth and early nineteenth century, American women began to employ man-midwives because they were more interventionist, but that they had to negotiate with the mother's friends and family, see: Judith Walzer Leavitt, *Brought to Bed: Childbearing in America, 1750–1950* (Oxford: Oxford University Press, 1986).

paperwork that the arrival of man-midwives did not change many aspects of birthing, especially when we consider that as we saw in previous chapters it was not the homosocial experience that other historians may have imagined it as. Indeed, female midwives often did much of the work at births, even when man-midwives were called on.

Like other aspects of childbearing, decisions about the practitioners that would be present at delivery was debated in family correspondence. Like the ways that male family members guided the purchase and acquisition of material things, they were also active in choosing 'good' midwives and nurses. Another theme of this book – that certain aspects of bearing children were highlighted and celebrated in family paperwork and other aspects minimised – is seen most clearly in the discussions that individuals had about practitioners. In particular, families became increasingly interested in the personal characteristics and identities of man-midwives in a way that they were not and had not previously been concerned with the biographical details of female practitioners. The exception was when female midwives and nurses were accused of malpractice. Instead, they were often designated 'the midwife' or 'the nurse' in account books, diaries and correspondence. Man-midwives, like the Chamberlens, a dynasty of man-midwives living in London of Huguenot descent who are most famous for having invented the forceps, represented themselves as having all-rounded expertise as family physicians rather than just experts in birth. These men became so-well known in certain elite circles that their eccentricities and mannerisms were celebrated. We know far less about individual female midwives. Even Jane Sharp and Sarah Stone, the only female midwives that are known to have published medical books in England, are difficult to identify in parish registers and family paperwork.[9]

Historians of medicine have pointed to a gradual co-opting of women's medical knowledge and skills in writing about generation from the medieval period to the eighteenth century.[10] From the late sixteenth century, as we have heard, men positioned themselves as having a superior knowledge of the secrets of generation and, as the seventeenth century progressed, importantly, they claimed to be better practitioners. Indeed, Mary E. Fissell suggests that man-midwifery was a logical development given the ways that generation was

[9] Jane Sharp, *The Midwives Book Or the Whole Art of Midwifry Discovered*, ed. Elaine Hobby, Women Writers in English 1350–1850 (Oxford: Oxford University Press, 1999), xi. For questions of the authorship, see: Katharine Phelps Walsh, 'Marketing Midwives in Seventeenth-Century London: A Re-examination of Jane Sharp's *The Midwives Book*' *Gender & History* 26, no. 2 (2014): 223–241.

[10] Mary E. Fissell, *Vernacular Bodies: The Politics of Reproduction in Early Modern England* (Oxford: Oxford University Press, 2004); Monica H. Green, *Making Women's Medicine Masculine: The Rise of Male Authority in Pre-modern Gynaecology* (Oxford: Oxford University Press, 2008); Lianne McTavish, *Childbirth and the Display of Authority in Early Modern France*, Women and Gender in the Early Modern World (Aldershot: Ashgate, 2005).

increasingly folded into technical, educational and institutional impulses of the Enlightenment project to improve infant and maternal welfare for the benefit of the State and its colonial power.[11] The shift to seeing man-midwives as more authoritative than female ones in the eighteenth century then is simply the next tangible development in this trend.

The story of man-midwifery in England is the broader story of generation in this period writ large. When women took pains in procreation, it was expected as part of their domestic role and redounded to the family name more broadly. When men did generative work, it was either obscured in family paperwork (when it appeared too similar to what women might be expected to do within households) or celebrated as being directly related to their own individual characteristics. Men entering the birthing room therefore was simply a more obvious and tangible reflection of a broader trend of men knowing about, directing and controlling childbearing. Whilst Wilson has claimed that the arrival of man-midwives in birthing chambers 'undermined an underlying pattern of gendered space' in which women deliberately excluded men and the family during birth,[12] looking at where and how women gave birth shows that men were active in shaping this 'space' long before the eighteenth century. Family correspondence reveals that women often went to their natal home to give birth, and that they insisted on their husbands being in the house when they delivered. The seventeenth-century birthing chamber may have been mostly female but the rooms below were filled with male family members, meaning that the incursion of man-midwives might not have been the dramatic cultural shift that other historians have claimed it was.

Good and Bad Midwives

From the 1630s onwards, the authors of childbearing guides began increasingly to write about the importance of selecting a 'good' midwife. Before the seventeenth century, childbearing guides were notably more neutral and often focused on procedures of care rather than the relative virtues of practitioners. *The Byrth of Mankynd* (1540), for example, told midwives that they should 'dilligently observe and wayte' during delivery and not to force the child out,

[11] Lisa Forman Cody, *Birthing the Nation: Sex, Science, and the Conception of Eighteenth-Century Britons* (Oxford: Oxford University Press, 2005); Mary E. Fissell, 'Man-Midwifery Revisited', in *Reproduction: Antiquity to the Present Day*, ed. Nick Hopwood, Rebecca Flemming and Lauren Kassell (Cambridge: Cambridge University Press, 2018), 319–332; Sasha Turner, *Contested Bodies: Pregnancy, Childrearing, and Slavery in Jamaica*, Early American Studies (Pittsburg: University of Pennsylvania Press, 2017).

[12] Amanda Flather, *Gender and Space in Early Modern England*, Royal Historical Society Studies in History (Woodbridge: The Boydell Press, 2007), 55.

but did not expand on what would happen if a midwife were to apply force.[13] John Jones' 1579 *Arte and Science* encouraged the practice of washing babies in warm water after birth, without spending too much time detailing the harm that might come from cold water or not washing newborns.[14] Other texts were directed towards women themselves that helped prepare them for what midwives would do during delivery. The 1636 *Sick Womans Looking Glass* noted that pregnant women should 'let' the midwife administer 'oyle of lillies, marjerom, and bayes' to her privities. The midwife 'putting up her finger, shall feele the mouth of it [the womb] retracted and closed up'.[15] From the mid-seventeenth century, however, midwifery guides became very vocal about the dangers and perils of childbirth, and the threat of poor care.[16] Whereas earlier guides advertised themselves as being useful to birthing women, now guides explicitly sought to instruct midwives in their craft.

The 1636 English translation of Jacob Rüff's *De Conceptu et Generatione Hominis* was retitled *The Expert Midwife.* For those selecting a midwife or training to become one, the emphasis on expertise in midwifery served to simultaneously conjure up images of an anti-midwife who was ignorant, careless and/or mercenary.[17] The guide worried that poor practice had already 'cost the lives of many'. Childbirth was 'so dangerous, and so full of perill' that the skills of a midwife could determine the outcome. In his chapter on 'the Office of Midwives', Rüff imagined a skilful midwife who knew 'the time', observed the pains, was able to 'comfort and cheare up the labouring woman' and direct prayers.[18] In Edward Poeton's manuscript dialogue between two midwives from the 1630s, he offered to help women who were 'not well furnished w[i]th knowldg concerning the misteries of yt profession'.[19] His insight, he claimed, came from male-authored childbearing guides – 'the matter is other mens'.[20] This was despite the fact that his own wife was a midwife. Whilst Poeton's characters were literate, skilled, accomplished

[13] Thomas Raynalde, *Byrth of Mankynde. Newly translated out of Laten into Englysshe. In the which is entreated of all suche thynges the which chaunce to women in theyr labor, and all suche infyrmitees whiche happen unto the Infantes after they be delyuered* (London, 1540), fol. xxv.

[14] John Jones, *The Arte and Science of Preseruing Bodie and Soule in Healthe, Wisedome, and Catholike Religion* (London: 1579), 32.

[15] John Sadler, *The Sick Womans Private Looking-Glasse* (London, 1636), 73, 88.

[16] Fissell, *Vernacular Bodies.*

[17] Jacob Rüff, *The Expert Midwife, or An Excellent and Most Necessary Treatise of the Generation and Birth of Man* (London: 1636), sig. A3r.

[18] *Ibid.*, sig. A3r.

[19] Edward Poeton, 'The Midwives Deputie or a help for such as are not well furnished with knowledge concerning the misteries of that profession, gathered out of sundry authorized and authentict authors by Edward Poeton of Petworth Licentiate in physic and chyrurgery', BL, Sloane MS 1954.

[20] *Ibid.*, fol. 3r.

midwives, they were merely literary devices to position himself as an obstetrical authority, even at the expense of his wife and assumed that there would be a great many midwives who were in dire need of his instruction.

The idea that many midwives were poorly skilled was often referenced in texts about the licensing and organisation of midwives from 1616 onwards too. Ecclesiastical licensing of midwives was the norm until the eighteenth century (apart from during the interregnum).[21] Dr Peter Chamberlen the elder furthered himself as the 'Governor' of a new 'Society' of midwives in a 'humble petition of the midwives in and about the city of London' that was presented to the king. They shared this prevailing fear that 'manny women labouring with child and their children do perish' as a result of poor practice.[22] The petition was unsuccessful. Peter's nephew, also called Peter, would petition the King again in 1634, calling again for a midwives' society. This time there was rather more opposition from midwives themselves, published in *An Answer* (1649).[23] A new development signed a complaint led by Mrs Shaw and Mrs Whipp in which they accused Chamberlen of refusing to attend poor women and seeking excessive rewards. A short tract represented him as trying to 'get himself created vicar generall of the Midwifes in city & suburbs'.[24] The appropriation of women's medical skills and knowledge into a male and learned corpus was not new to the mid-seventeenth century, however, we see clearly that the intensified interest in midwives was.

Nicholas Culpeper took on the task of directing midwives in their art even further in his 1651 *Directory for Midwives.* The preface was dedicated to 'The Midwives of England' who he 'wisheth success in their Office'. The *Directory* marked a major shift in the ways obstetrical knowledge was authored. As Fissell notes, Culpeper did away with the normal meek apologies for 'intruding' into women's business, and he was strident in his descriptions of all the things that could cause havoc in women's bodies originating from the womb.[25] Whereas Eucharius Roeslin, Rüff and Jones had simply described good practice, Culpeper set out 'Rules' for midwives to follow. They were not 'so many that they will burden your Brain, nor so few that they will be insufficient for your Necessity'. Importantly, following them would mean midwives did not have to send for a 'Man-Midwife', which was a 'disparagement

[21] Sarah Fox and Margaret Brazier, 'The Regulation of Midwives in England, c. 1500–1902', *Medical Law International* 20, no. 4 (2020), 308–338.

[22] College of Physicians Annals III, 3 June 1617, fols. 28b, 29a, cited in: Jean Donnison, *Midwives and Medical Men: A History of the Struggle for the Control of Childbirth* (London: Historical Publications, 1988), 13.

[23] College of Physicians Annals III, 1634, 141b, 143b, 144b, 145b, cited in: *Ibid.*, 13.

[24] Philalethes, *An Answer to Doctor Chamberlaines Scandalous and False Papers* (London: 1649), 2.

[25] Fissell, *Vernacular Bodies*, 119.

not only to your selves, but also to your Profession'.[26] Culpeper's text was laden with suggestions that it was the norm for midwives to do a bad job, foreshadowing the ways in which man-midwives constructed claims about their own superior knowledge and practice in the eighteenth century.

Over the seventeenth century, owing to authors like Culpeper, medical texts progressively devalued the skill and knowledge of midwives. So much so that from the 1650s, authors' definition of a good midwife narrowed and was eventually defined by their subservience to male practitioners, the family, the Church and community more broadly. The 1656 *Compleat Midwifes Practice* outlined how women ought to choose midwives who were neither too young nor old, were 'in good habite of body', free from disease or disability and had small hands with short nails. They ought to be 'Courteous, 'sober', 'chast[e]', 'prudent', 'wary' and 'cunning'. Perhaps most crucially though, they should not be arrogant, complaining or covetous.[27] Families should want to hire a midwife that was a social manager and obsequious rather than authoritative and firm. Indeed, it was dangerous for a female practitioner to be too confident in her expertise. *Aristotle's Master-piece* idealised midwives who never imagined themselves to be perfect and constantly added to their 'Knowledge by study and experience'.[28] By this, he meant that he expected them to defer to physicians regularly and thought this was the cause of 'so many Women and Children' dying.[29]

Percivall Willughby, a man-midwife, also used the amorphous threat of the death of 'poor innocent infants [and mothers]', which he perceived as at epidemic levels due to the poor industry of midwives, in particular the practice of tying labouring women to chairs, which he said caused injuries that prevented future conception.[30] Midwives should be 'Wise and Silent not apt to talk foolishly of what she sees in the Houses where she hath to do', yet another insight into the ways in which birthing practitioners were meant to uphold the narratives that families wanted to be told about them.[31] His *Observations* would 'inform common midwives with such ways as I have used with good success', although his text remained unpublished until the Victorian period.[32] Midwives also had to be outwardly and obviously pious. She should 'know,

[26] Nicholas Culpeper, *A Directory for Midwives, or, A Guide for Women* (1675), sig. A3r.

[27] *The Compleat Midwifes Practice* (London: 1656), 75.

[28] *Aristotle's Master-piece; Or, The Secrets of Generation Display'd in all the Parts thereof* (London: 1684), 101.

[29] *Ibid.*, 101.

[30] Percivall Willughby, *Observations in Midwifery by Percival Willughby*, ed. Henry Blenkinsop (Warwick: H. T. Cooke, 1863), 9.

[31] Robert Barret, *A Companion for Midwives, Child-bearing Women, and Nurses Directing them how to Perform their Respective Offices: Together with an Essay, Endeavouring to Shew the Influence of Moral Abuses upon the Health of Children* (London: 1699), 3.

[32] Willughby, *Observations in Midwifery by Percival Willughby*, 3.

that God hath given to all things their beginnings, their Increasings, their Estate of perfection, and declination'.[33] A key part of the midwives' role was increasingly represented as subservience – to God, to higher-trained male medical professionals and to the family. These delicate and pedantic boundaries mirrored the ways wives and mothers were expected to be knowledgeable about fertility, bodies and medicine but not too knowledgeable; skilled but not too skilled; and that they would tirelessly labour to procure positive procreative outcomes, without obvious credit. Midwives were also caught in this cultural bind. The fact that midwives occupied a socially laudable position in communities and households as well as a medical one has been prominent in histories of midwifery as evidence of their power in early modern society. This does not fully take account of the complexity of medical encounters in the period that rarely involved merely a patient and practitioner but always took place in a complex web of social, familial and community interactions and pressures. Social obligation or expectation did not necessarily bring authority or even influence.

This idea that good midwives would be discreet, adept social managers and administer care only so far as their (quite limited) capabilities allowed is a prominent theme in the oaths that midwives were asked to swear in order to obtain licences in the early modern period. The parallels between the expectations that midwives would be highly skilled as well as meekly work to perpetuate the family and enhance its social reputations, and the ways families imagined ideal mothers would also toil tirelessly and without much fuss, is by no means accidental. It spoke to male fantasies of domestic harmony and the discomfort with acknowledging the pain, peril and work that women had to do to obtain these ideals. Margaret Parrey was granted a licence in 1588 by the Bishop of London after she swore she would be 'dilligente faithfull and redye to helpe everye woman traveling of Childe' regardless of wealth; ensure women named the correct father of their child; ensure that women did not claim 'anye other womans childe for her owne'; prevent any babies from being harmed; request additional assistance from midwives when necessary; rely on prayer rather than sorcery; not provide advice or assistance to women wishing to end pregnancies; not try and extort too high of a payment from families; never allow women to give birth without at least 'two or three honest women' present; ensure men were not allowed into the birthing chamber 'unlesse necessarye or grete urgent causes shall constreyne you soe to doe'; if the child died, bury it in a 'secrett place' safe from disturbance; make sure other midwives were practicing appropriately and report them to authorities if they were not; be 'honeste'; report those midwives that did not have licences to the

[33] *The Compleat Midwifes Practice*, 76.

authorities; and finally, check that anyone serving under her was also 'righte honeste and discrete'.[34]

In this way, female midwives shouldered the weight of regulating and representing their whole profession, and the oaths they took often insisted on accepting being policed by families, the Church and state, and, in turn, policing other midwives. Another oath from 1649 consisted of fifteen promises that repeated many of the same hallmarks of practice.[35] She had to be 'diligent and faithfull, and readie to helpe every Woman labouring of Childe, as well as the poore as the riche'. Four items concerned preventing and managing bastardy: the midwife was asked to extract the name of the father; insist on having two or three witnesses to any woman seeking to give birth secretly; not advise or knowingly allow a woman to take measures to abort her child; and the midwife had to prevent the death or injury of the child. Others were religious – she should use 'honest behaviour unto the woman being lawfully admitted to the roome' and facilitate the baptising of the child into the Church of England. Four promises concerned what might be termed 'policing' the profession. Item 11 asked midwives to report other midwives who did not abide by the oath to the bishop or chancellor, and item 13 asked them to notify if they knew any midwives who were practicing without a licence. Item 9 asked them to keep their 'Office' secret from men unless 'urgent cause' necessitated it, presumably more about not divulging the details of birth rather than disguising their profession, and item 14 demanded they not appoint any apprentices 'but such as you shall perfectly know to be of right honest and discreet behaviour, as also apt, able, & having sufficient knowledge and experience'.[36] Midwives oaths show that despite the veneration of subservience, it was also hoped that midwives would minister in ways that continually adapted to the social and bodily needs of women and their families before, during and after delivery, which demanded skill and considerable knowledge.

It was not just male medical authors and oaths that sponsored fears about the dangers of unskilful practitioners. Female medical authors also added to this discourse. Sharp's 1671 *Midwives Book* reflected on the many 'Miseries Women endure in the Hands of unskilful Midwives; many professing the Art (without any skill in Anatomy, which is the Principal part effectually necessary for a Midwife)'.[37] And Stone's 1741 *Observations* repeated Culpeper's warning from 1651 that without proper training and instruction, country midwives would be forced to call male practitioners in uncomplicated

[34] James Hitchcock, 'A Sixteenth Century Midwife's License', *Bulletin of the History of Medicine* 41, no. 1 (1967): 75–76.
[35] Evenden, *The Midwives of Seventeenth-Century London*, 207.
[36] Reproduced in full in *Ibid.*, 206–207.
[37] Sharp, *The Midwives Book Or the Whole Art of Midwifry Discovered*, 5.

deliveries.[38] But for her, these 'boyish Pretender[s]' were an even greater threat than inadequate female midwives. She feared that they were likely to cause the death of healthy infants, expose the modesty of the pregnant woman and damage the midwife's reputation. She relayed in visceral and persuasive terms how babies had been born 'with their Brains working out of their Heads', butchered by hooks and knives.[39]

Both male and female midwives were represented as potentially murderous and dangerous in cheap print too. A 1699 ballad, *A Hue and Cry After A Man-Midwife, Who has Lately Deliver'd the Land Bank of Their Money,* described the new figure as a 'Doctor, Projector, Man-Midwife and C———' who 'Cunningly manag'd a subtle Device'. Through his deception, he 'strangles more Necks, than the Rope and the Gallows'.[40] In *A New Ballad of the Midwives Ghost*, the midwife in question murdered 'Bastard-Children' and buried them around a London house that was subsequently haunted.[41] Another midwife, Mary Hobry, supposedly murdered her own husband.[42] Elsewhere, midwives were represented as guilty of collusion and manipulation, particularly when it came to paternity. In the 1680–1690s ballad *Lass of Lynns New Joy*, the midwife colludes with a newly delivered woman and her mother to persuade a new husband that the baby is actually his rather than the result of a previous dalliance.[43] *Advice to Young Gentlemen* warned men not to be taken in by the 'Oration' that midwives made after the birth of a child that 'the poor Infant is so like the Dad' when really it was the product of pre- or extra-marital affairs.[44] The prevalence of inept, mercenary, and sometimes murderous, midwives – male and female – as characters in print culture in the latter part of the seventeenth century speaks to the perceived significance of practitioner

38 Sarah Stone, *A Complete Practice of Midwifery. Consisting of Upwards Forty Cases or Observations in that valuable Art, selected from many Others, in the Course of a very Extensive Practice* (London: 1737), vi.

39 *Ibid.*, xiii.

40 Edward Ward, *A Hue and Cry After A Man-Midwife, Who has Lately Deliver'd the Land Bank of Their Money*, EBBA 33185 (London: 1699).

41 *A New Ballad of the Midwives Ghost: Who appeared to several People in the House where she formerly lives in Rotten- Row in Holbourn, London, who were all afraid to speak unto her; but she growing very Impetuous, on the 16th of this Instant March, 1680, declarred her mind to the Maid of the said House, who with an Unanimous Spirit adhered to her*, EBBA 20763 (London: 1680).

42 *A Warning-Piece To All Married Men and Women. Being the Full Confession of Mary Hobry, The French Midwife, Who Murdered her Husband on the 27th January 1687/8. (As also the Cause thereof.) For which she receiv'd Sentence to be Burnt alive: And on Friday the Second Day of March, between the Hours of Ten and Eleven in the Morning, she was drawn upon a Sledge to Leicester-Fields, where she was burnt to Ashes*, EBBA 34436 (London: 1688).

43 *The Lass of Lynns New Joy For finding a Father for her Child. Being a Third Song of Marry and Thank ye too*, EBBA 21315 (London: 1682–1692).

44 *Advice to Young Gentlemen; Or, An Answer to the Ladies of London, To the Tune of, The Ladies of London*, EBBA 37687 (London: 1685–1688).

choice as well as their role in managing the emotional and practical demands of the households they served. But the questions that this literature asked about agency, control, power, knowledge and skill in managing generation were not new ones, but the ones that families had asked for decades.

The worry that female practitioners would do a bad job in managing childbirth and the consequences, not just for the health of mothers and babies, found its way into lots of different kinds of printed texts across the seventeenth century, and was backgrounded by the loud competition for clients and reputation that many healers were partaking in to stake out their claim within the marketplace. These discussions in early modern English midwifery guides reflect a wider intellectual trend in the period to subsume female procreative work – both by mothers and midwives (and as we shall later see by nurses and servants) – within expectations of basic female comportment.[45]

Selecting a Midwife

One wonders how in this cacophony of advice about what made a midwife 'good' and the possibilities of selecting a bad one how families ever landed on a practitioner they were happy with. Surprisingly, it was not a very common topic in family correspondence until the eighteenth century. Firstly, this was because it was hard to secure the services of midwives reliably in advance of birth because as specific (or accurate) as women were in calculating when their 'reckoning' was, they might deliver well before or after this date. Secondly, the visibility of these discussions about the expertise of birthing practitioners in medical and popular print appears to have led to more anxiety about the ramifications of bad midwives in the eighteenth century. In this period, the added possibility of hiring a man-midwife meant elite families were faced with new choices to make.

In some circumstances, elite families sought to select and retain a midwife in advance of birth to secure a particular practitioner. Wealthier families tended to pay a midwife to travel sometimes considerable distances and lodge with them for the weeks when the pregnant woman expected to give birth. Joan Thynne wrote to her husband in 1590, asking him and her sister to find a 'good midwife' for Easter 'or ten or twelve days after' because the midwife that had previously served her in Longleat, 'goody Barber', had died.[46] That they found a midwife living in London, a hundred miles away, points to the considerable distances that medical practitioners could travel to serve clients. Elite families relied on recommendations from other family members or

45 McTavish, *Childbirth and the Display of Authority in Early Modern France*, 1.
46 Alison D. Wall, ed., *Two Elizabethan Women: Correspondence of Joan and Maria Thynne 1575–1611* (Devizes: Wiltshire Record Society, 1983), 6.

similarly wealthy and ascendant friends. In 1698, John Mordaunt reported to his wife that 'Mrs North' had been 'very well [deli]ver'd of another Daughter' by a midwife from Lynn 'who, they commend very much'.[47] Midwives were often hired based on recommendation in much the same way as families recommended pregnant women eat certain things or alter things about their routine. Lower down the socio-economic scale, Rebecca Harley of Clapham, thirty-two, asked Richard Napier in 1617 whether she should 'leave her old midwife' who was a 'paynfull & a laborious woman' because all three of her previous babies had died in or shortly after delivery. She hoped a change might shift her 'ill lucke'.[48] In smaller communities, there would most often have only been one or two midwives who delivered the majority of babies. Not everyone might have the choice practically and financially that Rebecca did to simply change midwives.

When a midwife proved inept, violent or negligent, families typically sought the advice of other practitioners or even, at times, courts. These records of dispute reveal much about the contours of medical decision-making in the period and how individuals trusted particular medical practitioners. Mistress Newton of Bidnam consulted Napier in 1600 with her uncle, complaining that an 'unskilfull midwife' had 'rent' [ripped] her womb beyond repair. Goody Parker of Weston also asked for Napier's assistance when her bladder was 'perished by the mydwiffes negligenc'.[49] Similarly, when Anne Knutsford, a midwife, was accused of 'lying, swearing and cursing' in Nantwich, one witness, Elizabeth Cliffe, described her as a 'very good midwife' and indeed 'one of the best in these parts' but she behaved in a way that was 'unbecoming of her sexe and profession to reveale the secrets of women in the time of their extremity'. Thomas Proudman relayed how she was a 'ready handed woman in her profession' but 'given to vaine cursing and swearing'.[50] Such conflicts reveal that some individuals distinguished between the embodied skills of a midwife in facilitating delivery and their bedside manner. Both of these things made someone a 'good' practitioner and lacking one could render them undesirable and untrustworthy. A midwife could be good at delivering infants, but not good at managing the social relationships that made birthing a positive experience for families.

Men tended to be particularly taciturn in their diaries or account books about the details of the midwives that they hired. Whereas physicians were often

[47] John Mordaunt to Penelope Mordaunt, 27 October 1698, Warwickshire Record Office, Warwick, CR 1368, vol. 1, fol. 2v.

[48] CASE45627, CB. [49] CASE11088, CASE38861, CB.

[50] Karen O'Brien, 'Sexual Impropriety, Petitioning and the Dynamics of Ill Will in Daily Urban Life', *Urban History* 43, no. 2 (2016): 177–199; Samuel S. Thomas, 'Early Modern Midwifery: Splitting the Profession, Connecting the History', *Journal of Social History* 43, no. 1 (2009): 123.

named fully, midwives were often simply 'the midwife' in these records. Robert Woodford recorded early in the morning on 29 August 1638 that his wife Hannah 'began to fall in travell' [labour] and 'so the midwife was sent for, and came'.[51] The Thynne family book of receipts from 1599 to 1560 listed a reward 'to the Midwife bringing my Lady abed' of a son.[52] It was not just parents that paid the midwife or gave her gifts, but grandfathers too. William Jessop wrote to his daughter, Ann Hulton of Hulton Park in 1668, asking if she would 'give something as from me to y[ou]r Midwife & Nurses employed when litle Jess was borne I think it might doe well and I should take it well giuen', without bothering to find out or list their individual names.[53] A Gloucestershire man, John Clifford, recorded giving a sugarloaf to the midwife at his grandson's christening in February 1676.[54] When Sir Daniel Fleming of Westmoreland's daughter, Barbara Tathum, gave birth in March 1691, he recorded that his unmarried daughter, Alice, gave the midwife (called 'Grace-Wife') two shillings and six pence, and the baby, her god-daughter, one pound. Daniel himself gave the midwife and nurse five shillings.[55] The midwife returned to her home fifty-five miles from Kendal in Wigan shortly after. Fleming recorded the name of the midwife of each of the births of his children, including in 1673 when his wife died ten days after giving birth to a little boy. Mistress Scott delivered eight of the Fleming's children, Ann Rigg delivered two, Ann Array delivered one and 'Huff-wife [th]e midwife' also delivered one. Although Mistress Scot appears to have been the family's favourite, there was surprisingly little handwringing about getting a different midwife.[56]

These glimpses indicate that elite families had considerable buying power in selecting whoever they wanted to deliver their babies and in a style that fitted them. The perceived close and emotional relationship between these practitioners and the family mattered until it was inconvenient for the family in question. Added to this, although midwives were important members of the household for the time they were employed, men were not particularly interested in the details of their work. Although they were often largely uninterested in the individual

[51] Robert Woodford, 29 August 1638, *The Diary of Robert Woodford, 1637–1641*, ed. John Fielding (Cambridge: Cambridge University Press, 2012), 233.

[52] 'Miscallaneous receipts and disbursements of the Thynne family, 1559–1560', Longleat House, Longleat, TH/BOOK/146, fol. 55.

[53] William Jessop to Ann Hulton, 26 September 1668, Lancashire Record Office, DDHu 47/34.

[54] John Clifford 'Account book', 3 February 1675/1676, Gloucestershire Record Office, Gloucester, D149/A26.

[55] Daniel Fleming, *The Estate and Household Accounts of Sir Daniel Fleming of Rydal Hall, Westmorland, from 1688–1701*, ed. Blake Tyson, Record Series Volume 13 (Lancaster: Cumberland and Westmorland Antiquarian and Archaeological Society, 2001), 125.

[56] Daniel Fleming, 'A Booke of my owne Receipts and Disbursem[en]ts 1656–1688', Cumbria Record Office, Kendal, WDRY/Box 119.

and personal characteristics of the midwives they hired, they did find these women through recommendation. We see when considering the fuss that surrounded man-midwives that female ones had quite a different experience. Women's good work did not necessarily follow them in the same way.

The casebooks of three early modern midwives reveal that many families did tend to visit the same midwife habitually. An anonymous London midwife recorded the deliveries she attended between 1694 and 1716. She delivered a number of her own family members. On 17 March 1711, she 'Laid' her daughter 'of a son'.[57] She also delivered her daughter-in-law and her cousins of their children.[58] The frequent mention of the links between patients – in 1713, for example, she 'Laid in Ms Daingrfilds sister' – suggests she got business through recommendation.[59] A Cumbrian midwife practicing in Kendal between 1669 and 1675, Elizabeth Thompson, also kept a book recording births. She carefully recorded the profession of the father, whether a shoemaker, shopkeeper, apothecary or vicar. Her clients came from a wide range of professions and social statuses, including three children of Christopher Phillipson of Crooke, a prominent Westmorland gentleman.[60] This reinforces Doreen Evenden's finding from London midwives' testimonies that patients were often connected by the professions of their husbands, and midwives had substantial repeat business.[61] Katherine Manley, a Whitby midwife, similarly kept a casebook, containing 3,316 deliveries between 1720 and 1764, suggesting that women did often use the same midwife for a succession of deliveries.[62]

These casebooks suggest that when man-midwives fashioned themselves as offering wholistic care during childbearing, they were not really departing from tradition, but they borrowed the model of work that female midwives had been enacting for years before. Man-midwives, for the most part, had university degrees and stressed this as being crucial to being a good and well-rounded practitioner. Female midwives had and continued to provide women assistance in managing maternal health after birth and cooperated with other practitioners

[57] 'Diary of an anonymous midwife', MS Rawl D. 1141 (1694–1716), Bodleian Library, Oxford, fol. 8r. She again delivered her daughter of a son 25 September 1713, fol. 11r.

[58] She delivered a 'cousin' of a daughter 1 February 1712, fol. 9r and Cousin 'Jackson' 22 January 1714, fol. 11bv. Daughter 'Ofener' is delivered 19 February 1714, fol. 24r, 21 May 1717, fol. 15v and again 14 April 1716, fol. 26v.

[59] *Ibid.*, undated entry c. 1713, fol. 11br.

[60] 28 May 1671, 6 August 1672 and 8 July 1674.

[61] Doreen Evenden, 'Mothers and Their Midwives in Seventeenth-Century London', in *The Art of Midwifery: Early Modern Midwives in Europe*, ed. Hilary Marland (London: Routledge, 1993), 9–26.

[62] Mistress Katherine Manley, 'Diary, 1720–1764', Whitby Museum, WHITM:SOH170. For a discussion of this casebook, see: Joan E. Grundy, *History's Midwives Including a C17th and C18th Yorkshire Midwives Nominations Index* (Urmston: Federation of Family History Societies, 2003); Delphine Isaaman, 'The Diary of a Yorkshire Midwife 1720–1764' (diploma in History of the Family, London, University of London, 1990).

to provide the best care. Elizabeth Thompson and Katherine Manley used their books to record several medicinal recipes that were not always directly related to childbearing, suggesting that midwives might minister to multiple members of the family and in more wholistic ways than we might have previously imagined. Thompson kept a recipe for a plaster in the back of her records, now fragmented.[63] Manley included a receipts 'to hinder miscarriage', 'for a sore breast', an 'oyntment for a sweld brest', one for 'twisting of the guts' and a 'wound water' in the back of her book.[64] An anonymously penned book of Catholic prayers attributed to a nurse or midwife similarly contains a number of remedies directed towards parturient women and babies, including a receipt 'for hasting delivery' and 'for after Paines in women newly Delivered'.[65] Midwives sometimes visited Forman and Napier on behalf of their own patients when they were unable to travel – another indication that they took on a myriad of medical tasks for women rather than just delivering babies. In 1602, 'the midwife of newport' visited Napier on behalf of Mistress Garner. Elisabeth Colman's midwife, Goody Bird, came to Napier in 1609 for assistance immediately after the birth.[66] It should not be surprising that midwives did more than just deliver babies. Firstly because of the pluralism and fluidity of early modern medical practice, and secondly because of the ways (as we shall see) man-midwives sold themselves as practitioners. Man-midwives represented themselves as departing from tradition, even as they borrowed the model of work from their female counterparts and co-opted for their own gain.

Families wrote much more about their medical decision-making when they were considering hiring a male midwife rather than a female one. Elizabeth Freke recalled in her meditations how the man-midwife that had been employed during her first pregnancy with Ralph in 1675 had judged that the baby was 'long dead in me' and started to put on his 'butchers habit' to extract the unborn infant in pieces. Just before the man-midwife began the operation, God 'raised me up a good woman midwife who came in att this juncture of time and for aboutt two or three howrs in her shift worked till by my Gods mercy and providence to me I was saffly delivered'.[67] Mary, Marchioness of Worcester, worried that the midwife her daughter, Elizabeth Lady Bruce, had employed previously was 'quaking', or fearful, and that Dr Chamberlen would be more appropriate.[68] Like other decisions about the material preparation for

[63] Elizabeth Thompson, 'Diary', Cumbria Record Office, Kendal, WDCR/11/60–61.

[64] Manley, 'Diary'.

[65] 'Prayers of nurse or midwife', National Records of Scotland, Edinburgh, GD45/26/149.

[66] CASE20190, CASE35488, CB.

[67] 2 June 1675; Elizabeth Freke, *The Remembrances of Elizabeth Freke, 1671–1714,* ed. Raymond Anselment (Cambridge: Cambridge University Press, 2002), 41

[68] Mary, marchioness of Worcester, to Elizabeth Lady Bruce, c. 1680–1690, Wiltshire and Swindon History Centre, Chippenham, 1300/724/748.

childbirth, men as heads of household were often responsible for adjudicating this choice. In the eighteenth century, Sir John Gordon requested that the Duke of Newcastle allow his wife to be attended by a 'man midwife', either Doctor Bamber, Doctor Middleton or Doctor Nesbit. This was to be in addition to a female midwife, Mrs Cannons.[69] Gordon did not clarify the respective role of these practitioners, although as we shall see, it appears not to have been an uncommon practice to hire a female midwife as well as a male one.

Isabella Wentworth entered into lengthy and fraught negotiations with her son, Thomas, to pay for the hefty fees of 'Dr Chamberlin', Hugh Chamberlen, the last of five generations of man-midwives, to deliver his wife, Anne, of their first child in 1713. Although Anne was most likely in favour of this option, the enthusiasm and persistence suggests that it was more Isabella's request than anyone else's. Tellingly, she asked Thomas not to share her letter or hopes with his wife.[70] Three days later, she wrote again, this time more urgently, stressing that 'the time ~~drags~~ draws now very near' and Chamberlen would make Anne, who lost her own mother in childbirth, 'very esy'. Isabella paints him as a superior and self-important man who 'is very proud' and used to being 'very much Coarted'. He supposedly loved 'a glass, of good wyne' and was a 'very great man', although it was unclear in this latter observation whether she was referring to his stature or reputation.[71] Her following letters employed a number of persuasive tactics to get Thomas to agree to Chamberlen. She described how Anne had shed tears over his resistance. She supplied plentiful testimonies of other aristocratic women who had used his services with great success. Lady Roysten 'sayde that most had him in the house for it kept the wemen Midwifse in Awe'.[72] Isabella's own niece had already had 'five Lovly boys' by Chamberlen.[73] Lady Lansdell had been brought to bed 'of bothe her children' and Lady Massom consulted him for a number of health issues.[74] To justify his exorbitant fee (a figure she revealed rather late in these exchanges), Isabella stressed that Chamberlen was not merely a midwife but a 'Dockter to the family' and had as much 'pracktiss for Physick as for the other', and in this role he not only managed delivery but the care of the newborn (a job that we have already seen midwives had always done). He was not, she was at pains to say, as the stereotype suggested, overly interventionist. Isabella described how he had refrained from using any instruments because there might be 'harm'.[75] As yet another tool of persuasion, Isabella frequently mentioned that Anne's own mother had died in childbirth,

[69] Sir John Gordon to duke of Newcastle, 31 December 1746, The National Archives, Kew, SP 36/90/2/92, fols 92–93.
[70] Isabella Wentworth to Thomas Wentworth, 23 January 1713, BL Add MS 22225, fol. 352.
[71] *Ibid.*, 30 January 1713, fol. 355v.
[72] *Ibid.*, 3 February 1713, fols 361–362.
[73] *Ibid.*, 3 February 1713, fols 361–362.
[74] *Ibid.*, 9 February 1713, fol. 365.
[75] *Ibid.*, 3 February 1713, fols 361–362.

and that selecting a man-midwife would help prevent history repeating itself. She told her son that the cost of Chamberlen was worth securing an heir. She said if the baby was a boy, 'consider thear is twoe Livse depending upon him [Chamberlen]', not just his wife's.[76] What she failed to say in these letters was that they would also hire a female midwife for the birth and that Chamberlen would cost ten times more than her whilst she did most of the work.

Chamberlen's payment structure was two-tiered. It was possible that man-midwives also borrowed this structure from some female midwives, and particularly the practitioners that elite families employed to live in for weeks surrounding delivery. If parents wished to wait and see whether he was available, he charged thirty guinneys (£31.50).[77] If, however, they wanted to ensure he would be there when the woman went into labour, they could secure his services with a hundred guinneys (£105.00).[78] Isabella pushed for the latter, with a female midwife for ten guinneys. At last, Thomas wrote to Chamberlen formally contracting his services and Isabella was overjoyed. Isabella said they could only 'imagin how much better it is having him then a woman', and a recent happy client, Lady Lansdell, had proclaimed that she would pay 500 Guinness 'rether then not have him'. The Duchess of Buckingham '& many moar that he Lays [delivers]' also attested to his skill.[79] From Isabella's letters, one might assume that Dr Chamberlen would be the only practitioner serving the family during the birth. Certainly, he was the only one she wrote about. In fact, they also employed a female midwife who did the majority of the work. The 'woman Midwife' arrived at 10 pm, shortly after labour began, and assisted until 4 am, when Anne was close to delivery. This was when Chamberlen made his big appearance. As soon as she saw the doctor, 'she found a great alteration for the better' and, although it was 'the strongest part of her Labour', she did not 'indure soe much as with the woman', and was shortly delivered. The narrative is strikingly similar to the one Stone painted of rural midwives that called in men 'when the Work is near finish'd; and then the Midwife, who has taken all the pains, is accounted of little value, and the young men command all the praise'.[80]

The exchanges about Chamberlen in the Wentworth family letters would at first glance wholeheartedly confirm Wilson's argument that the shift to man-midwives in eighteenth-century Britain was driven by a particular brand of female elite sociability. Isabella reeled off the list of other ladies that had used

[76] *Ibid.*, 9 February 1713, fol. 365.

[77] This is equivalent to around £3,357 in 2017, according to the National Archives Currency Converter, www.nationalarchives.gov.uk/currency-converter/, last accessed 5/6/2019.

[78] This was equivalent to £11,017.47 in 2017, according to the National Archives Currency Converter.

[79] Isabella Wentworth to Thomas Wentworth, 13 February 1713, fol. 367.

[80] Stone, *A Complete Practice of Midwifery*, x.

his services to aide her case. Isabella's insistence on Chamberlen, however, was much about complying with family expectations and standing than it was about homosocial conviviality. That Isabella perceived Chamberlen to be a better and more qualified practitioner is hardly surprising given the rhetoric man-midwives fostered, and the longstanding attempts of male authors to position themselves as authorities on childbirth. Certainly, the fact that Chamberlen could offer forceps (something Wilson notes often appealed) did not feature prominently in Isabella's letter. Indeed, the 'Dockter to the family' did not seem to offer anything inherently different from a female midwife. Although it is often noted in correspondence that man-midwives were also doctors and therefore more dextrous and adaptable in their practice, they were simply following in the footsteps of female midwives who were intimately involved in the families and communities they served. Male practitioners, however, were seen as offering double the expertise, albeit for sometimes ten times the price. They supposedly combined the superior medical knowledge associated with university-trained physicians with the experience of more irregular practitioners, making them the superior choice. Nancy Tulley, for example, visited a 'Dr midwife' in 1701 after being told by a physician she was pregnant and taking medicines to 'bring the child to maturity'. The man-midwife, using his specialist knowledge, told her she was not pregnant, and got her to stop taking the medication that had made her 'soe monstrous fatt that shee would have dyed of fatt'. Then she said she was in 'such good order' that the 'Dr midwife' was sure she would go on to have children.[81]

Female midwives were never celebrated in the way their later male counterparts were like Chamberlen. This was not because they were any less qualified or because they necessarily came from a more lowly social group than man-midwives, although men like Chamberlen were careful to represent themselves as particularly befitting for elite families. Female midwives were the daughters, wives and widows of parish ministers, barber surgeons, clothworkers, shoemakers, innkeepers and yeomen.[82] They were often literate, and sometimes licenced. They performed important legal, religious, social and medical functions within their communities, and yet by the early eighteenth century, female midwives were increasingly represented as unlearned and incompetent in managing the grave task of birth. The spectre of the bad midwife was dominant in medical writing from the 1650s onwards, and mirrors the ways in which women's efforts in procreation were similarly embedded within a web of

81 William Chaytor to Peregrina Chaytor, 4 March 1701, North Yorkshire Record Office, Northallerton, 9/14/35.

82 David Cressy, *Birth, Marriage, and Death: Ritual, Religion, and the Life-Cycle in Tudor and Stuart England* (Oxford: Oxford University Press, 1997), 60.

social, emotional and financial imperatives set by the family. It was these same values and priorities that dictated where women would give birth too.

Going 'Home' to Give Birth

The retreat of women into a chamber to give birth has been prominent in accounts that argue childbearing took women away from the family and that birth was a moment where the ties of femininity were stronger than those of family, community or even faith. Accounts have envisioned this as a moment where a woman and her friends (gossips) took over domestic space and excluded men. Many women, however, chose to give birth not in their marital homes but in their own or their husband's family home, and although male family members were not usually permitted in the birthing chamber, they were often downstairs. We have heard how items like linen and clothes for birth helped to cement the social and emotional boundaries of family, as well as how male and female family members were invested in imagining and predicting the character and appearance of unborn babies. Women, by travelling to give birth in their own or their husband's family home, made their infants literally and symbolically part of the family and its perpetuation. In more practical terms, it also allowed them to take advantage of the emotional and practical support of kin. Anne Clifford recorded that Lady Margaret Coventry 'deliver'd of a Daughter in her fathers house', the earl of Thannet in Hothfield.[83] Elizabeth Freke gave birth at 'my fathers att Hanington' along with her aunt and Sir George Norton.[84] Katherine Danby travelled to be with her mother and father to give birth in 1633.[85] The Staffordshire gentleman and landowner Thomas Congreve, who kept a detailed account of business and family affairs, also recorded that his daughters, Isobel and Elizabeth, often returned to their parental or their uncle's home to give birth.[86] In 1608, Isobel stayed with her father for the ten weeks before she gave birth and for two months afterwards while she recovered.[87] Althea Talbot gave birth to her second child in 1608 while residing with her mother, Anne, countess of Arundel.[88] This was not just an elite practice. Thomas Congreve recorded that his wife's butler,

[83] 4 June 1656; Anne Clifford, *The Diaries of Lady Anne Clifford*, ed. D. J. H. Clifford (Stroud: The History Press, 2003), 139.

[84] 2 June 1675; Freke, *The Remembrances of Elizabeth Freke*, 41.

[85] Alice Wandesford to Sir Thomas Danby, 30 July 1632, North Yorkshire Record Office, Northallerton, MISC 2087/1232.

[86] Thomas Congreve, 'Commonplace book including diary entries, 1585–1611', Staffordshire Record Office, MS D1057/0/1. Elizabeth gave birth to a child on 5 March 1608 at Thomas' brother's house, fol. 75r.

[87] *Ibid.*, fol. 63r. She arrived on 22 September 1608 and left sometime towards the end of November.

[88] Talbot family papers, 1608, Lambeth Palace Library, London, MS 3205, fols 135–143.

Jane Pattricke née Blackemore, went to 'her fathers howse to lye in'.[89] Anne Dey, the servant of Elizabeth Congreve, went to her brother Edward's house to give birth.[90] Thomas (as their master) was deeply involved in the personal affairs of his servants. His daughter was a gossip at Jane's birth, and after Anne's birth, he hosted all the 'wieves' at his estate, Stretton Hall.

Family members often moved across the country to be with women when they gave birth. In 1607, Congreve and his wife, Margaret, travelled to Powick in Worcestershire to be with their eldest son, Frances, and his wife, Dorothy, when she gave birth.[91] Margaret also travelled to Elizabeth's home for her second birth.[92] Mary, countess of Warwick, was requested at the deliveries of her niece, Lady Ann Barrington. She reported, 'I went directly theithar' when Ann's pains began and 'stayed with her all night, she having a most terable sharpe labour. I was exsidingly afraide of her and with much earnestness and many teares begde a safe delivery for her.'[93] Jane Joselin was present for the births of all her daughters' first babies, and she offered assistance after birth.[94] The Scottish woman Margaret Cunningham described how her husband's neglect forced her to beg the vicar and his wife for a 'birthe chamber' and care when he threw her and her servant out of the house for sleeping naked together in the same bed in 1604. This was part of her account of her miserable marriage to Sir John Hamilton between 1598 and 1607, written either to justify her legal separation from him or her subsequent remarriage to Sir James Maxell in 1610.[95] For Margaret, the lack of provision of a place within the household to give birth in and support from her husband was key evidence in warranting a separation.

Families did not always discuss which friends or family members would be at births in detail in correspondence and diaries. However, like the choice of practitioner, when someone who was expected to be at the bedside was snubbed or conflict arose, this was worthy of note. Henry Newcome recorded in his diary on 1 March 1662 that his wife had not been called to Mrs Houlbrooke's labour, which was 'a pretty vanity of my spirit to be concerned as I felt myself to be this day'.[96] A defamation case from the Durham Consistory Court between Barbara Errington and Alice Coleman in June 1621 suggests that declining to invite certain individuals could be a real

[89] Congreve, 'Commonplace book', 1 March 1610, fol. 71. [90] *Ibid.*, 27 March 1610, fol. 71v.
[91] *Ibid.*, 14 February 1607, fol. 77v. [92] *Ibid.*, September 1607, fol. 82v.
[93] Mary Rich, countess of Warwick, 26 August 1668, in Charlotte Fell Smith (ed.), *Mary Rich, Countess of Warwick (1625–1678): Her Family and Friends* (London: Longmans, 1901), 281.
[94] Alan Macfarlane, *The Family Life of Ralph Josselin, a Seventeenth-Century Clergyman: An Essay in Historical Anthropology* (Cambridge: Cambridge University Press, 1970), 114.
[95] Lady Margaret Cunningham, 'A parte of the life of Lady Margaret Cunningham Daughter to the Earle of Geencairn', National Library of Scotland, Edinburgh, MS 906, fol. 4r.
[96] Cited in: Cressy, *Birth, Marriage, and Death*, 58.

insult. In a witness statement, Alice Lambton, claimed that Coleman had arrived late at the childbirth of another woman. When there, she 'began to find fault' with the women already present for not inviting her sooner. Errington reportedly told Coleman that if she 'had been a good neighbour her neighbours would have called her'.[97] There were clear social expectations around birth but families rarely agonised over non-related people who would be present at births, suggesting that the primary importance of such rituals was in cementing familial bonds.

Pregnant women often expressed their fervent desire for their husbands to be in the same house when they gave birth, indicating again a desire to be physically close to family when birthing. Peregrina Chaytor, for example, was deeply worried that she would be separated from her husband when she was pregnant in 1697. She was staying in London and worried that the journey to her home in Croft, Yorkshire, would be a 'great hassard' whilst so heavily pregnant, although the company of her husband would make the delivery 'e [a]sy'.[98] She desperately tried to seek another appropriate place to give birth, although was concerned that it was too expensive to find temporary lodgings and that the cold air rising from the Thames would damage her health. She could not give birth where she was staying because the lack of closet made it unsuitable. Someone called 'Mrs Brown' offered her Sir Richard Temple's apartment for twenty shillings a week, but this was thought to be too noisy. Another option was 'Mr Grey's' apartment, as he was due to depart for Barbados imminently, but his dates were unfixed and his resolve shaky. The instability of arrangements, lack of home comforts and loneliness of being away from her husband and their children made Peregrina uneasy. She complained to her husband that 'we se[e] littell company soe am lonely anuff for I am not well able to walk'.[99] Eventually, she decided to take Brown's apartment, but in her next letter complained that the noise was 'so ill for my head that I think I must ether lyin [lie in] in the room above or have my bed removed in to another part of the room tho they must go away when I am brought to bed for we must have boeth rooms above for that time'. Her lodger was unknown to her and rumoured to be in legal trouble, something she found worrying.[100] All of this was exacerbated by her husband's absence, and at times his infrequent correspondence. In one letter, she expressed that his letters were 'more pleasing to me then any deversion hear'. Given being cheerful was so important in healthy pregnancy and birth, this was not a flippant remark.

[97] Durham Consistory Court Deposition Book, DDRV, vol. 11, fols 152–154, 158. I thank Elizabeth Foyster for providing me with her transcript of this case.

[98] Peregrina Chaytor to William Chaytor, 29 July [1697], North Yorkshire Record Office, Northallerton, ZQH 9/12/51.

[99] *Ibid.*, 29 July 1697, ZQH 9/12/51.

[100] *Ibid.*, 14 August 1697, ZQH 9/12/52.

Another expressed that if he were there, his presence would quite literally be medicine or 'the best cordiell'.[101] It seems that Peregrina did secure her husband's presence at her delivery. There is a fragment of a draft letter to a male correspondent from William Chaytor in which he excused himself from business because 'my wife sent for me up shee being soe near her time and she came before her time and the child is since dead'. Another draft to an unknown 'Madam' reveals the infant 'took the gripes' four days after birth and died when it was eleven days old.[102]

Anne, countess of Leven, similarly pined for her husband while pregnant in November 1695, and was worried that he would be unable to be there for the birth. Her mother, Margaret, the countess of Wemyss, sought over several letters to calm her and told her to be 'wise and kinde to the childe in y[ou]r belly as not to grieve as much as you did last'. The emotional distress brought about by separation could threaten maternal and infant health. Anne's husband's 'presence' at her birth would be 'pretious'.[103] When Catherine Danby gave birth in 1632, her mother wrote to her son-in-law congratulating him on the birth of a second son, noting that her 'paines and weaknes' prior and during the birth were 'a[u]gmented by your absence'.[104] She fretted that if the child became unwell, they would have to baptise it in his absence, which would be all the more troubling. In these reflections, one senses that male presence and involvement in birth was perceived as essential in anchoring delivery and newborn babies in their proper context: in the family.

Husbands were also central actors in the ceremony of christening. Gossips, or 'godsiblings', were not always female (despite later cultural associations). Isabella Twysden listed her brothers as gossips at her delivery.[105] Simon Forman was entreated to be a gossip for a man called 'Fardell' in 1598.[106] This term could occasionally also mean family confidants – Henry, earl of Bath, and his wife Rachel called their respective friends gossips.[107] A three-tiered woodcut representing the experience of delivery that was printed in the frontispiece of the 1724 edition of Sharp's *Midwives Book*, retitled *The Compleat Midwife's Companion*, clearly shows the birthing room as female only (first tier), the baptism/churching ceremonies as male and female (second

[101] *Ibid.*, 19 August 1697, ZQH 9/12/53.
[102] Henry Chaytor to Sir William Chaytor, 19 September 1697, North Yorkshire Record Office, Northallerton, three unattributed drafts, ZQH 9/12/55.
[103] Margaret, countess of Wemyss, to Anne, countess of Leven, c. 30 November 1695, GD26/13/401/24 and c. 29 December 1695, GD26/13/401/25.
[104] Alice Wandesford to Sir Thomas Danby, 30 July 1632, North Yorkshire Record Office, Northallerton, MISC 2087/1232.
[105] Isabella Twysden, 'Almanack', 6 March 1645, 'the gossops were my bro: Tho: and Fra: Twysden, and my La: Hartlye, Jamme stode for hir', BL Add MS 34169, fol. 3.
[106] CASE4145, CB.
[107] Letters between Henry, earl of Bath, and Rachael Bourchier, countess of Bath, U269/C267.

tier), and the celebrations accompanying delivery and the baptism and churching ceremonies also as a mixed gender affair (third tier) (Figure 4.1). The seemingly private and solely female nature of the birthing chamber has been central in other accounts of childbirth in early modern England, and particularly the ways in which space was temporarily rearranged in women's favour. As this chapter has shown, however, not only were families and, in particular men, central in driving the choice of birthing practitioner, women often travelled to their natal or husband's natal homes to deliver. Giving birth, like other medical encounters in early modern Europe, provoked individuals to travel to receive the care they thought would be most beneficial.[108] By insisting on the presence of their husbands and fathers, women of different social levels often prioritised family connections over homosocial ones.

Conclusion

As women approached their reckoning day, they had to shoulder the domestic and social expectations of the family, including the possibility that the pregnancy that families had been investing in for many months would end not in the birth of a large, lusty baby but in their own or their child's death. It is perhaps in the genre of manuscript and printed maternal legacies that women most visibly displayed the ways that birthing served their husband's family and name.[109] When Peregrina Chaytor got closer to birth, she urgently wrote to her husband, setting out her desires and hopes for what might happen if she died. Even in these final difficult weeks and months before birth, women took pains to record parts of their experience that confirmed the ideas that families had about themselves and their identity. Peregrina hoped that her husband would 'take a true care of and be a verry kind father to' their children, particularly Tom, who she indicated had been treated too severely in the past. She hoped if at all possible that they should each have 'som[e] provesion and be put to imployments'. They ought to be led to understand their duty in God. She set out the ways in which she hoped her children, one alive and another not yet born, would be provided for, including the gifting of a locket if the baby was a girl. More instructions followed about how and when the estate should be sold. She hoped he would 'not take amis[s]' her directions, an apology which echoed the expectations of conduct writers that women would be ever

108 Carolin Schmitz, 'Travelling for Health: Local and Regional Mobility in Early Modern Rural Spain', in *Connected Mobilities in the Early Modern World: The Practice and Experience of Movement*, ed. Paul Nelles and Rosa Salzberg (Amsterdam: Amsterdam University Press, 2023), 87–110.

109 For a summary of the genre, see: Jennifer Louise Heller, *The Mother's Legacy in Early Modern England*, Women and Gender in the Early Modern World (Farnham: Ashgate, 2011).

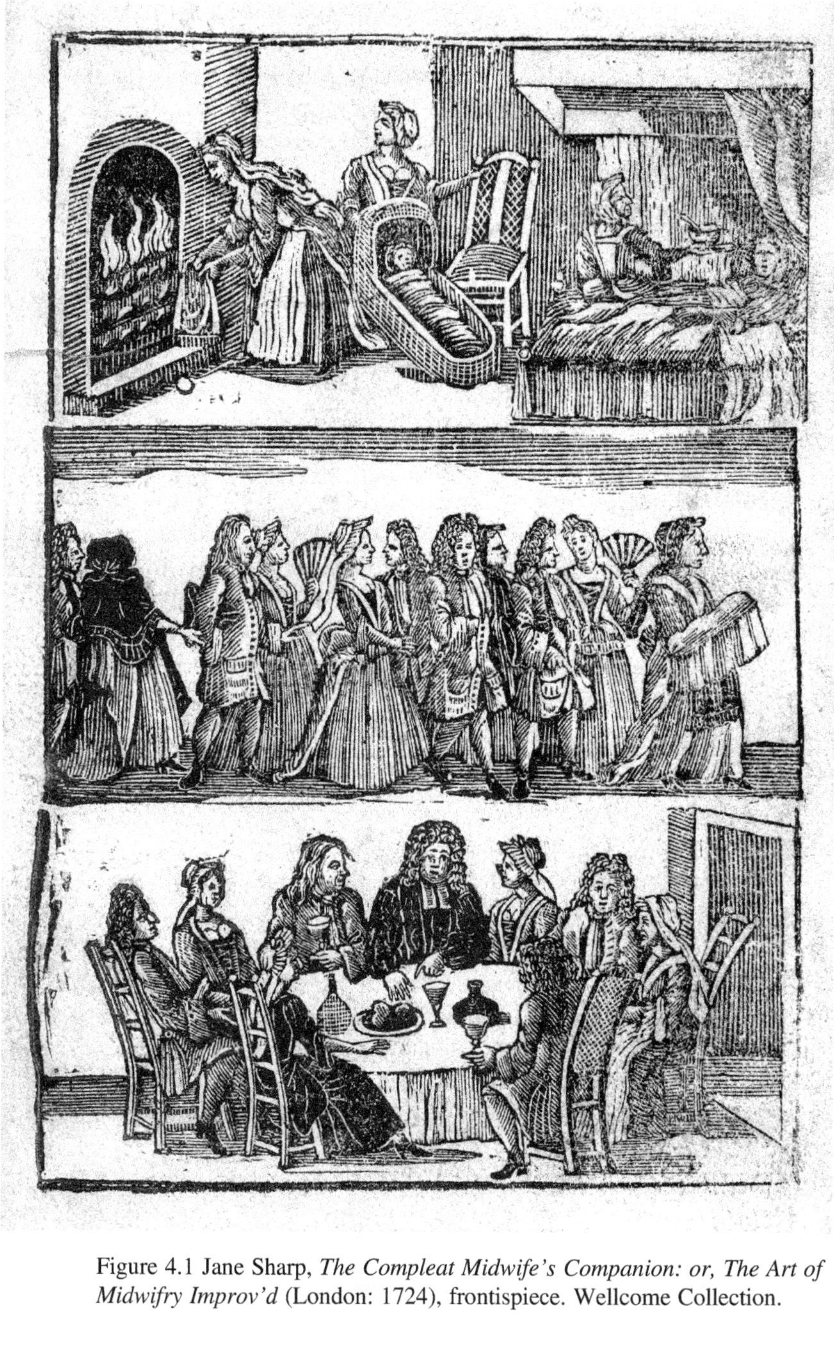

Figure 4.1 Jane Sharp, *The Compleat Midwife's Companion: or, The Art of Midwifry Improv'd* (London: 1724), frontispiece. Wellcome Collection.

submissive, even as to give up her body and soul for the furthering of her family. Peregrina's letter is a far cry from the convivial and profligate spending sprees and lying-ins that reformers worried women might engage in. Peregrina places her delivery within the context of her family, rather than within a female sociable world, even as she faced giving birth outside its confines. As the choice of practitioner and the decisions families made about where women would give birth indicate, bearing children was often aggressively familial and exclusionary. Like the material goods that families gathered, these aspects of preparing for birth were often represented as being 'given' to women as a sweetener for the pain and peril to come, but this idea concealed the ways in which gifting, borrowing and negotiating served a greater purpose: it cemented and delineated the family and provided tangible records of duty and approval.

5 'Safe' Delivery and Recovering from Birth

> Oh Lord, this daie is a gloomie daie, a bitter time and terrible houre, a daie (or night) of anguish and tribulation, of sorrowe and perturbation, vnto the verie soule of thine hand-maid: for the babe is come vnto the place of the birth, and lo, it seemeth that thou for my sins has shut vp the dores of my wombe, and caused the babe to stand still like to be stiffled.

This prayer composed by Thomas Bentley was to be read aloud during labour either by the birthing woman herself or those around her. One can imagine the low chants of the birthing woman's female family members, instructing her that not only was her child created by God but the descent of the baby in the birthing canal was governed by Him too. Below them, male family members might hear melodic traces of Bentley's description of the utter agony of birth as well as her screams. The mother might read out: 'How long shall I suffer the paines of the birth, and the anguish of the travel? How long Lord shall my bowels thus sound like an harpe, my bones and sinews be racked asunder, and mind inward parts be thus greevouslie tormented for my sins?' She longed for the baby to be born alive so that she could 'set it on my knees, and giue it sucke with my brests'.[1]

This prayer was in a popular anthology of prayers and meditations for women called *The Monument of Matrones*. Bentley was a student at Gray's Inn and a church warden, and his compilation offered women prayers for each stage of the lifecycle, although childbirth made up a notable third of the prayers in the volumes.[2] Whilst the prayer makes it clear that delivery was unthinkably painful, the prayers after birth were decidedly more celebratory.

[1] Thomas Bentley, *The Fift Lampe of Virginitie: Conteining sundrie forms of Christian praiers and meditations, to bee vsed onlie of and for all sorts and degrees of women, in their seuerall ages and callings; as namelie, of Virgins, Wiues, Women with child, Midwiues, Mothers, Daughters, Mistresses, maids, Widowes, and old women* (London: 1582), 115. See also: Colin B. Atkinson and William P. Stoneman, '"These Griping Greefes and Pinching Pangs": Attitudes to Childbirth in Thomas Bentley's The Monument of Matrones (1582)', *Sixteenth Century Journal* 2 (1990): 192–203.

[2] Colin Atkinson and Jo B. Atkinson, 'Subordinating Women: Thomas Bentley's Use of Biblical Women in "The Monument of Matrones" (1582)', *Church History* 60, 3 (1991): 289–300.

Indeed, one might judge them to expressly and explicitly forget the pain and peril of pregnancy and birth. One to be said at a woman's churching, for example, thanked God for 'thy so great benefits shewed vnto me, in pulling me out of the pit-brinke of death, easing and releeuing all my wofull sorrowes, labours, pangs, and most greeuous throwes, bitter anguishes, & vnspeakable paines'. Despite being close to death, once the child was born, she would 'forget all hir paines, not remembering them anie longer, and to rejoice, for that she hath brought foorth a child into the world'.[3]

If one was just to read Bentley's poems, without recourse to family paperwork or practitioners' casebooks, one might assume that the difference in tone between pre- and post-natal poems reveals that the period after delivery was a wholly celebratory one and that the difficulties of getting and staying pregnant and birthing were quickly forgotten, especially after churching, a ceremony in which newly delivered women gave thanks to God and supposedly went back to her normal physical, emotional and social self. Indeed, many historians have emphasised the conviviality of the days, weeks and months after birth. Laura Gowing notes that the 'focus of the social ritual which surrounded new mothers shifted from pain and fear to thanksgiving and celebration'.[4] Adrian Wilson has postulated that only 1.5–2.5 per cent of births were 'complicated' (either obstructed or with 'major complications') in the seventeenth century, and the older claim that early modern women were particularly aware of the dangers of delivery is misplaced.[5] Emphasising the social experience, David Cressy notes that the 'performance' of baptism and churching ceremonies 'secured a ritual closure to the extended process of childbearing'. He notes that these ceremonies connected the 'semi-secret domestic world of women and childbirth with the public ecclesiastical and communal business of religion'.[6] This chapter suggests that looking at family paperwork renders Bentley's vision simply an ideal. Recovering from childbirth was often long, painful and although not always life-threatening, it could be life limiting, in ways that did not always reflect well on families. The women in Bentley's poems were 'new female Protestant heroes' and their behaviour represented proper behaviour. Medical writers shared this vision of recovery from birth and anticipated that within months, women would be physically and emotionally capable of conceiving again. Even though elite families had far more in their arsenal than those lower down the

[3] Bentley, *The Fift Lampe of Virginitie,* 120.
[4] Laura Gowing, *Common Bodies: Women, Touch and Power in Seventeenth-Century England* (New Haven, CT: Yale University Press, 2003), 172.
[5] Adrian Wilson, *The Making of Man-Midwifery: Childbirth in England, 1660–1770* (London: Routledge, 1995), 18; Adrian Wilson, 'The Perils of Early Modern Procreation: Childbirth with or without Fear?', *British Journal of Eighteenth Century Studies* 16 (1993): 2.
[6] David Cressy, *Birth, Marriage, and Death: Ritual, Religion, and the Life-Cycle in Tudor and Stuart England* (Oxford: Oxford University Press, 1997), 197.

socio-economic spectrum, these religious and medical expectations were still out of kilter with the reality of women's bodies and minds after birth. The assumption in prescriptive works that birth ought to be painful but bearable and that women needed no more and no less than a month to languish after birth before returning to their former selves formed a kind of script that individuals writing diaries and letters were influenced by.

This chapter critically interrogates what recovery meant to early modern writers and families in generation, and how they experienced it. The preacher Caryl Joseph encapsulated the ambition of medical experts in the period when he described 'perfect recovery' from disease as there being 'no scar, nor print, no dregs, nor appearance of his former disease seene upon him'.[7] Hannah Newton has argued that complete removal of disease and full restoration of strength were obvious and achievable destinations for early modern people after a period of ill health or instability.[8] In contrast, scholars in disability studies have pointed to the ways in which the normativity of 'able-bodiedness' can foster untenable fantasies of health and ability, and that in some senses, all bodies are 'wounded' and fall short of ideals.[9] Complete and timely recovery from childbirth was then a normative construct that people defined their experiences in compliance with or in opposition to. This chapter reinforces Newton's findings that recovery was what birthing women sought and, often, expected, but contrastingly shows that this framework did not always adequately explain their bodily, emotional and social experiences after birth. This could be frustrating and lead to domestic and familial disorder. Childbearing was of course not an invariably difficult or torturous experience in the early modern period, but we do women a disservice when we imbibe and reiterate the narratives of prescriptive religious and medical authorities uncritically. It was in the interests of the Church and families to represent childbearing as unproblematic. In the same vein, to elite families, the details of recovery from childbirth were often far less interesting than the question of when women might be able to conceive again and perpetuate the family further.

Torment, Peril and Pain in Birth

The pain that women experienced was a central theme in the accounts that devout female diarists created for posterity and the family archive. Here, their

7 Cited in Hannah Newton, *Misery to Mirth: Recovery from Illness in Early Modern England* (Oxford: Oxford University Press, 2018), 231.

8 *Ibid.*

9 See, for example: Allison P. Hobgood and David Houston Wood, 'Ethical Staring: Disabling the English Renaissance', in *Recovering Disability in Early Modern England* (Athens: Ohio University Press, 2013), 1–22; Simi Linton, *Claiming Disability: Knowledge and Identity* (New York: New York University Press, 1998); Tobin Siebers, 'Disability as Masquerade', *Literature and Medicine* 23, no. 1 (2004): 22–65.

forbearance often served to highlight their devotion to God and to carrying out their maternal and familial duty. Alice Thornton described the 'great & excessiue torment & Perill of my Life' she experienced in birthing her second child, Naly. The baby's neck and shoulders became 'stuck' for a full hour.[10] When she gave birth to her fourth child, Katherine, in 1656, she noted that she was in labour for a whole week 'very strong, in somuch that I indured more in that time & in the extreamity then of my other' and she resigned herself to the fact she might die.[11] In the meditations of Elizabeth Egerton, countess of Bridgewater, she described the pain that she expected to feel. She begged God would have 'compassion on me in the great paine I am to feele in the bringing forth of this my Child'. She hoped he would not levy any more than she was able to 'beare'.[12] In contrast, single women told courts that they had been unaware they were pregnant and that their infant had simply slipped from them without pain or commotion. These births, in Gowing's terms, were 'shamefully easy'.[13] Like suffering in illness or infirmity, for the hotter sort of Protestant, the pain of childbirth might be contextualised as a direct test from God and a sign of being part of the elect, and was to be welcomed, accepted and borne patiently.

In family correspondence written by men, however, this pain was often taken for granted or seen as inevitable. Often these letters summarised the whole experience of labour as one in which the woman had been 'safely delivered', a phrase borrowed from the prayer said at the 'Thanksgiving' ceremony 'it hath pleased Almighty God of his goodness to give you safe deliverance' in childbirth. The phrase 'brought a bed' or 'to bed' was also often used. Both left out the details of what women felt or experienced during their pangs, how long the delivery was or whether it had caused potential lasting injury that might complicate their recovery. Charles Cheyne, for example, told his brother-in-law in 1656 that his wife was 'well and safely brought to bed of a daughter'.[14] When Oliver St John, of the aristocratic Bedfordshire family, had a daughter, Francis Thornhough, his brother-in-law, congratulated him on the 'safe delivery' of a child.[15] Nehemiah Wallington described in his diary how his wife, Grace, had been 'in great paine' with childbirth, which continued for a full day until 'it pleased God to

[10] Alice Thornton, 'Meditations', BL, Add MS 88897/1, 135. [11] *Ibid.*, 144.

[12] Elizabeth Egerton, 'Devotional Pieces by Elizabeth, Countess of Bridgewater', BL, Egerton MS 607, fol. 25r–25v.

[13] Laura Gowing, 'Secret Births and Infanticide in Seventeenth-Century England', *Past & Present* no. 156 (1997): 99.

[14] Charles Cheyne to Viscountess Mansfield, 18 May 1656, University of Nottingham Library, Portland Papers, PW1/84.

[15] Francis Thornhough to Oliver St John, 13 October 1674, Bedfordshire and Luton Archives and Record Service, J1469.

give her safe deliverance of a Daughter'.[16] Framing birth in this way focused almost exclusively on the outcomes of generation – the survival of child and mother – with little interest in the journey to recovery and restoration that women faced. When Anne Wentworth wrote to her husband, Thomas, describing the birth of her first child, once she was granted the 'Liberty' by the famous man-midwife Doctor Chamberlen (which her mother-in-law petitioned for, as we heard in Chapter 4), she noted that her cousin and 'Sister Betty' perceived her to be 'much perter and brisker than I used to be & they tease me all day long to know what has happen'd to me to delight me so much.' Isabella's petitioning, it seems had, in Anne's opinion, worked out for the best.[17] Four weeks after she gave birth, she told him in a letter filled with other family details that she had done her 'Lying in' and was going to see Queen Anne, who was the child's godmother. She had been churched ten days prior.[18]

Birth lists in diaries, account books and recipe books also often prioritised facts over detail or experience in creating records of actual delivery. Isabella Twysden wrote in the blank leaves of her almanac that she was simply 'brought a bed of a boye' 'betwene one and 2. in the morning'.[19] George Langton recorded on 14 May 1690 that 'John was born about 4 of ye clock in ye morning & Christned ye 22th [sic]', and on 6 May 1696, 'between 12 & 1 in the morning', his son Bennet was born. Sir Edward Dering recorded on 8 February 1656 that his 'wife was deliuered of a boy', and then on 12 February, 'He was named Charles.'[20] Being safely delivered, or even just delivered, was not the same thing as being recovered, which Thornbough hinted at in his follow-up wish that God would 'still continue good unto' Oliver's wife 'in restoring her to her former strength'.[21]

[16] Nehemiah Wallington, 'A Record of Gods Marcys', 13 October 1622, *The Notebooks of Nehemiah Wallington, 1618–1654: A Selection*, ed. David Booy (Aldershot: Ashgate, 2007), 55.

[17] Anne Wentworth to Thomas Wentworth, 24 March 1712/1713, BL, Add MS 22226, fol. 109. See also 13 March 1712/1713, fol. 97 and 17 March, 1712/1713, BL, Add MS 22226, fol. 101.

[18] 27 March 1712/1713, *ibid.*, fol. 115.

[19] Isabella Twysden, in John Booker, *Mercurius Coelicus: sive Almanack, et Prognosticon, Vel* speculum, almanac (London: 1647), BL, Add MS 34169, fols 2r and 3r. It appears that either Isabella retrospectively recorded these events from 1644/1645 in her 1647 almanac, or that she had these previous entries bound in instead of the normal blank leaves that printers offered.

[20] George Langton's almanac, Richard Saunders, *Apollo Anglicanus, The English Apollo: Assisting All Persons in the Right Understanding of this Years Revolution, as also of things past, present, and to come* (London: 1690), Lincolnshire Archives, Lincoln, MASS 28/1, unfoliated; George Langton's almanac, *Cardanus Rider, Riders (1696) British Merlin: Bedeckt with many Delightful Varieties, and Useful Verities, Fitting the Longitude and Latitude of all Capacities within the Islands of Great Britain's Monarchy* (1696: London), Lincolnshire Archives, MASS 28/2.

[21] Francis Thornhough to Oliver St John, 13 October 1674, Bedfordshire and Luton Archives and Record Service, J1469.

Childbearing guides of the period rarely ruminated on what labour felt like beyond being simply painful, either because it was uninteresting or an uncomfortable prospect. Given the duration and intensity of most deliveries, it seems striking that most authors described contractions as ‘throws’ or ‘pains’ without more expansion. These sensations were described in ways that might make a reader who had never seen or felt labour before assume that these pains were constant and unchanging throughout delivery. This may of course have been because male authors had never set foot in a birthing chamber. Elsewhere, even when the writers claimed to have attended many births or even experienced birthing themselves, these pains were presented as being minor enough to not hinder normal activity. Jane Sharp pithily described how when women had ‘come to their Labour’ and they felt their ‘Throws coming’, they should ‘walk easily in her Chamber’, lie down, keep herself warm and then move to facilitate the ‘waters coming down and the womb to open’. Other women should not let her lie in bed too long, and they should ‘refresh’ the labouring woman with broth, eggs, bread or wine; ‘cheer her up with good words’ and stroke her ‘belly above her Navel gently with her hand’.[22]

Several things, however, seem to be missing from this account. One cannot help but wonder how an early modern woman, or midwife, distinguished between early pains and what we now might term ‘active’ labour? If a woman was to take herself to the birthing chamber and keep herself warm, who exactly was meant to refresh her, cheer her and stroke her? Was it the midwife, the women around her or a nurse, or as we have heard in Chapter 4, did it not really matter to medical writers as long as this care was carried out? The continual reference to the necessity of cheering women hints at the emotional difficulties of labour and delivery that women no doubt faced, without a recognition of how frightening and traumatic this experience might be and how recovery involved not just physical restoration but a more wholistic return to self. When the author of *Every Woman Her Own Midwife* described how ‘pangs of childbearing’ would ‘increase more and more’ just before delivery, and it was at this point that the midwife should anoint the womb with oil of camomile and white lilies, one is left wondering what this stage of labour might look or sound like?[23] Why are authors so pithy on this subject in comparison to the ink spilt on setting out the most desirable diet and conduct of pregnant women leading up to this point?

[22] Jane Sharp, *The Midwives Book Or the Whole Art of Midwifry Discovered*, ed. Elaine Hobby, Women Writers in English 1350–1850 (Oxford: Oxford University Press, 1999), 145.

[23] *Every Woman Her Own Midwife, or, A Compleat cabinet opened for child-bearing women furnished with directions to prevent miscarriages during the time of breeding* (London, 1675), 10.

The authors of childbearing guides it seems were overly optimistic about women's sprightliness during delivery. *Aristotle's Master-piece* described how when the 'time of Birth' was 'drawing near', the woman should 'prepare a Pallet-Bed or Couch, and place it near the fire', along with a change of linen and a 'small Cricket or little Log' to rest her feet against. This was to allow 'the Midwife and her Assistants' to easily pass around 'and help on every side as occasion requires'. She should 'expect the coming down of her water' and the 'Womb to open and dilate it self'.[24] There was no mention of what it felt like for a womb to 'open and dilate' or to sense a baby descending. William Sermon's encouragement that midwives should ask their patients 'Whether they have pains, and in what manner they are where they begin, and where they end' but that they ought to remember that 'it would be almost a miracle to see a woman delivered without pain' points to why the gradients and complexities of sensations were of little interest to the authors of childbearing guides.[25]

Pain, in this sense, was represented as instrumental in delivery. Added to this, it was figured as a key part of birth as redemptive for Eve's sins.[26] Not only did the rhythmic pressure of contractions drive the baby out, but these sensations were often the baby 'kicking' its way out too. Robert Barret instructed midwives to 'make as much use as you can of the woman's own pressure' because if you 'discourage or prevent her bearing down, all her pains will vanish; and so the child perish locked up in the passage'.[27] When Elizabeth Bessy, a midwife, was accused of misconduct by Agnes Fisher whose baby had died shortly after delivery in 1631, Bessy defended herself by saying that Agnes herself was responsible for the child's death because she had refused to lean into her pains. The birthing woman was 'so dull and slow in her pains and so unapt or unwilling to help herself and to set forward the production of her child', causing the baby to be born 'very weak and feeble'.[28] By refusing to centre the details of the sensations of labour, the authors of childbearing guides relegated pain as an inevitable, necessary and unremarkable part of having a baby.

This is why childbearing guides were not overly concerned with trying to lessen or manage aches. It was only in the eighteenth century with the popularity of laudanum and other opiate concoctions that physicians became

[24] *Aristotle's Master-piece; Or, The Secrets of Generation Display'd in all the Parts thereof* (London, 1697), 160

[25] William Sermon, *The Ladies Companion, or, The English Midwife* (London, 1671), 97.

[26] Genesis 3:16, King James Bible.

[27] Robert Barret, *A Companion for Midwives, Child-bearing Women, and Nurses Directing them how to Perform their Respective Offices: Together with an Essay, Endeavouring to Shew the Influence of Moral Abuses upon the Health of Children* (London, 1699), 29.

[28] Patricia Crawford and Laura Gowing, eds., *Women's Worlds in Seventeenth-Century England* (London: Routledge, 2000), 193–194.

interested in trying to lessen labour pain. Even then there was substantial debate about whether it was appropriate for childbirth. William Giffard wrote in 1734 that laudanum ought only to be used to relieve 'those false and irregular pains which often afflict women' and not regular contractions that were productive for birth.[29] Thomas Dawkes, the surgeon, wrote in 1736 that it was important to distinguish between colic and 'true' labour pain, the latter of which was productive, the former could be relieved.[30] Even in the eighteenth century, there was a pervasive belief that pain was a normative, necessary and redemptive part of giving birth.

Indeed, one might say that pain was strongly linked to proper and legitimate birth in a way that delivering quickly and easily was linked to immoderate sexual conduct. This was perhaps one reason why elite families rarely sought analgesic measures for birth in ways that have survived the historical record. Added to this, although prior to the Reformation people of all levels of society may have made use of apotropaic objects like girdles, eagle stones or textual amulets hung around the neck or stomach, these were increasingly seen as popish and unbefitting for more ascendant and well-educated families.[31] Shifting from venerating Mary to Eve encouraged women to pray directly to Christ rather than an intercessor, which meant that saints relics were also frowned upon.[32] In some instances, obtaining or proffering relics for the purpose of relieving pain in childbirth could even warrant an accusation of witchcraft. In the 1590s in Scotland, Agnes Samson, a midwife, offered Euphemia Maclean a bored stone, a rock with a hole in the middle thought to have magical powers. She was told to put the stone under her pillow and her husband's shirt under her bed to ease her suffering during labour. Agnes also offered Euphemia a 'Inchantit mwildis', the finger, toe or knee joints of a disinterred corpse. These objects and Euphemia's acceptance of pain relief was evidence that she was a witch, a crime for which she was subsequently hanged.[33] The practice of using objects to relieve pain, however, as with other remnants of pre-Reformation worship in material culture and the landscape,

29 William Giffard, *Cases in Midwifery Written by the late Mr William Giffard, surgeon and man-midwife. Revis'd and publish'd by Edward Hody* (London: 1734), 329; Thomas Denman, *An Essay upon Natural Labours* (London: 1786), 17.

30 Thomas Dawkes, *The Midwife Rightly Instructed* (London: 1736).

31 Róisín Donohoe, '"Unbynde Her Anoone": The Lives of St. Margaret of Antioch and the Lying-in Space in Late Medieval England', in *Gender in Medieval Places, Spaces and Thresholds*, ed. Victoria Blud, Diane Heath and Einat Klafter, IHR Conference Series (London: University of London Press, Institute of Historical Research, 2019), 139–156.

32 Mary E. Fissell, *Vernacular Bodies: The Politics of Reproduction in Early Modern England* (Oxford: Oxford University Press, 2004), 50.

33 S. Lurie, 'Euphemia Maclean, Agnes Sampson and Pain Relief during Labour in 16th Century Edinburgh', *Anaesthesia* 59, no. 8 (2004): 834–835.

were not always rejected swiftly or cleanly.[34] Thomas Lupton's 1579 *Book of a Thousand Things* included a great many remedies for childbearing including objects that could be tied next to the body, similar to girdles.[35] In a 1694 pamphlet by a 'Physitian in the countrey' that advertised the many virtues of the maldiva nut (now more commonly known as coco de mer) supposedly a new import from the 'Indies', the author described how 'Persons of the best Quality in India' tied it around their neck and placed into wine or other alcohol to ward against poison and 'Infections'. Its other use was that it could speed up delivery, so much so that in Spain it was called the 'Egyptian midwife' owing to the long-standing narrative that Hebrew women gave birth quickly and easily.[36] The Conway family, if we recall, were keen to locate an eagle stone in 1658, but they begged for discretion lest people judge them for being superstitious.[37]

That is why it is hard to come by remedies to alleviate pain in domestic receipt books too: both because pain was seen as medically and religiously important. Instead, recipes were framed as being able to 'ease', 'help' or 'hasten' delivery. Not explicitly mentioning pain relief, one imagines, may have allowed elite women to circumvent the Church's valorisation of painful labour as redemptive, whilst simultaneously achieving some measure of relief. Elizabeth Egerton, who hoped God would enable her to withstand the pains of childbirth at the beginning of this chapter, kept 'the Earl of Chesterfeilds Powder' in her recipe book to be used when the child was 'stick in ye birth' or if a woman's 'paines' abated, if the child was dead or if the 'after birth stay behind'. It should be administered when the midwife 'thinks fit'. Egerton wrote 'this hath don[e] much good' underneath the recipe.[38] The unmentioned secondary impact would surely have been to bring the torturous pangs to a swifter end. Another was a 'Cordiall to be taken in labor and for after paines and any faintness in lying in for hesterical fits'.[39] Similarly, a remedy in Jane Jackson's book supposedly quickened delivery by using the horse grease to fumigate the woman's privities, rather than making more comfortable.[40]

[34] See, for example: Alexandra Walsham, *Reformation of the Landscape: Religion, Identity, and Memory in Early Modern Britain and Ireland* (Oxford: Oxford University Press, 2011).

[35] Fissell, *Vernacular Bodies*, 50.

[36] *Some observations made upon the maldiva nut shewing its admirable virtue in giving an easie, safe, and speedy delivery to women in child-bed/ written by a physitian in the country to Dr Hinton at London, 1663* (London: 1694), 6–7.

[37] Edward Conway to Major Rawdon, 12 October 1658, Sarah Hutton and Marjorie Hope Nicolson, eds., *The Conway Letters: The Correspondence of Anne, Viscountess Conway, Henry More, and Their Friends 1642–1684* (Oxford: Oxford University Press, 1992), 152–153.

[38] Lady Brilliana Harley, 'Medical recipes', Egerton MS 2214, fol. 4v.

[39] *Ibid.*, fol. 5r.

[40] Jane Jackson, 'A very shorte and compendious Methode of Phisicke and Chirurgery', WL, MS 373, fol. 52r.

Other recipes specify that they are to be taken during difficult or protracted labours, but similarly steer clear of mentioning pain. Anne Glyd, for example, included one concoction for 'a Woman To Take in Trauell' and 'in hard trauell'. Further remedies expressly intensified pain – 'To Caus pains when a woman cannot be deliuered', one of which was to have the woman drink a porringer of her husband's urine, which she noted she had done with success herself.[41] Others optimistically promised a 'good Labour' – one in an anonymous recipe book was to be taken 'morning and night, for three weeks before you are brought to Bed'.[42] In 1691, Robert Bunn asked the Somerset apothecary-surgeon, John Westover, for 'a medicine to facilitate her labour in childbirth' for two shillings and six pence.[43] Only the commonplace book of Edmund Kershaw, a middling-sort Lancashire man, contained a treatment for a woman to be 'deliuered of Childbirth without paine' that involved holding a root of basil and swallowing a feather 'wn shee is in trauell, she shall be deliuered by & without any paine'. Its resemblance to older pre-Reformation habits of tying objects around the body during labour is notable.

Pain was perceived as an acceptable part of birthing by early modern medical and religious authors. Even if it was torturously sore, labour pangs were seen as necessary and instrumental in delivery. Given the prominence of pain in descriptions of religious devotion and redemption, it is not surprising that there is little direct evidence of elite families seeking to dull the suffering of delivery. To do so would not only contravene divine will, but also potentially threaten one's heavenly ascent.

Expectations for Recovery

Although religious and medical writers expected birth would hurt, they also assumed that this pain and suffering would only last a month, and that it was concerning if women continued to bleed or feel unwell beyond this time. This was conditioned by the Judeochristian tradition of considering women impure for a month after birth and an accompanying ritual of cleansing. In England in the medieval and pre-Reformation era, the ceremony continued to be one of 'Purification' as well as one of thanksgiving for survival, but nevertheless marked the end of the experience of childbearing. After the Reformation, the 1552 Book of Common Prayer re-designated this ceremony as 'Thanksgiving' or 'Churching'.[44] Early modern medical authors gestured to Leviticus' and the

41 Anne Glyd, 'Her Book 1656', BL, Add MS 45196, unfoliated.
42 '17th century recipe book', Firestone Library, University of Princeton, RTC01, MS 214, 9.
43 William G. Hall (ed.), 'The Casebook of John Westover of Wedmore, Surgeon, 1686–1700', in *Wedmore Geneaology Pages*, www.tutton.org/, fol. 120v, last accessed 10/10/2020.
44 David Cressy, 'Purification, Thanksgiving and the Churching of Women in Post-Reformation England', *Past & Present* 141 (1993): 106–146.

Old Testament edict that women needed to bleed for a month or longer after birth and connected this to classical medical traditions. In doing so, authors avoided writing about this kind of blood loss in direct connection to the religious ceremony of purification whilst simultaneously stressing that excretion was central to survival and future health. Physicians largely believed that a woman was recovered once she had bled away the remnants of pregnancy. Although there were increasingly denominational differences in the period – notably with staunch puritans shunning Churching – we can see that the medical framework persisted in the ways families thought about postpartum bodies and 'their' month.

The blood lost after birth was called lochia and was described in manuals as highly toxic. It was menstrual blood that remained in the womb and 'filled daily more and more till the Birth' with the infant's sweat and urine to create a 'foul liquor.[45] Medical authors used the same terms to describe this bleeding after birth as they did for menstruation: 'them', her 'terms', 'flowers', 'courses' or the 'flux', and they were interested in setting out rules for how long or how much women should shed. Sharp explicitly drew on both religious and classical authorities. She cited Leviticus and the proposition that women would bleed for thirty-three days after giving birth to a boy and sixty-six after a girl, but also gestured to Hippocrates' calculation that women would bleed for thirty days for a male child and forty-two for a female.[46] The French physician Jacques Guillemeau calculated that women ought to lose thirteen pints as she had nine periods worth each of a 'pint and a half' to lose. She ought to bleed a pint in the first days after delivery, but he too thought Hippocratic time frames were also instructive.[47] When this bleeding was profuse or extended beyond the month it was deemed problematic. 'Flooding', sudden, heavy haemorrhagic blood loss, therefore, was described by Pechey as 'a more dangerous accident' than any other in bearing children. This was because even after 'nothing remains behind in the Womb' (placenta or lochial blood) but the blood 'notwithstanding continues to flow', depleting the woman in question of her vital spirits. He recommended blood-letting to draw blood away from the womb.[48] These kinds of treatments entrenched an understanding of recovery from childbirth as primarily involving the loss of matter from pregnancy, and

[45] John Pechey, *A General Treatise of the Diseases of Maids, Bigbellied Women, Child-bed Women, and Widows together with the best methods of preventing or curing the same* (London: 1696), 84.

[46] Sharp, *The Midwives Book Or the Whole Art of Midwifry Discovered*, 179.

[47] Jacques Guillemeau, *Child-birth or, The Happy Deliverie of Women Wherein is set downe the government of Women* (London: 1612), 222. See: Cathy McClive, *Menstruation and Procreation in Early Modern France* (London: Routledge, 2015), 89 for a discussion of eighteenth-century calculations of the quantity of menstrual blood that needed to be shed after childbirth.

[48] Pechey, *A General Treatise of the Diseases of Maids*, 158.

then the cessation of excretion once this blood had been removed. These conflicting calculations often sat side-by-side without resolution. In these prescriptive accounts, although this process was meant to take a month, they rarely explicitly mentioned the ceremony of Churching, which marked the end of this period of menstruation.

Lochial bleeding was instigated by the removal of the 'after birth', 'after burden', 'secundine', 'womb cake' or placenta. *Aristotle's Master-piece* and *The Compleat Midwifes Practice* told midwives they could get the placenta out by 'wagging and stirring' it.[49] Sharp warned against cutting the navel cord of the baby too hastily without holding it steadily because the womb was liable to snatch it back and 'hid there with the Secundine'.[50] The retention of the whole or part of the placenta was particularly concerning in the eyes of medical writers. Pechey described how difficult labour, the thickness of the baby's caul (amniotic sac), the mother experiencing 'violent passions of the Mind', poor posture during delivery, the overly large and 'lusty' size of the child, 'Coldness of Air', or if perfumes were administered that 'allured the womb upwards' too soon after the birth could all cause the womb to hold fast to the whole or part of the placenta.[51]

The consequences of a retained placenta or insufficient bleeding after birth were perceived to be dire by medical writers. Being improperly or partially 'cleansed' of lochia after birth was, in Pechey's terms, 'one of the worst Symptoms that can befall a Woman in Child-bed'.[52] Immediately after delivery, 'they should come down plentifully'. If they did not, the woman would suffer from a 'putrid fever', nausea, fainting spells, shaking, frenzy, a desire to 'eject something' along with a 'sense of heat and pain'. Finally, the corrupting matter within her would emit a 'cadaverous smell'.[53] The 'Coldness of the extream parts' was the last sign before convulsive fits led to death.[54] Simon Forman explained that frenzy arose out of those who 'have not their Courses well', which made the womb 'ful of melancholy and burnte blod' which ascended to the brain.[55] To kickstart or intensify bleeding, the patient could be given wormwoom, glysters and other 'opening herbs'. She might be chafed from the 'groines down to the very ankle-bone', have her blood let and not given too much to eat to save her life.[56] All this meant women were warned that they were 'in as great danger if not more, after the young is born' than during labour and delivery, but again only until they had bled sufficiently.[57]

49 *Aristotle's Master-piece*, 140.
50 Pechey, *A General Treatise of the Diseases of Maids*, 155–156. 51 *Ibid.*, 155.
52 *Ibid.*, 161. 53 *Ibid.*, 156. 54 *Ibid.*, 165–166.
55 Cited in: Philippa Carter, 'Childbirth, "Madness", and Bodies in History', *History Workshop Journal* 91 (2021): 37.
56 *Aristotle's Master-piece*, 90–91.
57 Pechey, *A General Treatise of the Diseases of Maids*, 155–156.

The somewhat myopic focus of childbearing authors on excretion to recovery from childbirth makes sense when we consider the ways in which menstruation was framed as fundamental to women's health more generally in the period.[58] A woman's 'flowers' could provide an additional form of excretion in recovering from disease and could hasten the Hippocratic-Galenic moment of 'crisis' – a positive point in recovering from illness.[59] So too did bleeding mark a transitional turning point in the restoration of health and self after birth.

For this reason, women and their families expressed considerable concern in their diaries and correspondence when bleeding either ceased prematurely or was deemed to be insufficiently heavy. Awareness of this imperative also frequently compelled them to seek the help of medical professionals. The Anglican minister Isaac Archer noted in his diary two weeks after the birth of his son, William, that his wife Anne was 'grievously sick, and faint' because of 'some noxious and venomous impurities that nature should have cleansed her of'.[60] Her condition was grave and her were parents sent for and the family prepared for her death. Anne took boiled herbs and 'by degrees her fitts went away, and nature did it's (sic) office, without any other physick'.[61] In 1638, Hannah, the wife of the Northamptonshire puritan lawyer and diarist Robert Woodford, consulted Dr Gourdon 'for advice' a month after she gave birth; he prescribed a purge.[62] Hannah's birth had been complicated. Robert recorded in his diary that the midwife had determined that the infant had lain 'crosse' the womb 'a great while' in delivery. A day later, Robert thanked God that his wife's 'physic' had been successful.[63] John Cotton wrote to the Bedfordshire physician John Symcotts in c. 1656 asking him for 'abstersive [purgative]

[58] Wendy D. Churchill, *Female Patients in Early Modern Britain: Gender, Diagnosis, and Treatment* (Farnham: Ashgate, 2012), 93–123; Gianna Pomata, 'Menstruating Men: Similarity and Difference of the Sexes in Early Modern Medicine', in *Generation and Degeneration: Tropes of Reproduction in Literature and History from Antiquity to Early Modern Europe*, ed. Valeria Finucci and Kevin Brownlee (Durham, NC: Duke University Press, 2001), 109–152. See also: Patricia Crawford, 'Attitudes to Menstruation in Seventeenth-Century England', *Past & Present* 91, no. 1 (1981): 47–73; Jennifer Evans, '"Gentle Purges Corrected with Hot Spices, Whether They Work or Not, Do Vehemently Provoke Venery": Menstrual Provocation and Procreation in Early Modern England', *Social History of Medicine* 25, no. 1 (2012): 2–19; McClive, *Menstruation and Procreation in Early Modern France*; Sara Read, *Menstruation and the Female Body in Early Modern England*, Genders and Sexualities in History (Basingstoke: Palgrave, 2013).

[59] Pomata, 'Menstruating Men', 137–138.

[60] Isaac Archer, 13 June 1672, 'Diary', Cambridge University Library, Add 8499 G, 154. For more on the role of 'Nature' in early modern medical cultures, see: Hannah Newton, '"Nature Concocts and Expels": Defeating Disease', in *Misery to Mirth*, 33–64.

[61] Archer, 'Diary', 154.

[62] Robert Woodford, 10 October 1638, *The Diary of Robert Woodford, 1637–1641*, ed. John Fielding (Cambridge: Cambridge University Press, 2012), 246.

[63] *Ibid.*, 11 October 1638, 246.

Physicke' three weeks after his wife had given birth 'for though shee finds her selfe very well, yet I thinke after such a time it will not bee a misse to use evacuation'.[64]

Twenty-four-year-old Anne Jackson, the wife of a minister, consulted John Hall, a Stratford-upon-Avon physician and son-in-law of Shakespeare, in May 1630 because 'after childbirth, as she was not well purged'. She had suddenly fallen 'into a severe frenzy with no other illness appearing'. She was 'enraged, chiefly with those whom previously she had most loved, though she spoke much about religion'. He did not visit her in person, so prescribed by message a series of purges, and towards the end, instructed her to place a chicken cut in half on top of her head and radishes sprinkled with rose vinegar and salt on her feet 'to draw away the humours'. This regimen apparently had 'happy success' and she supposedly returned to complete health.[65] Cecily Hopper sought Hall's help because 'the products of conception' were 'retained and corrupted' within her. She was expelling them in 'foul-smelling pieces'. Hall copied out a passage from Rüff's *De Conceptu*, explaining that this foul smell was ascending to her 'stomach, heart, liver, diaphragm and in consequence to the brain', causing headache, collapses and cold sweats with the threat of death.[66] With a plaster and an ointment for the womb, she was 'freed' from all her symptoms within 24 hours.[67] Likewise, Mrs Chandler, the second wife of a prosperous merchant, William Chandler, consulted Hall five days after giving birth with 'an erratic fever' and 'frequent shivering, hot spells and rigors day and night'.[68]

Women consulted the astrologer-physicians Richard Napier and Forman regularly to trigger or intensify bleeding too. Joan Dean consulted Napier in April 1633 three months after she had given birth but had already sought treatment in the form of blood-letting and purgatives. She complained that she had not bled since 'she lay in'. It is unclear whether she meant that she had not resumed menstruating or she thought that she had yet to bleed away the full remnants of pregnancy. She was 'Very cold' and 'Full of melancholy & has mind for nothing nor husband nor child.'[69] Goody Prior's 'natural courses' [period] had stopped a week after birth in 1632, when she consulted Napier.[70] Mercy Fish gave birth in early May 1628 and had only had one or two periods when she consulted Napier towards the end of June, despite being let blood to

[64] John Symcotts, 'Symcotts family medical letters and case books 1628–92', X 125, 326, Bedfordshire and Luton Archives and Records Service, Bedford, fol. 17.

[65] CASE149, Greg Wells, trans., *John Hall Master of Physicke: A Casebook from Shakespeare's Stratford* (Manchester: Manchester University Press, 2020), 230–32.

[66] Carter, 'Childbirth, "Madness", and Bodies in History', 47.

[67] CASE151, Wells, *John Hall Master of Physicke*, 234. [68] CASE28, *ibid.*, 101.

[69] CASE76882, CB. [70] CASE75795, CB.

facilitate menstruation. She had fits and pain in her side and 'knoweth not what'.[71]

Medical authorities' expectations of recovery meant that lochial bleeding beyond a month was also perceived as a problem. Mary Barnes asked Hall for help for 'excessive red menstrual flow a month after giving birth'. Hall's prescription of hartshorn shavings with a drink in the morning meant she 'immediately felt relieved, completely restored and cured'.[72] Elizabeth Randolph described how there was 'too much Flux of her Courses' after giving birth, along with 'Wind in the Stomach.' She was prescribed alum in red wine, an astringent applied externally and internally to slow the bleeding. In one case, Hall was explicit that Lady Sandys consulted him 'after her Purification' or Churching, yet she continued to bleed through haemorrhoids.[73] In 1691, John Pitte purchased medicine 'for his wife for the imoderat flux of her blood or childbead purgations' for one shilling from the Somerset apothecary-surgeon John Westover.[74]

Alice Thornton similarly recorded in her manuscript meditations how concerned she was that she continued to bleed 'four or five ounces of blood' through haemorrhoids every day twenty weeks after giving birth to her fifth child. It is worth bearing in mind that lots of different kinds of vicarious bleeding could be considered to be menstrual or lochial. Thornton consulted a physician and travelled to Scarborough to take the waters in the hope this would go some way to remedy the 'excessive losse of blood and spirits, in childebed'.[75] Her physician warned that her condition was potentially fatal and would prevent her from conceiving again. Thornton termed her long, difficult struggle back to health her 'childebed', including labour *and* the period of time in which she was unwell after birth, pointing to the ways that temporalities of prescriptive frameworks did not adequately describe women's experiences of recovery. Bleeding too little and too much after birth were both worrying in the view of medical authorities, but for very different reasons. Retaining the placenta and lochia led to fever and frenzy,[76] whilst those who bled too much became depleted and weak. Bleeding too long after childbirth threatened to rid women of their spirits and energy.

Domestic recipe books also contained remedies both to intensify bleeding the month after birth, and halt it following this period, corresponding to the priorities of steadily excreting for a month and then stopping set out in

[71] CASE66415. See also: CASE63685, CASE66124, CB.

[72] CASE55; Wells, *John Hall Master of Physicke*, 130–131. [73] CASE37, *ibid.*, 114–115.

[74] John Westover, 2 January 1691, 'The Casebook of John Westover of Wedmore, Surgeon, 1686–1700', William G. Hall (transcriber), www.tutton.org/content/Westover_journal.pdf, fol. 107v, last accessed 25/03/2025.

[75] Thornton, 'Meditations', 155–156.

[76] Carter, 'Childbirth, "Madness", and Bodies in History'.

childbearing guides. Frances Springatt and others' recipe book contained 'Mrs Tassells cawdle to bring away the After berth or any part left behind' and one to stop 'An immoderate flux of the Redds'.[77] As lochia was understood as menstrual blood, it is difficult to separate the wealth of remedies that sought to regulate periods alongside that which might manage bleeding after birth. Jane Jackson's 'Against too much flowres of women or the superfluitie thereof' and two others that promised to do the same thing might have been used both by women seeking an end to long and heavy periods, or those seeking to manage lochial bleeding. Similarly, one to 'cause a woman haue her flowers to haue her flowers that bee destroyd' could have had a similar double use.[78]

Postpartum bodies were, in the words of *Aristotle's Master-piece*, expected to be 'disordered' as if they 'were out of frame' until they had bled sufficiently.[79] This understanding was so dominant, however, that it often did not leave space for the ways that women might continue to *feel* disordered or out of frame after this month despite meeting the requirements of recovery contained in prescriptive ideals. A month after Mary Verney gave birth, her physician, Dr Denton, wrote to her husband, Ralph, to tell him that she was 'churcht [churched] & well, but lookes ill enough'.[80] Being 'well' in this context meant she had stopped bleeding.[81] Denton's comments expose the dominance of humoral understandings of health to recovery from childbirth. Mary no doubt felt as ill as she looked, but as long as she had returned to her former self in a humoral sense, her physician was unconcerned. As we shall see, prolonged and precocious recoveries were perceived as abnormal.

Prolonged Recoveries

Although women were meant to bleed after birth for four to six weeks, during which time they expected to feel progressively better before the excretion ceased, a great many did not experience recovery in this way. Recovery was complicated and could be impeded by all manner of social, emotional and physical interruptions. Pain, discomfort, disability and fatigue could plague women for months and months after delivery. Three weeks after Mary Verney gave birth to a son in 1647, she told her husband that although the baby was well 'for my self I am so very weak that ontell (until) yesterday, since I was brought to bed, I have neavor been able to sitt up ann hower at a time'. She was

77 Frances Springatt & others, 'Recipe book, 1686–1824', WL, MS 4683, fols 204v and 231r
78 Jackson, 'A very shorte and compendius Methode of Physicke and Chirurgery', fols 89r and 101r.
79 *Aristotle's Master-piece*, 157.
80 Dr Denton to Ralph Verney, 4 July 1647, Frances Parthenope Verney, ed., *Memoirs of the Verney Family during the Civil War* (London: Longmans, 1892), 272.
81 Read, *Menstruation and the Female Body in Early Modern England*, 164.

'so tormented with pains' in her head that if she sat up for more than a quarter of an hour, 'it puts me into such sweates as I am not able to endure itt'. If only her headache would subside, she thought she would be able to 'recover' her 'strength apace'.[82] After the birth of her first child, which died hours after birth, Thornton suffered from a fever and ague that lasted three months, after which she suffered from jaundice for another six months. In total, she was unwell for '3 q[uarte]r of a yeare full out'.[83] Even after she considered herself to have recovered, she noted that it was a full three months after this that she was able to conceive.[84] Two days after being churched, Mary Smith, of the Bristolian Smyth family, had an 'unlucky fall' and injured her back. She was confined to 'bed and chamber almost another monthe, I was so yell [ill] I feared some bone was amisse, but now I find it brused'. In a letter to her brother, she told him 'this beinge the furst day I haue bein out of doors sense crismas'. Even when she left the house, she stressed to her brother 'I think I shall feele it agood while' and apologised for her poor handwriting, which was a result of her afflictions.[85] Recovery from childbirth, these women recognise through experience, was not solely bound up with whether or not they had bled sufficiently. It took much more than excretion to return women to their former selves within their families and communities.

Elizabeth Walker, wife of the puritan minister, Anthony, suffered from a sickness that lasted 'almost a quarter of a Year' and brought her 'very low' after giving birth. She was so sick that she had one or two people watching over her every night and had a constant stream of neighbours and relatives visiting. Anthony, Elizabeth's husband, published extracts of her diary that he claimed to have stumbled upon after her death. He was so impressed with her forbearance and exemplary life that he was compelled to share 'such Tryals' so that they might be 'useful to other Women, Wives, and Mothers in like Tryals'. Elizabeth had, in her husband's opinion, 'travailled in pain', birthing and caring for her infants in a way that was without fanfare or virtue signalling.[86] Anthony described how she was uncomfortable with having to stay in bed beyond her lying in and soon as she was left alone, she would sit up and pray. Elizabeth was the antithesis of bawdy women in ballads who used the month after lying-in to indulge and collude with friends.

[82] Mary Verney to Ralph Verney, 24 June 1647, *Memoirs of the Verney Family during the Civil War*, 267–268.

[83] Thornton, 'Meditations', 130. [84] *Ibid.*, 134.

[85] Mary Smith to Thomas Smith, 30 March c. 1630, Bristol Record Office, Bristol, AC/cC53/6. This could have been the daughter that she gave birth to on 8 August 1633.

[86] Anthony Walker, *The Virtuous Wife: or, the Holy Life of Mrs Elizabeth Walker, late wife of A. Walker, D. D. sometime Rector of Fyfield in Essex Giving a modest and short account of her exemplary piety and charity. Published in the glory of God, and provoking others to be like graces and vertues* (London: 1694), 93–94.

Men were also aware that prolonged recoveries were worthy of comment and concern. The Plymouth surgeon, James Yonge, recorded that his wife had a 'sickly and tedious lying-in' as a result of 'taking some cold' in his diary.[87] Charles Trelawny, an army officer and Tory politician, apologised to Sidney Godolphin, First Lord of the Treasury, in November 1700 for 'soe long neglecting, to owne the favour of your too (sic) letters, but when I tell you, that the indisposition of my other Side, was the cause, I'm sure you'll forgiue me'. His wife had 'been very much out of order, euersince she was brought to bed'. The child had been 'at death & door more than once since she was born, and is at this minute upon the Rack w[i]th convulsive fits'. The infant's illness had made its mother 'almost mad'.[88]

Women often described how grief could completely decimate their minds and bodies as they were recovering from birth. Thornton was 'at deaths doore' herself while recovering from the birth of Elizabeth in 1655 as a result of the illness of her other daughter, Naly. Naly 'fell into a desperate fit of convulsions ... her breath stoping & grew blackish in her face'. Alice ailed so dramatically in response that 'my Aunt & friends did imagine I could not liue', and they conspired not to tell her how sick Naly was in case that hastened her death. The family removed Naly's cradle away from Alice's room into the parlour to stop the infant's cries distressing Alice.[89] Again, a fortnight later, while breastfeeding her newborn, a maid cried out of the nursery that Naly was 'dead or diving'. The distress that it caused Alice meant that her mother forbid her breastfeeding any more and she was forced to dry her breasts.[90] In 1690,7 when William and Peregrina Chaytor's baby died from gripes in the belly when it was four days old, it made 'a deep impression upon a tender mother'. Some time after the death, she was still 'not yet in a Capasity' to return letters. Her husband wrote instead and in a draft letter wrote that a potential correspondent's 'sentiments of her sorrow will much contribute to her recover'.[91] Others did not always afford grieving mothers the same sympathy. Christopher Wandesford instructed his daughter Catherine Danby sharply to 'take care to comfort' her husband and 'not ad[d] to his loss by your over grieving' when her baby died in July 1634.[92] When Lady Ann Fanshawe's newborn died in 1645, it 'cost' her 'so dear that was ten weeks before' she could be left alone. Anne gave birth in February but it was May when she first left her 'chamber

87 James Yonge, 7 January 1681, *The Journal of James Yonge [1647–1721]: Plymouth Surgeon*, ed. F. N. L. Poynter (London: Longmans, 1963), 147.

88 Charles Trelawny to Sidney Godolphin, 7 November 1700, BL Add MS 28052, fol. 100.

89 Thornton, 'Meditations', 138. 90 *Ibid.*, 139.

91 William Chaytor to unknown, Draft letter to 'Honor[e]d Madam', September 1697, North Yorkshire Record Office, Northallerton, ZQH 9/12/55.

92 Christopher Wandesford to Katherine Danby, 20 July 1634, North Yorkshire Record Office, Northallerton, MISC 2087/1327.

and to church' at St John's College, Oxford. Even then, she was forced to sit and rest in the college gardens, 'being very weak'.[93] Again in 1657, after a difficult birth, ten weeks before she expected, Anne described how her father's illness complicated her own recovery. She was so ill 'I was like an anatomy' and 'I never stirred out of my bed in seven months, nor during that time ate flesh, or fish, or bread, but sack, posset drink, and pancake or eggs, or now and then a turnip or carrot.'[94] The link between grief and postpartum complications was so strong that when Mary Rich was lying-in after birth, her relatives concealed her father's death from her 'tell I was upe againe', so as not to jeopardise her health in her already vulnerable condition.[95]

The health of mothers and infants were intertwined in ways that meant restoration was unstable and quickly threatened, but at other times described as making women more resilient to other assaults. In February 1679, after a long labour and a succession of miscarriages and a stillbirth, Anne Archer gave birth to a son but her and her husband's 'joy' was instantly dampened by the infant's illness.[96] When the little boy died in July, his wife took a 'feaver and ague' through grief, and then his youngest daughter also became ill. His wife's condition started to mirror the daughter's. As the 'child grew worse', his wife grieved and it 'sett her back'.[97] When their youngest daughter died fourteen days later, Isaac reflected that rather than threatening his wife's health further, her pre-existing illness had prepared her for the 'loss'. Had she been well, the grief would have killed her.[98] In a similar vein, when Lady Anne Conway's two-year-old son Heneage died, Henry More tried to comfort her by saying the sickness and grief she was experiencing would 'conduce so much to the clearing of your body, as well as the above sayd method for the perfecting of your minde, that your health may prove much thereby bettered, and your life more comfortable than hitherto'. He compared her to a tree that once it was 'safe, it may blossom and beare fruit better than before', or in other words, she would be more fertile. Whether Anne felt the difficult pregnancy, arduous birth and then traumatic premature death was part of a restoration from illness or childbirth is less clear, although fertility looms large in More's assumptions about recovery.[99] A reply in November in which she apologised for not writing sooner,

93 Lady Anne Halkett, in John Loftis (ed.), *The Memoirs of Anne, Lady Halkett and Ann, Lady Fanshawe* (Oxford: Oxford University Press, 1979), 31–32.
94 *Ibid.*, 86.
95 Mary Rich, 'Some Specialities in the Life of M Warwicke', BL Add MS 27357, fol. 18.
96 Archer, February 1678/1679, 'Diary', 185–186. 97 *Ibid.*, July 1679, 188–189.
98 *Ibid.*, 14 August 1679, 191.
99 Henry More to Lady Anne Conway, 23 October 1660, Hutton and Nicolson, *The Conway Letters*, 69.

gestured to her 'desperate sickness' as well as 'a griefe proportionable to so great a losse' that she was not so well able 'to overcome'.[100]

Emotional distress or even madness was another affliction that women might suffer from after childbirth that was rarely represented as being particularly common after birth in childbearing guides. Despite this, it not only hampered recovery but could mean that women harmed themselves and their babies beyond possible repair. Mercy Fish of Bigglesworth consulted Napier a month after giving birth because she 'rageth sorely & talketh more idlely then before & waxeth worse & worse & will hardly be kept in her bed'.[101] She was as 'Sick as life will hold', could not sleep, and was hot and sweaty. Three weeks later, she still 'lyeth in' and was 'frentick', 'mad & distracted'.[102] Sibil Fisher was light-headed, 'settes her teeth' and 'one night did nothing but swear and curse'. She had to have her hands and feet bound because she was 'so strong that they cannot Deale with her'. She was 'well laid', despite a first unskillful midwife, but a week afterwards, accused her second midwife of being a witch.[103] Sibil never returned to herself. Fifteen years later, Napier simply called her 'Goody Fisher of Cocknoll lunatick'.[104]

Similarly, Mistress Kent of Beckley, a quarter of a year after she 'lay in in childbed', was tormented by her own thoughts, in this case visions of crimes she may have committed, like sleeping with her brother-in-law's son. Medical intervention, including blood-letting, had not helped.[105] Agnes Olny of Tebworth was 'hot in her body' and 'full of aches' as a result of a 'bad midwife' who had been too hasty and used an iron hook to deliver her baby when she saw Napier in 1600. Agnes was now incontinent.[106] Two years later, she was still not better but was 'worse and worse'. She was now a 'frentick woman', 'furious' and had 'no use of her wits'. Napier hoped that this 'sick little woman' would be 'freed from this distraction of mind and also be greatly and powerfully consoled, and with compassion and blessing'.[107] 'Ever uppon childbearing' Anne Syred had fallen 'into her mad fit tearing & breaking & burning things'. Napier noted in 1617, three years after she had given birth, that she 'defile herself', bit and scratched people.[108] At times, these torments could threaten the health of newborn babies both as a result of neglect or maternal violence. Mistress Mary Crowly, who had given birth three months previously, and had three other children, was unable to suckle because of a 'disquiet of the mind' and had 'No joy for anything.'[109] Alice Goodcheape became 'light headed' a week after giving birth, and the next day 'put her fingers into the child's mouth & tore it'. The next night, 'she smothered it with

[100] *Ibid.*, Anne Conway to Henry More, 28 November 1660, 180–181. [101] CASE66223.
[102] CASE66253, CB. [103] CASE15411, CB. [104] CASE49971, CB.
[105] CASE48121, CB. [106] CASE11071, CB. [107] CASE16959, CB.
[108] CASE44800, CB. See also: CASE23730, CASE23753, CB. [109] CASE35006, CB.

her hand'. The record in Forman and Napier's casebooks added that she was found guilty of infanticide. The practitioner prescribed her an unguent and a syrup.[110] Temperance Negoose wanted to drown herself in 1619 because of 'Grief touching' the death of her child, a month after giving birth.[111] Mistress Joan Plot consulted Richard Napier in 1629 because five weeks after birth she was 'mopish' and cared 'not for her husband nor child but goes into a corner to weep'. The cause was because she was still 'sorely tormented about her child that died a year since'.[112]

Childbirth could leave women 'out of frame' or 'order' for the rest of their lives. Anne Dormer, a Buckinghamshire woman who wrote over 50,000 words in letters to her younger sister (Elizabeth Trumbull or Katherine) between 1685 and 1691 about her unhappy marriage and consistently poor health, noted that her 'childing' had contributed to her difficulties. Anne described how she did not have 'great paines only a languishing kind of unaccountable illness which keepes me pale and leane'. She compared her body to a horse 'to tug through all I haue endured of illness and childing'.[113] She could not eat, had difficulty moving and was unable to sleep properly: 'if I get but one good [night of sleep] me thinks I am so well I can complain of nothing'.[114] Anne gestured to the torments of her husband, Robert, who teased and humiliated her regularly to explain her continual poor health. Childbirth played a role in her continuing poor health.[115]

Although sore or inflamed breasts hampered women's ability to return to their normal activities, it was represented by childbearing guides as largely ancillary to the larger process of recovery from childbirth. Pechey instructed women to leave swellings in the breast 'if no other Symptom attend them', as they were the cause of 'the over eagerness of the milky Ferment'.[116] Breast milk was understood as blood from pregnancy purified in the breasts, and therefore, it was perceived by medical writers as not needing to be excreted in the same way as lochia that was not concocted. But the diaries and letters of women indicated that sore breasts could be a major and painful condition that left them affected for months or even years after birth. Florence Smyth, for example, was 'still much tormented w[it]th payne under her breast, & be very weake' months after giving birth in 1637.[117] Likewise, Hannah Woodford, wife of Robert, continued to suffer with sore breasts for three months after

[110] CASE713441, CB. [111] CASE48556, CB. [112] CASE68796, CB.
[113] Anne Dormer to Elizabeth Trumbull (or Katherine), 9 August c. 1685, Add MS 72515, fol. 157v.
[114] Dormer to Trumbull, 10 September c. 1685–1691, fol. 167v.
[115] Leah Astbury, 'When a Woman Hates Her Husband: Love, Sex and Fruitful Marriages in Early Modern England', *Gender & History* 32, no. 3 (2020): 523–541.
[116] Pechey, *A General Treatises of the Diseases of Maids*, 175.
[117] Thomas Smithe to Thomas Smyth, 28 March 1637, Bristol Record Office, Bristol, AC/C 55/2.

birth. Shortly after the delivery of the Woodford's second child in 1637, Robert recorded in his diary 'Litle John sucks well blessed be the Lord and is mending thanks be to god.' His wife, however, was 'troubld with sore & tender breasts'. Over these months, Robert wrote almost daily in his diary about his wife's breasts and prayed to God 'heale them and make her a Joyfull mother'. Such problems, although not perceived as life-threatening, could persist and prevent the return to normal life, and even meant that Hannah had to be churched at home on 3 September 1637.[118] On 31 August, the family asked Mrs Rushworth, a friend and former servant, to suckle the child.[119] Despite sending 'Nurse Woodnot', presumably Hannah's nurse, away on 11 September, she continued to ail.[120] Finally, on 2 October, Robert recorded that the people caring for his wife predicted that her breasts would split or 'break' with inflammation. It is unclear whether these people were midwives, family friends, unlicensed healers, physicians or a mixture.[121] Robert continued to comment on the condition of Hannah's breasts throughout the year and on 10 December remarked that she was too unwell to attend church.[122] Clearly, the bodily changes brought about by pregnancy, birth and caring for a newborn could continue to condition women's lives long after their lying-in month was up.

Grace Wallington, Nehemiah's wife, similarly suffered from sore and inflamed breasts for a full six weeks after delivery. A month after birth, she was unable to suckle because of pain and hardness, and as a result they considered getting a 'norse into the country' because she was 'in such paine' that 'she coulde take no rest for many days and nights together and was in great paine for sixe weeks together'. Eventually, with the help of medicines, her breasts were 'healed'.[123] Recipe books are similarly littered with remedies for breast injuries like one for 'Soar nipples' in an anonymous commonplace book.[124] An anonymous recipe book compiled between 1675 and c.1800 included a recipe 'For sore or chapt nipples', taking a piece of chalk, shaping it like a nipple, dipping it in tar and then putting them onto the breasts after the child 'hath dun sucking'. A concoction with quince seeds boiled in plantain water could be added. Not only would it provide relief for new mothers but could be kept a 'good many years' and would do the infant's 'mouth good'.[125] Jackson included a remedy 'For the rankling of a womans brest by ouer much milke' that involved soaking a plaster in vinegar and laying 'it thereto', and

[118] Woodford, 3 September 1637, *The Diary of Robert Woodford*, 107.

[119] *Ibid.*, 31 August 1637 and 1 September 1637, 104. [120] *Ibid.*, 11 September 1637, 111.

[121] *Ibid.*, 2 October 1637, 120. [122] *Ibid.*, 10 December 1637, 150.

[123] December 1624; Wallington, *The Notebooks of Nehemiah Wallington*, 412.

[124] 'Commonplace book, ca. 1713–1740', Clark Library, UCLA, MS.1982.001, unfoliated.

[125] 'English Recipe Book, c.1675–c.1800', WL, MS 7721, 247.

another for a breast that was 'cankled'.[126] The Godfrey-Faussett family receipt book contained a 'Salve for a sore Breast' that involved clarifying mutton in a quarter pint of rape seed oil and white wine. A cloth dipped in the concoction was laid to the breast hot.[127] Elizabeth Egerton included a remedy 'for a sore breast' that demanded linseed be tempered with milk, unleavened white bread and butter and then laid to the breasts. Another 'For heate or swelling' asked for new laid eggs be broken and placed onto violet leaves before application.[128] Lady Brilliana Harley's recipe book also had a remedy for a sore breast and 'For heate or Swellinge in a womans breast'.[129] One remedy for sore breasts in an anonymous book recommended letting the child 'suck ye mother quickly after they are brought to bed', which would prevent the milk curdling.[130] This was in contrast to the unequivocal stance of childbearing guides that women ought to wait days or even weeks after birth to breastfeed and that the first milk should be drawn out. *Aristotle's Master-piece* was unusual in suggesting that this early milk might be 'drawn off' by the baby. Importantly, this was not the beginning of feeding but an initial purge.[131]

The disconnect between the concern hinted at by women in family paperwork and the dismissal of the seriousness of sore and inflamed breasts in printed medical literature carried over into the discussion of tears and prolapses too. Daniel Sennert explained that if not treated quickly, a prolapse would become 'hard' and difficult to remove but it was 'not deadly'. If it was present without a fever and convulsive fits, which would suggest the ailment was the result of humoral imbalance, it was '*only* it is troublesome and nasty'.[132] Sharp concurred, reinforcing that 'it is not mortal, though it be filthy and troublesome'. Recipes for 'pain', or in one instance, 'greevance' after childbirth in domestic collections are further evidence to suggest that these were more than simply troubling symptoms for women.[133] We see from the casebooks, however, that tears and fistulas could leave women incontinent for life, and was even explained as contributing to their madness. Injuries sustained in delivery could be life-changing and serve to torment women months and even years hence.

One cannot help but wonder about the myriad of ways that early modern women's bodies were altered by childbearing that did not affect their health in

126 Jackson, 'A very shorte and compendius Methode of Phisicke and Chirurgery', fols 60r and 102r.

127 'Receipt book, late 17th century–mid 18th century', WL, MS 7997, unfoliated.

128 Harley, 'Medical recipes', fol. 132. 129 *Ibid.*, 132.

130 'English Recipe Book, c.1675–c.1800', 176. 131 *Aristotle's Master-piece*, 159.

132 Daniel Sennert, *Practical Physick the Fourth Book Three Parts* (London, 1664), 51. My emphasis.

133 Jackson, 'A very shorte and compendius Methode of Phisicke and Chirurgery', fol. 83v. One remedy is for 'soreness of ye womb after child bed', 'English Recipe Book, 17th–18th', MS 7721, 220.

an externally measurable way. Jackson included a remedy for 'swelling in the feete after labour'.[134] In a letter to a correspondent known only as 'Pens', Margaret Hamilton imparted her experiential advice about how to make a protruding navel go back in. Her own 'was a letel so' a 'long tyme befor[e] I left of beiring of childrene' but she had never used anything to try and cure it. But she thought it could be cured soaking a plaster in castel soap, crushed capons and placed on to leather.[135] Childbearing guides too often contained recipes for ointments for the belly 'least it become wrinkled or deformed' but this was expressly not cosmetic but to strengthen it and help it to 'return to the old form'.[136] Sharp explained how women's 'bellies' would be 'plaighted, and full of wrinkles ever after' childbearing, but this might be altered by anointing the stomach with oil of sweet almonds, lillies, goat suet and sheep suet.[137] In the early modern period, anti-cosmetic tracts often warned that altering the body for aesthetic reasons was a crime against God.[138] Removing sagging skin or dropping breasts clearly fell under this latter category, whereas removing wrinkles in the belly to facilitate the ability for a woman to conceive again was a more acceptable intervention.

Reading against the grain in family paperwork reveals that elite individuals were very much aware of medical and religious expectations of recovery, and sought treatment and intervention when their bodies and minds did not behave in expected ways. Underlying much of the advice and the stories that women told about themselves, being able to conceive again promptly was a recurring signifier of recovery from childbirth. This imperative dovetailed with the emphasis on humoral imbalance as the cause of disease and ill health, causing the authors of childbearing guides, and sometimes medical professionals, to be not overly interested in whether women felt well a month after birth. Emotional distress compounded by grief and even madness could continue to define women's lives long after delivery. Breast problems might scar women permanently. Whilst Newton has called for a more positive turn in medical history, it also appears as crucial that we do not assume the idealised vision expressed by medical and religious authorities to map on to experience.[139] In unpicking the normative frameworks that underpinned prescriptive print, we can also start to be critical of individual and familial accounts of birth. Families fashioned narratives of recovery in ways that complied with

[134] *Ibid.*, fol. 102v.

[135] Unknown note, Papers of the Oglivy family, Earls of Seafield, National Records of Scotland, Edinburgh, GD248/566/84.

[136] *Every Woman Her Own Midwife,* 14

[137] Sharp, *The Midwives Book Or the Whole Art of Midwifry Discovered,* 312.

[138] Farah Karim-Cooper, *Cosmetics in Shakespearean and Renaissance Drama* (Edinburgh: Edinburgh University Press, 2006), 34.

[139] Newton, *Misery to Mirth*, 4.

these expectations. This is especially important to bear in mind given prescriptive accounts were framed in relation to redemptive and martyry understandings of sacrificial motherhood. Inconvenience or discomfort was part of the course of bearing and raising a child.

A Good Death

Nowhere is the desire to shape an appropriate and favourable birth story more apparent than in the work that families did to eulogise women who died in childbirth. In doing so, they created a 'lasting image' of their family member as chaste, silent and compliant.[140] This in turn redounded to the family's piety and orderliness. Thornton devoted several pages of her meditations to examining the conduct of her sister during her arduous and ultimately fatal birth in 1645. 'She had bin very ill a long time before her delivery, and much altered in the heate of her bodie being feavorish.' Her labour was long and she was 'exceedingly tormented with paines' so that she could not sleep or eat for two weeks. She eventually gave birth to a baby boy, named Francis (who died when he was several months old from smallpox). Her condition deteriorated after the birth and she and those around her became increasingly aware that her life was slipping away. She spent her time in 'discourse of goodnesse excellently pieous, godly and religious instructing her children and servants, preparing her soule for her deare Redeemer, as it was her saing she should not be long for Him [God]'. Neither was she concerned about the prospect of leaving her husband or children, such was her commitment to God. According to Thornton, she whispered 'Lord Jesus, receive my spirit' before taking her last breath. Accounts of deaths in childbirth like Danby's often emphasised the pain that these women endured with unfathomable forbearance whilst submitting wholly to God.[141]

When Frances Tufton Drax died in childbirth in 1665, her sister-in-law Elizabeth Tufton was asked to write a 'full' and detailed account of the labour and birth for Frances' sister, Cicely Hatton. Elizabeth promised to 'relate to you as many perticulars of it as I can'. On Monday, Frances sent for Elizabeth, one of her gossips, since she had 'had paines' over the weekend. 'Mis Baker', either a friend or maid, 'beleeued it was not her labor, and soe made nothing of it'. When Elizabeth arrived, she found Frances 'in greate paine' and at night 'her water broke'. When the midwife arrived, she decided that the 'Child came wrong'. Elizabeth had 'preuailed with' Frances' husband to get Dr Peters from Canterbury, who was 'very famous for his skill' in the house for the delivery,

[140] Lucinda M. Becker, *Death and the Early Modern Englishwoman* (London: Routledge, 2003), 177–199.
[141] Thornton, 'Meditations', 86–91.

but 'wee were desirous' to wait to call him until they were sure the infant's life could not be saved. We have heard in Chapter 4 how male surgeons and man-midwives were often associated with butchery and poor procreative outcomes in this period. Male surgeons were often called in if a labour was protracted to dismember the child and save the mother's life. The pains continued and the midwife, 'finding by some tokens that the Child was deade', asked Dr Peters to use his skill 'for it was past hers' to extract the baby. She noted that Frances was 'uery discouraged' and just hoped the doctor would inflict 'little paine'. While the doctor made 'use of his meanes', Elizabeth and others 'prayed either in the same roome, or the next to it all the while'. The procedure took hours and 'wee were forced to giue her Cordialls euery minuit'. Peters protested that he had tried 'all ye ways hee could imagine', and Frances, growing 'faint and light headed, begd of the Docter for Christs sake, to let her dye at rest'. Elizabeth and others took her to her bed where she suffered for three days before dying surrounded by the women invited to the birth, including Elizabeth, her husband and brother. Evocatively, Elizabeth describes the 'flood of those things that came from her', robbing her of her spirits and energy, and eventually life.

After she died, she was 'opened' and the baby found 'right at the birth', or in other words right at the mouth of the womb and ready to be born. Peters claimed that it was his hard work that had 'forced it to that place' and without his skill she would have died much sooner. On closer inspection, however, it appeared that 'her bones within especially her Back bone was soe bowed as he said it was impossible to make passage so much as for a limbe of the Child'. For Elizabeth, this was proof both of Frances' strength and forbearance through her torturous pains, and of Dr Peters lack of intuition. There are several telling moments that this description of labour was more than simply an account for a grieving sister but rather served a larger purpose within the family. Elizabeth apologised to Cecilia's pardon if the story was in any way 'imperfect'. Indeed, she noted she would have been very 'unwilling' to have been the first to set this 'malancholy story' down, indicating another family member had already written about the birth and death.[142] Birthing and dying in an exemplary fashion was important in being seen as a godly family.

Elizabeth's account of birth was unusual in its length and detail. It provides the historian a glimpse at all the hidden work that individuals did during labour that are regrettably impossible to recover because they were deemed largely

[142] Elizabeth Tufton to Cecily Hatton, November 1665, Northamptonshire Record Office, Northampton, MS FH 4412. Anne Clifford wrote about the death of Frances Drax, who was her granddaughter, in her diary too. See: Anne Clifford, 22 November 1665, *Anne Clifford's Autobiographical Writing, 1590–1676*, ed. Jessica L. Malay (Manchester: Manchester University Press, 2018), 140.

ancillary to the broader narratives about fruitful families. There was a constant stream of visitors coming in and out of the birthing chamber notably Frances' husband and her brother, as well as the women who over the course of days cheered her, gave her cordials and ministered to her. The negotiations and conflict between the midwife, Dr Peters, her gossips and family members reveal a birthing chamber that was busy, tense and constantly shifting, far from the dark, peaceful, warm and quiet environment that was supposedly ideal.

Sir John Clerk, the Scottish politician, lawyer and composer, was similarly concerned to write a detailed account of his wife's death in childbirth in 1700. In the account, Margaret had been unwell for more than a month when she went into labour at midnight on 20 December. He departed her side as husbands were not routinely present in the chamber for birth. Towards the morning, she 'felt her pains coming fast upon her' and requested John's father travel from Edinburgh to be in the house and pray for her since she was convinced that she was dying. Although those around her reassured her that she 'had not one bad symptom about her', John noted that it later became apparent that she had felt some of the 'symptoms, in child bearing' that her mother had had when she died in childbirth with Margaret. She gave birth a day later to a little boy, but when 'every body had run into my Room to carry me the good news, she fell into fainting Fits'. John himself was ill and incapacitated and was helped by the women attending Margaret and 'staggered into my dear Wife's Room' to make a 'last Visite'. Margaret told him that she was happy and hopeful to die. Other family members, including her brother and 'her Friends', came to visit and be with her. They called a doctor and two surgeons to assist her, but they were 'too hasty in their operations' and used too much force to extract the placenta, which meant she lost a lot of blood. A minister was called, and although she was told not to speak, 'expressed great fervency in prayer by her eyes and hands lifted up to heaven'. Although in the last hours of her life she screamed in agony, just before death, she turned in the bed and called on 'God to receive her soul'.[143] This wholly redemptive narrative cemented Margaret as one of the elect for posterity.

This tradition of creating accounts of death in childbirth was no doubt encouraged by the popular genre of printed legacies published by pregnant women anticipating their demise and seeking to instruct their children in godly conduct.[144] Elizabeth Jocelin died nine days after giving birth to a daughter,

143 John Clerk, *Memoirs of the Life of Sir John Clerk of Penicuik, Baronet*, ed. John M. Gray, vol. 13, Scottish Historical Society (Edinburgh: Edinburgh University Press, 1892), 39–42.

144 Teresa Feroli, '"Infelix Simulacrum": The Rewriting of Loss in Elizabeth Jocelin's *The Mother's Legacie*', *English Literary History* 61, no. 1 (1994): 89–102; Jennifer Louise Heller, *The Mother's Legacy in Early Modern England*, Women and Gender in the Early

Theodora, in October 1622. Her handwritten directions to her husband and children in the eventuality of her death were transcribed and published by the theologian Thomas Goad, as *The Mothers Legacie, to her Unborne Childe*, 1624.[145] Jocelin's preparations to meet her maker were so extensive and thorough that she even bought her own winding sheet when she felt the baby quicken many months before she delivered and actually died. Dorothy Leigh, a puritan woman from Cheshire, penned a similar text in 1616 titled *Mothers Blessing*. In it she professed to be 'trobled and wearied with feare, lest my children should not find the right way to heauen' and therefore sought to provide them with guidance in her absence.[146] In these texts, women never recovered from pregnancy and birth but they submitted to meeting God meekly. These stories of submission and sacrifice were additionally beneficial for the maintenance of familial authority and godliness within wider communities.

Whilst these women died expressly in labour and delivery, other women might perish days, weeks or even months after birth from related injuries and complications. The haberdasher and early demographer John Grant distinguished between deaths in childbirth and those within a month of delivery in his 1662 *Bills of Mortality*. He points to the complexity of the category of recovering when he explains that formerly 'Accompts' or accounts point to 3 in 200 women dying in 'Child-bed' a year, but that these statiticians were only considering those who passed away from the 'harndess of her Labour' and not those who had retained lochia and placenta and died within a month of birth.[147] Judging whether a woman has died from childbirth or from unrelated causes is something that bothers contemporary demographers too. B. M. Willmott Dobbie estimates that between 24.4 and 29.4 women died in childbirth per thousand baptisms between 1583 and 1758 in England, but reflects on the difficulty of 'for how long after childbirth may death of the mother be of consequence?'[148] Dobbie decides that any death before the baptism of the child counts as a maternal death because this was a reliable date that parish registers might provide. Most infants were baptised within a week or two of birth, suggesting this date is wholly inadequate even by early modern medical expectations that women would be incapacitated for a month after delivery.

Modern World (Farnham: Ashgate, 2011); Wendy Wall, 'Isabella Whitney and the Female Legacy', *English Literary History* 58, no. 1 (1991): 35–62.

145 Elizabeth Joscelin, *The Mothers Legacie, to Her Unborne Childe* (London: 1624).

146 Dorothy Leigh, *Mothers Blessing, or the Godly Counsel of a Gentlewoman Not Long Deceased Left Behind for Her Children* (Essex: 1616), sig. A2r–v.

147 John Graunt, *Natural and Political Observations Mentioned in a following Index, and Made upon the Bills of Mortality* (London: 1662).

148 B. M. Willmott Dobbie, 'An Attempt to Estimate the True Rate of Maternal Mortality, Sixteenth to Eighteenth Centuries', *Medical History* 26 (1982): 79–90.

More recently, Chris Galley and Alice Reid of the Cambridge Population Group have drawn on current World Health Organization guidelines that see any death while a woman is pregnant or within forty-two days of the end of pregnancy as a maternal death, but rely on burial and baptism records to estimate numbers.[149] Judith Lewis suggests six weeks as an appropriate time frame to expect the body to still be affected by birth, but draws attention to records of aristocratic women dying between 1603 and 1938 six to four years after delivery from causes clearly related to childbearing.[150] These demographic studies, however, do not access how and when women felt the experience of bearing babies was over. A death a year after delivery from madness brought about by a difficult labour and grief might have been considered very much a death related to generation.

Conclusion

The host of ways that childbirth changed the bodies and minds of women point to the difficulties of talking about complicated versus uncomplicated birth in early modern England or relying on the frameworks espoused in printed medical guides. Indeed, postpartum health has become a substantial focus in recent years, with some medical professionals calling for this period to be considered the 'fourth trimester'. More than half of pregnancy-related deaths occur at least seven days after delivery, and most of these deaths are attributed to what would now be considered preventable causes. This period is even more dangerous for people of colour in the United States and the UK.[151]

Early modern women expected to be incapacitated for a month after childbirth in which they would bleed steadily and eventually feel well before being churched. But this did not always match up with experience. Some women recovered far quicker, others languished for months and years after bearing children. This too was commented on in family correspondence. When Thomas Smyth wrote to Edward Phelips in 1641, he relayed that his wife, Florence, was so well a week after birth that they 'dispatch[ed] away her midwife'. This was cause for celebration and news he hoped that would 'setle my cousens mynde'. He thanked God for his wife's 'easy partinge with her fruit when tis ripe'. She had recovered so quickly he joked that he would be

[149] Chris Galley and Alice Reid, 'Sources and Methods: Maternal Mortality', *Local Population Studies* 93, no. 1 (2014): 68–78.

[150] Judith Lewis, "'Tis a Misfortune to Be a Great Ladie": Maternal Mortality in the British Aristocracy, 1558–1959', *Journal of British Studies* 37, no. 1 (1998): 26–53.

[151] Sara E. K. Phillips, Ann C. Celi, Alexandra Wehbe, Jasmine Kaduthodil and Chloe A. Zera, 'Mobilizing the Fourth Trimester to Improve Population Health: Interventions for Postpartum Transitions of Care', *American Journal of Obsetrics and Gynecology* 229, no. 1 (2023): 33–38.

'trying my skill for another boy'.[152] By 1641, it had become a running joke that Florence and Thomas were doomed to only ever produce girls. When Thomas Smith, another male relative, wrote to Smyth in 1637, he toyed 'if you hold one [on]' in his current efforts, 'you'll be able to people a whole country out of your daughters'.[153] Mary Hatton wrote to her brother Christopher in 1676 explaining that her 'sister comes so quick' that she would probably have another child within a year.[154] When women recovered within the expected time frames from delivery and got pregnant again, men and families took this as evidence of their own virility and ascendancy, in ways that reinforce that maternal effort was often subsumed within expectations of everyday domestic labour.

[152] Thomas Smyth to Edward Phelips, October 1641, Somerset Heritage Centre, Somerset, DD/PH/224133.
[153] Thomas Smithe to Thomas Smyth, 28 March 1637, Bristol Record Office, Bristol, AC/c54/5.
[154] Mary Hatton to Christopher Hatton, 1678, BL, Add MS 29571, fol. 341.

6 'Ordering' Infants

Jakob Rüff's *De conceptu et generatione hominis* (1554) contains a woodcut depicting a lying-in scene. The mother lies prostrate in bed, taking a bowl of pottage or caudle from a woman (a nurse, midwife or just one of the women attending the birth). Nearby, another woman holds the newborn and takes it out of or places it in a bathtub. In the foreground, a little girl holds a doll in her hand and rocks a cradle that is waiting to receive her new sibling. In the background, two women talk (Figure 6.1). This woodcut owes much stylistically to paintings of the birth of Christ. Although images of the nativity, perhaps owing to a post-Reformation move away from the Virgin Mary, did not appear regularly in English childbearing guides, the scene was a familiar one. Here, the other actors that helped to create and sustain middling and elite families that we often know so little about come into focus. And yet, whilst this laborious, intensive and repetitive work to ease infants into the world was set out in painful detail in childbearing guides, who these women were, what they felt and the toll that this care took on their social and bodily lives was largely uninteresting to artists and writers of the period alike. Family paperwork reveals that a great many women were brought into the household during this period after birth to care for infants, although yet again, specific details of the care they carried out is often left out of these accounts that preferred to believe it was mothers that would carry out the majority of this work.

Chapter 5 pointed to the ways that newly delivered mothers might not be ready to celebrate their recovery a month after childbirth. This was made all the more complicated by the care that newborns required. Childbearing guides of the period set out a regimen for babies similar in style and structure to adult texts of the same nature. In this period, after birth, the six non-naturals – air, exercise, sleeping, nourishment, excretion and the passions – were central in coaxing the baby from its watery life in the womb to the cradle and beyond. This was often called 'ordering' the infant, owing to the ways in which this care was expected to regulate and control babies' bodies. As Sandra Cavallo and Tessa Storey have noted, 'worrying about the air, fussing about a healthy way to get a good night's sleep, and judiciously regulating one's passions were prerequisites of the day-to-day management of the body' for those hoping to

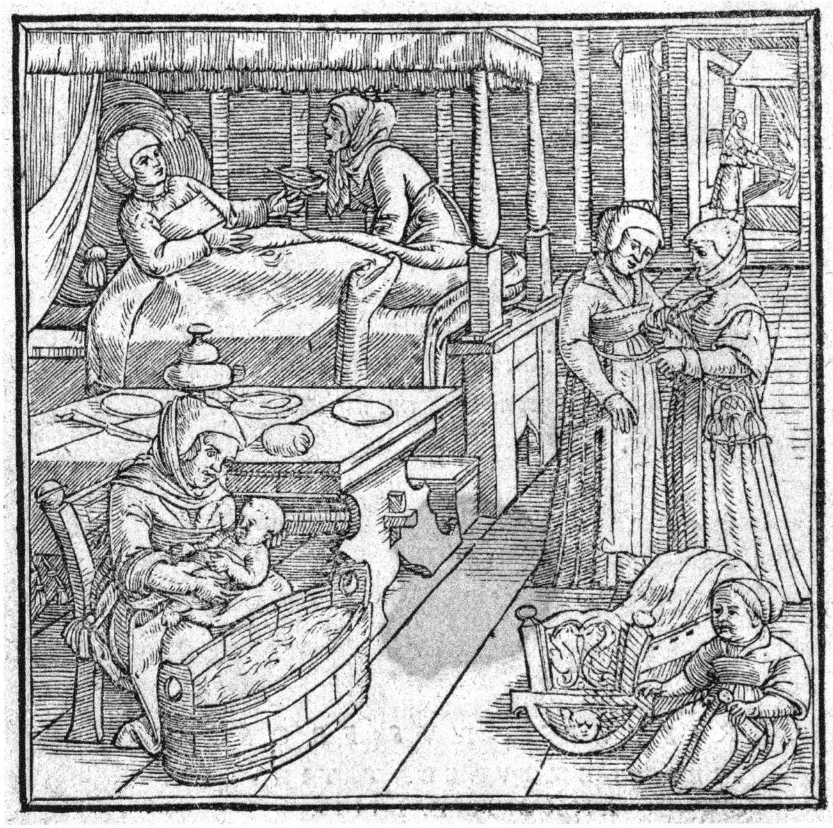

Figure 6.1 Jakob Rüff, *De conceptu et generatione hominis, et iis quae circa haec potissimum consyderantur libri sex* (Zurich: 1554). Wellcome Collection.

avoid disease in early modern Europe.[1] Newborns were no different. They had to cry, change colour, their navel cord had to be cut and their bodies searched for impediment. They were bathed, rubbed, moulded and clothed. They were rocked to sleep and, finally, they were fed. This process continued for months and years, albeit often by nurses and servants rather than family members, in a way that shows that birth and childbearing was an experience that conditioned and determined domestic life long after delivery.

[1] Sandra Cavallo and Tessa Storey, *Healthy Living in Late Renaissance Italy* (Oxford: Oxford University Press, 2013), 270. See also: Sandra Cavallo and Tessa Storey, eds., *Conserving Health in Early Modern Culture: Bodies and Environments in Italy and England* (Manchester: Manchester University Press, 2017).

It is often unclear, both in medical books and in family accounts, however, who did what care. Mothers, as we have read, were often incapacitated for days, weeks and months after delivery. Whilst childbearing guides and manuals on infant health provided extensive guidance on what was good for young children, there are few accounts of the mundane details of how people actually cared for newborns in family paperwork. Did families follow this advice? Could families follow this advice? Chapter 5 noted that families often lost interest in the details of generation once a child was born. This influenced the ways family members wrote, or did not write, about the work of ordering infants too. Although historians have argued that the time after birth was one of celebration, if childbearing guides are to be believed, this was a period of incredible industriousness. We know that babies were 'watched' to see if they thrived, but this chapter finds that looking and observing was only the beginning of the work involved after birth.[2] Examining family paperwork and employment records helps to uncover who these women were that dominate Rüff's postpartum scene.

In doing so, this chapter builds on the work of other historians who have proposed that the days, weeks and months after birth were not necessarily happy, restful and harmonious but potentially fractious, especially when new individuals were brought into the physical and emotional boundaries of the household to undertake care for mothers and babies. Historians of witchcraft, for example, have shown that many accusations happened in this period, and this may have been because employing nurses, midwives and others to undertake childcare, medical work and housework led to practical and emotional disruption. In this difficult time, it was easy to blame a servant or other newcomer for unfavourable outcomes like the illness or death of the mother, child or even animals. Relinquishing control over domestic duties could be a particularly powerful breeding ground for mistrust and suspicion.[3] For Lyndal Roper, witches became a 'kind of evil mother who harmed instead of nourishing her child' in new mothers' paranoid fantasies.[4] The elite families that created the paperwork examined in detail in this chapter were rarely involved

[2] Laura Gowing notes, for example, that the 'focus of the social ritual which surrounded new mothers shifted from pain and fear to thanksgiving and celebration'. During this time, the newborn was 'watched to see if it thrived'. Laura Gowing, *Common Bodies: Women, Touch and Power in Seventeenth-Century England* (New Haven, CT: Yale University Press, 2003), 172.

[3] Diane Purkiss, 'Women's Stories of Witchcraft in Early Modern England: The House, the Body, the Child', *Gender & History* 7, no. 3 (1995): 408–432.

[4] Lyndal Roper, 'Witchcraft and Fantasy in Early Modern Germany', in *Oedipus and the Devil: Witchcraft, Sexuality and Religion in Early Modern Europe* (London: Routledge, 1994), 207. Philippa Carter argues that the gendered pattern of witchcraft accusation and conviction is better explained by gendered patterns of work, leading to gendered distribution of risk in 'Work, Gender and Witchcraft in Early Modern England', *Gender & History* 37, no. 1 (2025): 91–108.

in witchcraft accusations (in making them or being blamed). Nor were they as common in England as elsewhere in Europe in the period. However, these findings point to the ambivalence that families felt about hiring help during a period of emotional and bodily vulnerability, and to the difficult and delicate work of restoring the health of newly delivered women and coaxing their newborns into the world. A theme of this book has been the ways in which certain aspects of procreation were meant to appear easy and effortless and to proceed in expected and normative ways that were understandable. For these elite families, the necessity of hiring midwives, nurses and wet nurses often conflicted with prevailing religious and medical prescriptions that mothers ought to take on this bodywork themselves. Maternal breastfeeding was often represented as the ultimate act of sacrificial motherhood. As discussed in Chapter 4, these individuals – their names, specific work and identities – were often only of note in family paperwork when there was a problem. It makes sense then that the practical details of who took on this care and how it was administered was often left out of family paperwork. Acknowledging this labour for what it was compromised the narrative that a family's fruitfulness had sprung from its own providential standing or from domestic orderliness. At the heart of this was an often-unquestioned belief that those lower down the social scale would prioritise the children of elite families often at the expense of their own.

The First Cry

Owing to their time in the womb in what the Scottish physician James McMath called 'the Slime of its Waters, or the Milky Liquor it swims in', newborn babies were excessively hot and wet.[5] So writers were concerned that infants had to shed this moisture as soon as possible and they focused on making sure the baby could excrete through tears, sweat and defecation. The baby's first cry was of the utmost importance. Crying was instrumental in securing survival but also could be useful to those in earshot to get a quick idea of the newborn's health. According to Welsh medical writer, John Jones, crying after birth communicated to others that the delivery had happened and the baby was alive. He noted that if the infant 'weep a little' at birth, 'then (as sayeth Avicen) it shal not be unwholesome, nor to many fathers irksome, but rather joyfull news', hinting at a shared and acknowledged soundscape of birth, difficult for historians to capture, but that might have been important in monitoring and

[5] James McMath, *The Expert Mid-wife a Treatise of the Diseases of Women with Child, and in Child-bed* (Edinburgh: 1694), 316.

understanding delivery for husbands, friends, family members and servants listening for groans, moans and cries.[6]

It was good news if the child's cries were 'loud and clear', the London physician John Pechey explained, because that signified that the baby had 'plenty of Spirits, and a strong breast'. If the cry was low or soft, 'it is a sign that the vital strength is small, and the Spirits few, and the Muscles of the Breast weak'.[7] Midwives were encouraged to stick their fingers into the throat and nose of babies to make sure they were clear of obstruction. Daniel Sennert, the German physician and alchemist, and Jane Sharp both noted that vigorous crying indicated the breast was strong.[8] Crying was understood by medical authors as a form of excretion. Timothy Bright in his 1586 *A Treatise of Melancholie*, for example, defined tears as the 'excrementitious humidity of the brayne, not contained in the vaynes'.[9] The compression of the brain forced moisture through the passages of the head and out of the tear ducts. In adults, blocked tear ducts were commonly treated with bloodletting, a medical treatment that assisted the expulsion of bad humours.[10] Crying emerges as an important way that babies shed the fluid or 'filth' they were surrounded in in pregnancy from their lungs, throats and noses, and fulfilled a crucial non-natural function of excreting.[11] This was particularly urgent in newborns because their brains were perceived as especially moist and had 'many excrements which Nature cannot send out its proper passages'.[12]

Another reason that crying was linked with vitality and viability in medical writers' eyes was because it showed that the baby had emotions that could be expressed. The English translation of Jacques Guillemeau's *Child-birth*

6 John Jones, *The Arte and Science of preseruing Bodie and Soule in al Health, Wisedome, and Catholike Religion Phisically, Philosophically, and Diuinely deuised* (London: 1579), 32.

7 John Pechey, *A General Treatise of the Diseases of Infants and Children Collected from the Best Practical Authors by John Pechey* (London: 1697), 2.

8 Daniel Sennert, *Practical Physick the Fourth Book Three Parts* (London: 1664), 229. Jane Sharp, contains exactly the same passage verbatim in Jane Sharp, *The Midwives Book Or the Whole Art of Midwifry Discovered*, ed. Elaine Hobby, Women Writers in English 1350–1850 (Oxford: Oxford University Press, 1999), 272.

9 Timothy Bright, *A Treatise of Melancholie Containing the Causes thereof, & reasons of the Strange Effects it Worketh in Our Minds and Bodies* (London: 1586), 144.

10 Johann Gottfried von Herder notably had blocked tear ducts that were treated by bloodletting. See: Frank W. Stahnish, 'The Tertium Comparationis of the Elementa Physiologiae: Johann Gottfriend von Herder's Conception of "Tears" as Mediators between the Sublime and the Actual Bodily Physiology', in *Blood, Sweat and Tears: The Changing Concepts of Physiology from Antiquity into Early Modern Europe*, ed. Manfred Hortsmanhoff, Helen King and Claus Zittel, Intersections: Interdisciplinary Studies in Early Modern Culture 25 (Leiden: Brill, 2012), 595–625.

11 Marion A. Wells, '"Full of Rapture": Maternal Vocality and Melancholy in Webster's Duchess of Malfi', in *Blood, Sweat, and Tears*, 685–713.

12 Nicholas Culpeper, *A Directory for Midwives, or, A Guide for Women* (London: 1662), 246–247.

described how babies cried out of 'necessity' and 'his owne feeling' and to 'shew, in what need he stands in helpe' forcing or 'wring[ing] from him cries and moanes'.[13] Babies cried to communicate a specific need that ought to be met, rather than out of preoccupation or boredom. A 'Prudent Mother or Nurse' would 'endeavour to find out what is the cause [of the crying] that being removed, the Child may be at quiet' – presumably a neglectful one would ignore or dismiss such motions.[14] Robert Barret recommended comforting children by ensuring it was 'clean and dry' and removing anything that was frightening or grieving it.[15] In such instructions, good mothering is represented as begetting good (and importantly settled) babies. Rather than acknowledging the expertise of mothers, nurses or midwives in knowing why a baby was crying and rectifying it, medical writers make a settled baby the bare minimum of good motherhood. Early modern English medical texts equated effort – running through different acts of care tirelessly to still the child – with positive procreative outcomes, all the while effacing the specificity of this care and the individuals that had to take it on. It was women, but often those not related, the midwife, nurse, wet nurse or servants that did this work.

Families often expressed great relief when newborns cried enthusiastically. A letter from Anne, Countess of Arundel, to her daughter, Mary Talbot in 1689, described how her three-day-old grandson was a 'most ernest crier', a promising portent despite the fact that he had refused to breastfeed.[16] In Sarah Stone's printed observations of her midwifery practice, crying was represented as being one of the earliest signs of infant survival and health. She described how sometimes man-midwives were so hasty in trying to extract infants that had become stuck in delivery that they failed to recognise the baby was still alive. The infants were 'debrained' only to be born 'crying, with their Brains working out of their head', a disturbing image that, for Stone, reinforced these male pretenders' lack of obstetrical intuition and tragic loss of life.[17] In cheap print about bad mothers, crying was similarly a literary trope that drove home the innocence, vulnerability and viability of babies as victims of infanticide. In the 1670 pamphlet *The Cruel Mother*, Mary Cook murdered her own infant.

[13] Jacques Guillemeau, *Child-birth or, The Happy Deliverie of Women Wherein is set downe the government of Women* (London: 1612), 1.

[14] Pechey, *A General Treatise of the Diseases of Infants and Children*, 7.

[15] Robert Barret, *A Companion for Midwives, Child-bearing Women, and Nurses Directing them how to Perform their Respective Offices: Together with an Essay, Endeavouring to Shew the Influence of Moral Abuses upon the Health of Children* (London: 1699), 81.

[16] Anne, countess of Arundel, to Mary Talbot, 21 August 1689, Lambeth Palace Library, London, MS 3205, fol. 143.

[17] Sarah Stone, *A Complete Practice of Midwifery. Consisting of Upwards of Forty Cases or Observations in that valuable Art, selected from many Others, in the Course of a very Extensive Practice*, Obs. XIII, (London: 1737), 39.

As she lifted it from the cradle, it gave a 'shrieke' and tried to see 'from whom the fatal bloody stroke came' before she cut its throat.[18] The 1610 pamphlet *The Bloudy Mother* detailed how Jane Hattersley tried to make away with her secret illegitimate child under her apron when her baby started crying to 'tell his preseruers' Good-man King and his wife, 'that she told a wicked and villainous untruth' and thereby saving its own life.[19]

Although in these examples crying was an obvious signal to others that the baby was healthy, medical texts warned that excessive or protracted crying could indicate that the baby was ailing. This was because the effort of sobbing was thought to be able to warp and distort the wax-like bones of newborns. Barret, the English physician and author of the 1669 *A Companion for Midwives* addressed nurses directly and noted that 'above all' other concerns, she should 'be very careful not to suffer the Child to cry too much' because the navel-string might fall off too soon.[20] Crying could also cause rupture. The author of *Paidon Nosemata* (1664) identified the 'External Causes' of 'Rupture and Broken Belly' as 'vehement motion, extraordinary Crying, holding of the Breath' along with 'abundance of Wind, and a Strong Endevour of disburthening the Belly'. [21]

Notably, rupture as brought on by crying in babies frequently appears in domestic recipe books as a condition requiring remedy. The book of Elizabeth Okeover compiled between c. 1675 an 1725 listed five remedies for convulsive fits, three for troubled or fretful young children and two for rupture in the belly.[22] The Jerningham family book, compiled in the late seventeenth century, contained a remedy for 'Burstness or any Rupture' that promised to cure a 'broken belled [bellied] child' with a plaster and drink that was made with 'the Common beere hee drinks'.[23] Added to this, parents of infants frequently sought the assistance of astrologer-physicians Simon Forman and Richard Napier for excessive crying, convulsions, being 'burst' or having ruptures. William Mallins sought Napier's advice in 1600 for his seventeen-week-old

[18] *The Cruel Mother; being a true relation of the bloody murther committed by M. Cook, upon her dearly beloved child* (London: 1670), sig. A3r.

[19] T. B., *The Bloudy Mother, Or, The Most Inhumane Murthers, Committed by Jane Hattersley vpon divers infants, the issue of her owne bodie & the priuate burying of them in an orchard with her arraignment and execution* (1610), sig. A3v.

[20] Barret, *A Companion for Midwives*, 80–81.

[21] J. S., *Paidon Nosemata. Or, Childrens Diseases, Both Outward and Inward. From the time of their Birth to Fourteen Years of Age. With their Natures, Causes, Signs, Presages and Cures* (London: 1664), 31.

[22] Elizabeth Okeover and others receipt book, WL, MS3712. Convulsive fits: 119, 203, 210, 212, 213; troubled or fretful children: 142, 142, 157; rupture in the belly: 91, 198. This recipe book has been discussed in more detail: Richard Aspin, 'Illustrations from the Wellcome Library: Who Was Elizabeth Okeover?', *Medical History* 44, no. 4 (2000): 531–540.

[23] 'Jerningham family recipe book, late seventeenth-century', Staffordshire Record Office, Stafford, D641/3/H/3/1, fol. 42.

son, Thomas, who 'skremes skriketh & cryeth [tha]t they cannot still him'.[24] Charity Caldam consulted Forman in 1597, three months after the birth of her child, because it cried too much.[25] Six-month-old William Perry was taken to Napier in 1600 because he 'shriketh & starteth'.[26] Thomas Brownsoll, nineteen weeks old, from Bedford similarly 'cryes and grones'. His parents suspected he had been 'beworded' or bewitched.[27] Mary King brought her 23-week-old to Napier in 1625 because of convulsions and because he was black in the face.[28] Eleven-week-old Harry Shefherd was taken to Napier in 1601 because he was 'burst in the bowels'.[29] While Anne, countess of Arundel, had initially interpreted the newborn's crying as a promising sign of his wellbeing, she wrote again to Mary a month after the baby was born explaining 'I hoped at the first he would haue left it' or ceased crying so much by now. Instead, as 'he growth', the crying fits were getting longer. He began to 'look black' and once or twice in the throes of these 'extreme fitts', the infant's 'Navell hath bled'.[30] The child's 'extremety of crying' disturbed his grandmother so much that she vowed she would not 'willingly be in the house again wher a poore child shall be so long deferred from christening in such a case'.[31] Alice Thornton's two-year-old daughter Naly fell into a fit of convulsions in 1655 just after Alice had given birth to Naly's younger sister, Elizabeth. When she cried, she was described as turning 'blackish in her face'.[32] As with many aspects of regimen and the maintenance of health in early modern English medical texts, there was a delicate balance to be met between the non-naturals. By crying too much, babies were both over exerting and over excreting.

A good substitute for excretion could be found in the administering of gentle purges. The 1656 edition of *The Compleat Midwifes Practice* suggested offering newborns wine because it 'cuts the flegm which the Child has in its throat' and the 'spirit of the Wine rising up to the head, comforts and strengthens it'. This could prevent epilepsy in infancy too.[33] The recipe book of Lady Sandys, wife of Sir Edwin, the Jacobean statesman and treasurer of the Virginia Company 1619–1620, contained a programme of care 'whilst the childe is anoynted'. Boiled aniseed, raisins, liverwort and hartstongue, strained, could be given to the baby in the morning and afternoon at 4 pm and again at night sweetened with brown sugar. The 'child then being purged' ought to have its blood let from the ears, be left to fast and then only given small amounts of sustenance. 'All these directions must be constantly used for

[24] CASE13003, CB. [25] CASE2837, CB. [26] CASE 13031, CB. [27] CASE15176, CB.
[28] CASE59664, CB. [29] CASE19275, CB.
[30] Anne, countess of Arundel, to Mary Talbot, 11 September 1608, Lambeth Palace Library, London, MS 3205, fol. 145.
[31] *Ibid.* [32] Alice Thornton, BL, Add MS 88897/1, 138.
[33] T. C., I. D., M. S. and T. B., *The Compleat Midwifes Practice, In the most weighty and high Concernments of the Birth of Man* (London: 1656), 98.

2 or 3 months, if any Good by expected.' Bloodletting from the ears ought to be continued till 'it be 11 or 12 days ould and not after'. The recipe was 'Probatum est' or 'It has been proven.'[34] Honey or sugar in water was a common concoction given to newborns, a practice that persisted into the eighteenth century; Stone recorded in her *Observations* that she gave an infant 'warm water and sugar'.[35]

What remains unclear in the advice about getting babies to cry and purging them in childbearing guides was who might do this care. Barret imagined immediately after birth that it would be a 'good Mother' who would hold the baby in her lap and keep it warm 'whilst the Midwife is busied in taking care of the Woman'. Then the midwife would turn her attention to tending to 'the Child'.[36] Sharp assumed it would be the midwife who would immediately 'handle' the baby and therefore ensure the baby's throat was clear. She ought to 'Take notice of all the parts of it and see all be right' immediately after birth. This was crucial for directing the baby's regimen as impediments or weaknesses could be remedied if understood. But in this same section, when discussing the child at seven months, she generically addresses the person who will wash the baby twice a week as 'you'. When it is seven, someone should simply 'give' the child 'nourishing meats and an indifferent plentiful diet to make it grow'. Not once did she intrude into the regiment to specify who might do what, nor does she clarify who 'you' might be.[37] Sometimes, as we have heard in previous chapters, childbearing guides were written explicitly for mothers. But it is never clear that this care could not be done vicariously by others directed by the mother and mistress of the house. Rüff's lying-in scene with the newly delivered woman lying-in bed observing the activity around her becomes especially relevant if we imagine a newly delivered woman watching, assessing and instructing others to carry out the tasks of holding, turning, searching, washing, clothing and feeding the baby. The relative invisibility of this care fits with the broader story of this book that women's procreative labour was taken for granted and subsumed within expectations of everyday domestic maintenance even if it was often extraordinarily demanding or taxing.

Turning, Cutting and Searching

The next stage set out by medical authors after crying was observing that the newborn changed colour. Newly delivered, babies were expected to be greyish

34 'Lady Sandys her receipts', Firestone Library, University of Princeton, RTC01, no. 208, fol. 14r–v.
35 Stone, *A Complete Practice of Midwifery*, Obs. XVI, 52.
36 Barret, *A Companion for Midwives*, 13.
37 Sharp, *The Midwives Book Or the Whole Art of Midwifry Discovered*, 271–274.

or white, but as soon as they cried, they ought to turn pink, the authors of childbearing guides stressed. This showed that the baby was making a transition to life outside the womb. Changing colour was perceived as portentous not just for its health but also future character. 'Children that look white and pale when they are born, are weak and sickly, and seldome live long', Sharp noted. If, however, the infant was 'a reddish colour all over the body, when it is first born, and this colour *change by degrees* to a Rose colour, there is no doubt of the child but it may do well'.[38] As with the interest in bodily signs during pregnancy, this regimen suggested that families could find clues in the way the baby responded or behaved in the earliest minutes and hours of life that would reveal whether or not it would live not just a healthy and long life, but a generally good one. Like big bellies or the movements of unborn children, this was yet another detail that could be knitted into the narratives that families told about themselves and their fruitfulness. Those in the birthing room, and possibly outside, could see the transformation from womb to cradle happening in front of their eyes. Pechey stated one must 'mind what is the colour of the new-born Infant' – ideally it would be 'reddish all over the body, for that by degrees turns daily florid' (ruddy or rosy).[39] It was this gradual shift that was an important indicator of future health and wellbeing. If a baby was precociously florid, it was the same as if it had been white; it would not live long, or would mature to be 'of an ill temperament, Cold, Dull'.[40] Medical writers effortlessly intertwined instructions that seemingly had specificity to the newborn period and immediate survival with broader and intangible assessments of the baby's, and by extension family's, future.

Watching the baby's skin tone dovetailed with the general instruction that those present at the birth ought to be attentive to 'searching' the infant's body. '[S]earch whether any thing be amiss in any part that it may be rectified as much as may be', Pechey instructed.[41] At the centre of this advice was both a desire to note and plan for bodily impediment and encourage excretion from certain orifices (the mouth, fundament and genitals) and close others (the navel cord) to regulate the flow of humours. Someone should bend and extend the child's legs to look at the way they moved. One of the problems that might be revealed by searching, was whether the baby was tongue-tied, and writers suggested remedying this immediately if it was discovered. If it was not done soon enough, it might hinder speech Sharp warned.[42] Not all parents clearly followed this

[38] *Ibid.*, 271–272. Author's emphasis.
[39] Pechey, *A General Treatise of the Diseases of Infants and Children*, 1. [40] *Ibid.*, 1.
[41] *Ibid.*, 2. [42] Sharp, *The Midwives Book Or the Whole Art of Midwifry Discovered*, 275.

schedule. John Woodford, son of the Northamptonshire lawyer, Robert, had his tongue cut by 'Mrs davison' a full two months after birth.[43]

After the baby's body had been searched thoroughly, medical writers insisted that the 'navel string' should be cut. Many texts warned about the dangers of pushing corrupted blood from the cord back into the baby's body. François Mauriceau noted 'tis a very bad custome some Midwives have, before they make the Knot, they drive all the blood out of the String into the Infants Belly, believing that by this means they fetch it to it self, and strengthen it when it is weak'. Once cooled, this blood 'quickly loses its spirits, and is half coagulated in the infants', and pushing it back would 'cause very great Accidents'.[44] Parents, nurses, midwives or servants should also look at the baby's 'fundament' or anus, to ensure the child could excrete properly. If it was found to be absent or obstructed, writers similarly recommended the baby be operated on. The East Riding gentlewoman Lady Margaret Hoby, who attended to her neighbours' ailments and births, was persuaded to operate on a newborn in 1601 who was born without a fundament to try and locate one. Tragically, it did not survive the intervention.[45]

The shape of newborns' heads might also reveal much about their future lives. John Jones provided a two-page guide on how to interpret the facial features and dimensions of the infant. Studying the head might reveal whether the child had 'dwarfism', 'pigmeis' or 'giantism'. Jones described how one's hands might be placed across the breastbone and head; between the breast and top of the legs and from the legs to the toes, measuring to pinpoint abnormalities. In summary, the 'lengthe of euerye one of iuste proportion is the bredth his armes stretched abroade between the two formost fingers endes'.[46] Jones argued through such measurements 'you may knowe the heauenlye Idea of best nature, shape, and temperature', for there was a connection between the 'forme of the body' and the mind, drawing on the much older tradition of physiognomy.[47] Jones criticised 'curious and daintie dames' who used devices

[43] Robert Woodford, 11 October 1637, *The Diary of Robert Woodford, 1637–1641*, ed. John Fielding (Cambridge: Cambridge University Press, 2012), 124.

[44] François Mauriceau, *The Accomplisht Midwife, Treating of The Diseases of Women with Child, and in Child-bed* (London: 1673), 355.

[45] Margaret Hoby, *Diary of Lady Margaret Hoby 1599–1605*, ed. Dorothy Meads (London: Routledge, 1930), 184. For a discussion of Margaret Hoby's medical activities, see: Effie Botonaki, 'Dissecting Bodies and Selves in the Early Modern Period', in *Flesh Made Text Flesh: Cultural and Theoretical Returns to the Body*, ed. Zoe Detsi-Diamanti, Katerina Kitsi-Mitakou and Effie Yiannopoulou (New York: Lang Publishing, 2007), 75–86; Lucinda McCray Beier, *Sufferers and Healers: The Experience of Illness in Seventeenth-Century England* (London: Routledge & Kegan Paul, 1987), 219–220.

[46] Jones, *The Arte and Science*, 31–34.

[47] *Ibid.*, 31–34; Silvia de Renzi, 'Resemblance, Paternity, and Imagination in Early Modern Courts', in *Heredity Produced: At the Crossroads of Biology, Politics, and Culture, 1500–1870* (Cambridge, MA: MIT Press, 2007), 61–82; Gabriella Zuccolin, 'The Speculum

to shape their 'babes bodies' away from their 'rounde and handsome' nature to be more 'slender'. Whilst he is unbothered about praising the activities of the women who carefully measured infant's heads and bodies (they are simply 'you') he is quick to condemn fashionable mothers who seek to manipulate their baby's bodies. Having a child was a 'healthy, seemely, and comelye' body was clearly something that elite women hoped for as it reflected on their parents' moral character and credit. But to obtain this through unnatural means was represented as distinctly ungodly. The message in childbearing guides seems contradictory in that mothers ought to do anything to ensure the health and wellbeing of their infants on the one hand but not do anything that might contravene divine will. This is similar to the way in which childbearing guides often warned midwives and parents against trying to ensure their sons had large penises by cutting the navel cord far from the body. This kind of intervention was morally wrong. Medical writers consistently made this move – naming and shaming a particular kind of mother, nurse or midwife for poor practice, while effacing the individual delivering what was perceived to be 'good' care.

The appearance and health of the infant body was also central to ascertaining the moral character of unmarried women accused of murdering their own children, albeit in very different ways. In such cases, it helped women prove their innocence if the body of their infant was small and unhealthy. Whether or not an infant was 'full term' was important in infanticide trials as it helped to work out whether it was possible that the woman in question had not killed it but suffered from a miscarriage or stillbirth. Medical evidence became increasingly important in legal settings in the eighteenth century, particularly in the Northern Circuit courts in England, but in the seventeenth century, infant bodies were not formal a source of evidence. Courts often, however, noted this information alongside other kinds of testimony about whether women had acknowledged their pregnancies or given birth alone.[48] When an unnamed woman was tried at the Old Bailey for 'making away her Bastard-childe', she was acquitted because 'upon hearing the Evidence, and examination both of the Midwife and Coroner, it appeared tobe [sic] onely a Miscarriage'. The midwife judged 'that she had not gone above sixteen weeks, and had never been quick, the abortive Infant being not above eight inches long, and no symptoms of Wounds or Bruises' could be found.[49] A similar case was

Phisionomie by Michele Savonarola', in *Universality of Reason, Plurality of Philosophies* (16–22 September 2007, Palermo, Italy), available through Open Research Online, https://oro.open.ac.uk/, last accessed 27/03/2025.

48 Mark Jackson, 'Suspicious Infant Deaths: The Statute of 1624 and Medical Evidence at Coroners' Inquests', in *Legal Medicine in History*, ed. Michael Clark and Catherine Crawford (Cambridge: Cambridge University Press, 1994), 64–89.

49 Killing; infanticide, 13 December 1676, The Proceedings of the Old Bailey, www.oldbaileyonline.org/record/t16761213-1?text=t16761213-1, last accessed 27/3/2025.

described in the 1651 lengthy and detailed pamphlet Newes from the Dead about Anne Greene, a twenty-two-year-old Oxfordshire woman accused of killing her newborn. Greene was tried and hanged for the crime before being revived by physicians in Oxford a day after her attempted execution. The author, Richard Watkins, noted that the baby was 'very unperfect, being not above a span in length, and the sexe hardly to be distinguished: so that rather seemed a lump of flesh, then a well and duly formed Infant', making it likely it had never lived.[50] It did not have any hair on its head either and the midwife testified that she 'did not believe that ever it had life'. Despite the midwives' testimony, she was found guilty of infanticide. The body of the infant, which was described as 'nothing but [a] lump of the same matter [menstrual blood] coagulated', was used in conjunction with Anne's own testimony (her claim that she had resumed menstruating a month before the child 'fell from her unawares')[51] to adjudicate her case.

Although the experiences of women like Anne Greene and the married women who bought and read childbearing guides could not be more different in many ways, they were both made to feel as if their baby's body was living proof of their own moral character when something was amiss. Medical texts and court cases shared an understanding of what a healthy infant would look like. It would be big, have lots of hair, lack deformity and would be 'duly formed'. It is unclear from these guides who searched babies. Medical authors were not in the practice of rewarding and valuing the medical work that women took on in procreation.

Bathing

As the lying-in scene in Rüff's book suggests, bathing babies immediately after birth was an important part of the work of 'ordering' infants. Bathing was

[50] Richard Watkins, *Newes from the Dead. Or A True and Exact Narration of the miraculous deliverance of Anne Greene* (Oxford, 1651), 6–7. This case has been discussed numerous times in scholarship. Anne Greene was hanged for infanticide but miraculously she survived and was granted pardon. Bent Juel-Jenses, 'News from the Dead: The Remarkable Story of Anne Greene', *Oxford Medical School Gazette* 14 (1962): 135–140; Scott Mandelbrote, 'William Petty and Anne Greene: Medical and Political Reform in Commonwealth Oxford', in *The Practice of Reform in Health, Medicine and Science, 1500–2000*, ed. Margaret Pelling and Scott Mandelbrote (Aldershot: Ashgate, 2005), 125–151; J. Trevor Hughes, 'Miraculous Deliverance of Anne Greene: An Oxford Case of Resuscitation in the Seventeenth Century', *British Medical Journal* 285 (1982): 556. There have also been two novels: Douglas Angus, *The Green and Burning* (London: Robert Hale, 1958) and Iain Pears, *An Instance of the Fingerpost* (London: Jonathan Cape, 1997).

[51] Laura Gowing has argued that the discourse of painless and quick births was an important strategy by unmarried women who were accused of committing infanticide to argue that their infant had not been fully formed or a stillbirth, Laura Gowing, 'Secret Births and Infanticide in Seventeenth-Century England', *Past & Present* 156 (1997): 87–115.

a tool that could be used to remedy 'such indispositions which he [the infant] sometimes brings into the world', Guillemeau described.[52] These were presumably the same impediments that had been identified while searching. Jones described how washing newborns in warm water would help them 'unto growsomenesse, largenesse, and talnesse'. The ideal mixture was made of one part 'new' cow milk and ten parts lukewarm water.[53] Other writers like Sharp, Nicholas Culpeper and Sennert advised washing the infant in warm wine to heat the body to help concoction and excretion.[54] Pechey demanded that newborn children 'be washed every day' and from the third to the seventh month twice a week. Once it was weaned, this was much less frequent.[55] He condemned the older practice of sprinkling babies with salt to make their skin 'more dense and solid' because this caused itching and other problems. Wine was a more appropriate substitute.[56] The water *had* to be warm, not cold. Jones recorded the tragic mistake of some priests that had plunged newborns too vigorously to the 'bottome of the font'. They did not know 'that all sodayne mutations be most daungerous'. He explained that 'if the naturall heate within, shoulde be ovwercome of the outward colde, the living creature must needes perishe, when as of the immoderate use of Elements death ensueth'.[57] Pechey too warned against the dangers of bathing infants in cold water. The 'barbarous people' of Germany dipped the 'warm Infant from the Womb in the next Brook' to make it 'more strong and lusty' so as to 'design' it for conflict. '[N]one but strong Children would survive such a dipping.'[58] Once again, medical writers drew distinctions between medical interventions that were seen as ungodly either through vanity or contravening divine will, and those that were simply part of good motherhood and household management.

In regimens for adults, bathing was a substitute for exercise that was prominent in adult regimens to help digestion. Babies ought not move too much lest their bones warp and bend. This was the key reason they were swaddled, as we shall learn in the next section. The 'frictions' of bathing, Pechey explained, 'help Concoction, and the distribution of nourishment' in newborns.[59] Likewise, the 1662 edition of *Directory for Midwives* explained that 'a cold and dry distemper of the guts from birth' caused a 'slimy flegm that wraps the dung', this is remedied by washing the child 'often'.[60] Alongside the purge that was administered after birth to 'carry off the stomach an bowels' of the 'filth Collected in the Womb', bathing was associated with keeping the

[52] Mauriceau, *The Accomplisht Midwife*, 353. [53] Jones, *The Arte and Science*, 32.
[54] Culpeper, *Directory for Midwives* (1662), 229; Sennert, *Practical Physick*, 229; Sharp, *The Midwives Book Or the Whole Art of Midwifry Discovered*, 372.
[55] Pechey, *A General Treatise of the Diseases of Infants and Children*, 9. [56] *Ibid.*, 3.
[57] Jones, *The Arte and Science*, 36.
[58] Pechey, *A General Treatise of the Diseases of Infants and Children*, 4. [59] *Ibid*. 5.
[60] Culpeper, *A Directory for Midwives* (1662), 152.

body 'open' and preventing cositiveness. Being 'bound' or constipated was bad for everyone, including adults, but it was particularly dangerous for infants. Bathing was a common 'cure' for this. Pechey prescribed it for children who were suffering from looseness, constipation, worms, the protrusion of the navel, 'falling of the Fundament', stones in the bladder, retention of urine, incontinence, chafing of the hips and wasting.[61] Babies were washed far more frequently than adults owing to their moisture. Generally, adults bathed yearly or every several months, except where it was prescribed as a cure for illness. Bathing was also prescribed as a cure for adults to remedy excessive heat or moisture.[62] How often people washed and bathed in early modern England is hard to calculate, but it was closer to yearly than weekly or monthly, except where it was prescribed as a cure for illness.[63]

In addition to frequent baths, infants also needed to be 'shifted' often, meaning they were unswaddled, the clouts that served as a kind of nappy removed and changed, and the 'piss and dung' cleaned, before being dressed again. Guillemeau described how 'the nurse or some other' ought to make sure there were no draughts and 'sit neere the fire, laying out her legges at length, hauing a soft pillow in her lap'. She should have 'something about her' to keep the wind from the infant, and when 'thus accommodated, she shall vnswatch and shift him drie'.[64] For Guillemeau, this should be done once in the morning, once at midday and once in the evening, with a further change recommended at midnight. If the infant was 'verie foule, she may wash him with a little water and wine luke warm' using a sponge or linen cloth.[65] Pechey's outline of the common illnesses that afflicted infants described how 'chafing in the Hips' was normally the result of the 'clouts' not being changed often enough. A powder of 'Litharge of Silver, Seeds and Leaves of Roses, burnt Allum and Frankincense' might relieve some of the symptoms.[66]

61 Pechey, *A General Treatise of the Diseases of Infants and Children*, 112, 114, 127, 133, 138, 141, 144, 146, 147–148, 159.

62 Fabiola I. W. M. van Dam, 'Permeable Boundaries: Bodies, Bathing and Fluxes: 1135–1333', in *Medicine and Space: Body, Surroundings and Borders in Antiquity and the Middle Ages*, ed. Patricia A. Baker, Han Nijdam and Karine van't Land (Leiden: Brill, 2007), 117–149.

63 Lawrence Stone notes that 'Men and women [in this period] rarely, if ever, washed their bodies, and they lived in the constant sight and smell of human faeces and human urine'; Lawrence Stone, *The Family, Sex and Marriage in England 1500–1800* (London: Weidenfeld & Nicolson, 1977), 159. Keith Thomas suggests bathing was more regular than Stone allowed in Keith Thomas, 'Cleanliness and Godliness in Early Modern England', in *Religion, Culture and Society in Early Modern Britain: Essays in Honour of Patrick Collinson*, ed. Anthony Fletcher and Peter Roberts (Cambridge: Cambridge University Press, 1994), 56–83. For bathing and health, see: Cavallo and Storey, *Conserving Health in Early Modern Culture*, 240; van Dam, 'Permeable Boundaries'. Tessa Storey and Sandra Cavallo point to the ways bathing became more fashionable as a health practice over the seventeenth century, Sandra Cavallo and Tessa Storey, *Healthy Living in Late Renaissance Italy* (Oxford: Oxford University Press, 2013), 240.

64 Guillemeau, *Child-birth*, 23. 65 *Ibid.*, 23. 66 Sennert, *Practical Physick*, 267.

This cycle of removing clouts, cleaning and drying the baby, and then reswaddling was frequent and laborious. Barret noted that 'cleanly' and assiduous nurses would do this three, four or more times a day. He specified that these good nurses would use clean 'Rags' each time, wiping the ears and armpits.[67] Sharp stressed that it was important that 'Piss and Dung' be removed promptly as it could 'put the child to great pain'.[68] The clouts, cloths and linens new babies required must have added an additional strain on the servants whose job was to wash clothes. It was also left unclear in childbearing guides when this regimen of shifting and cleaning could end. At some point, it was expected that infants would be able to 'hold' their excrement. If they never learnt how, it was either 'ill Custom', a bad habit that would cease of its own accord, or the result of a stone or humoral imbalance. If the latter, Pechey recommended giving the nurse or woman feeding the infant a hot and dry diet of meat, sage, fennel and marjoram. The baby should be bathed with oak leaves and sulphur to help dry it out further.[69] Childbearing guides suggest that the infant's needs could be easily discovered if nurses, mothers and others just simply paid attention, and that by subtle manipulation of bath ingredients and routine, could be easily remedied. Some baths heated whilst others cooled. Knowing which one to employ when was a kind of knowledge that those looking after babies were expected to have intuitively. And yet this attention – like the attentiveness that women were meant to pay to their bodies during pregnancy – was time consuming, indeed potentially all-consuming labour. Here lies a cultural tension between the medical skill and knowledge required to restore mothers and usher infants into the world and keep them healthy, and the representation of this bodywork as unskilled and menial in medical print.

Swaddling

After bathing, wiping and rubbing the infant, writers proposed that the mother, midwife or nurse should swaddle the infant. These two rituals of bathing and binding were intertwined: one encouraged excretion and the other supported and stemmed the flow of humours. This meant putting the baby in a shirt, cap (called a biggin), clouts, a blanket and rolls of plain fabric wrapped round and round the body until it was bound tightly. Wealthier families often invested in lace or embroidered bands to decorate the outer swaddle. This was done 'lest it should move its hands and feet too freely, and thereby distort the bones, which are yet flexible'. Swaddling also might rectify ills in the newborn's body by supporting and reshaping it.[70] Although many early modern medical writers

[67] Barret, *A Companion for Midwives*, 80
[68] Sharp, *The Midwives Book Or the Whole Art of Midwifry Discovered*, 374.
[69] Pechey, *A General Treatise of the Diseases of Infants and Children*, 21.
[70] *Ibid.*, 6.

warned that binding too tightly could be dangerous, none discouraged the practice absolutely. Sometimes if the child seemed frustrated by the bands, writers suggested making 'little sleeues' for the baby to allow it to move its arms.[71]

It was not just the infants' arms, legs and torso that were liable to bend and warp without proper support, but its head too. Babies' heads, medical writers argued, should always be covered although they were often unsure about how supportive or firm this should be. In Jones' 1579 treatise, he told mothers and nurses after bathing the infant to 'slicke vp the forehead or forfronte of the tower and ampier of Reason and Sapience', and then 'ouerclasping your hands' in front and behind the head, reshape it.[72] Barret cautiously suggested after bathing putting a 'Compress' under the 'Biggin', or bonnet, 'to keep the Brain warm' and support the 'Mould of the Head'.[73] Compress in the seventeenth century meant both a pad of material to warm and soothe and an action that involved squeezing and forming an object.[74] Guillemeau instructed if 'deformity' was present, it could be mended 'by bringing the said head vnto the forme of a boule [bowl], a little pressed and made flat on both sides'. The aim was that neither the 'forepart, nor hinderpart of the head, stand too farre out, not yet be too flat' and should be performed with 'head-cloths'.[75] At the same time, many of these authors expressed anxieties about being too heavy-handed with moulding. We recall Jones' anxieties about parents using 'instruments and trickes of their own trifeling' to shape their babies' bodies.[76] Others like Felix Wurtz in his 1656 treatise *The Children's Book* fretted that even placing the child's head in a cradle where it 'may be framed round' could harm the baby's dreams, thoughts and memories.[77] The French Royal midwife, Louise Bourgeois, alluded to the controversy of head shaping in 1609, noting 'it is a bad habit to clench the infants' head as is binding which gives them the long head one can observe in Paris infants'.[78] Writers drew subtle distinctions between care that was necessary and that which was perceived as meddling and vain. Once again, Jones makes a confusing distinction between acceptable intervention – shaping the baby's head with one's own hands – and unacceptable and ungodly care using instruments. This latter act caused 'obstructions and infirmities', 'stinking breathes, copper faces, redde noses, riueled skinne,

71 *Ibid.*, 6; Guillemeau, *Child-birth*, 23.
72 Helkiah Crooke, *Mikrokosmographia a description of the body of man* (London, 1615), 32.
73 Barret, *A Companion for Midwives*, 80. 74 OED. 75 Guillemeau, *Child-birth*, 11.
76 Jones, *The Arte and Science*, 34.
77 Cited in: John Ruhräh, *Pediatrics of the Past: An Anthology Compiled and Edited by John Ruhräh with a Foreword by Fielding H. Garrison* (New York: P. B. Hoeber, 1925), 203.
78 Louis Bourgeois, *Observations Diverses sur la Sterilité, Perte de Fruits, Feocondité, Accouchments, et Maladies de Femmes, et Enfants Nouveaux-naiz, suivi de Instructions a ma fille* (Paris: 1609), 96, cited in Michael Obladen, 'In God's Image? The Tradition of Infant Head Shaping', *Journal of Child Neurology*, 27, no. 5 (2012): 677.

tawnie coloure, and lesse fruitfulnesse'.[79] Although the differences between the bathing, clothing and moulding practices medical writers advocated were often subtle, they were represented as meaningful. Choosing the wrong regime might reflect poor motherhood.

In histories of the family, swaddling has taken on something of an emblematic status of the cruelty and inflexibility of parenting practices in the past. At best, it has been represented as reducing 'necessary' contact between parents and children, and at worst, a consciously cruel way of avoiding responsibility by immobilising newborns. Lawrence Stone provocatively stated that swaddling 'prevent[ed] the mother or nurse from cuddling, hugging and caressing the child', and that it enabled mothers to hook their infants on doorways to keep them out of the way, although there is no direct evidence of parents actually doing this.[80] Valerie Fildes, influenced by the work of John Bowlby and other proponents of attachment theory, argued that early modern parents were 'apparently indifferent' because they failed to hold and breastfeed infants.[81] Linda Pollock and others have challenged the theory that early modern parenting was devoid of affection, and yet the assumption that swaddling hampered parental engagement and touch is still part of this argument.[82]

In fact, swaddling was perceived as crucial in meeting the bodily and affective needs of newborns in early modern England. It was thought to serve to support the growth of the body, and settled babies so that they could sleep properly and did not become too distressed. It was therefore another part of the extensive regimen of newborn care that women took on in the days, weeks and months after birth. In many ways, the practices of swaddling although settling the infant, made more work for caregivers rather than less as the rhythmic binding and unbinding was time consuming. Parents made a substantial financial investment in swaddling bands and infant clothes.[83]

The material investment in blankets, swaddling bands and clouts during pregnancy that was discussed in Chapter 3 was realised in the after birth period. Babies were clothed in new and borrowed items in a way that materially and emotionally situated them in their new family and its social network. Purchasing blankets, swaddling bands or clouts while pregnant could even be

[79] Jones, *The Arte and Science*, 34.
[80] Stone, *The Family, Sex and Marriage in England 1500–1800*, 65, 115.
[81] Valerie Fildes, 'The History of Infant Feeding 1500–1800' (PhD thesis, University of Surrey, 1982), 72.
[82] Linda A. Pollock, *Forgotten Children: Parent–Child Relations from 1500 to 1900* (Cambridge: Cambridge University Press, 1983). For the persistence of this idea, especially in public history, see: Nicholas Tucker, 'Boon or Burden? Baby Love in History: Did Past Ages Care for, or Curse the Cradle and Its Occupant? Nicholas Tucker Sifts the Evidence', *History Today* 43, no. 9 (1993): 28–35.
[83] Heather Toomer, 'Seventeenth-Century Baby Clothes? The Problems of Identification', *Costume* 55, no. 1 (2021): 24–48.

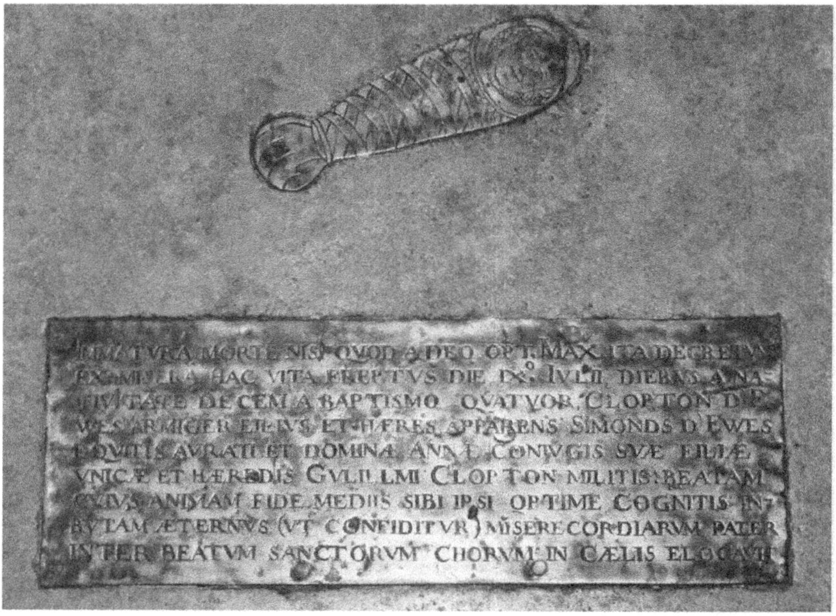

Figure 6.2 Baby brass of Clopton D'Ewes, son of Sir Simonds D'Ewes who died in 1631. St Peter and St Paul Church, Lavenham, Suffolk. Author's photograph.

exonerating evidence by unmarried mothers in court cases where they had been accused of committing infanticide.[84] Swaddling was so symbolically linked to parental love that this material investment in the newborn's future and wellbeing was deemed sufficient proof that the woman had hoped to keep the child. A baby in swaddling bands was a kind of visual shorthand for innocence and vulnerability in the period, yet another indication that the medical work of ordering infants was part of the same process by which babies were defined in relation to their family. Baby brasses like the one of Clopton D'Ewes (Figure 6.2) can be seen on the walls and floors of churches all over England commemorating family losses. Whilst some historians have argued that these little bundles signified that these children had died before they were baptised, Sophie Oosterwijk suggests that they were part of a broader liturgical and cultural tradition of representing the duties of parenthood and the pain of premature death.[85] The effigy of Clopton, an 'innocent soul' memorialised his

[84] Gowing, 'Secret Births and Infanticide in Seventeenth-Century England', 99.
[85] Sophie Oosterwijk, 'Chrysoms, Shrouds and Infants on English Tomb Monuments: A Question of Terminology?', *Church Monuments* 15 (2000): 44–64.

short life, the medical failures that led to his death and that he had left 'the most sad and disconsolate father that could possible be'.

Although the practice of swaddling was culturally linked to understandings of maternal affect, medical authorities were predictably less concerned who actually did the swaddling as long as it was done in a way that they thought was loving. Jones assumed it would be the mother who should take great pleasure in conceiving, carrying, delivering, holding and swaddling the child 'dayly on hir louing lappe, and to giue it sucke with hir own most tender breastes'. If one had to hire a wet nurse, it was important she was 'curteous, louing and kinde to hir suckling'.[86] A page later in his instructions on how to swaddle a baby, he simply talks about placing the baby on 'your lappe'. 'You' should 'plac[e] euery lime [limb] and joynt right for as yet it will be' that were 'pliant as waxe', before binding the infant in swaddling cloths, revealing the myopic focus of physicians on infant welfare.[87] Given, as we shall come to understand, a great many families were hiring help of some kind during this period, it seems highly unlikely that it was always mothers that were swaddling babies, particularly during the weeks after birth. Infant welfare and wellbeing were prioritised in the narratives families told about themselves, with little bother for the complicated bodily and emotional experience that taking on this childcare might have for servants, midwives and nurses.

Swaddling went out of favour in the eighteenth century and was increasingly perceived as curtailing rather than promoting bone growth. Thus, the English translation of Peter Moulin's *Directions for the Education of a Young Prince till Seven Years of Age* (1673) contrasted the upbringing of a prince with that of a poor boy. The prince was 'wrapt up in warm Cloaths, with great care, compass'd in Skreens and Hangings' and a nurse gave him suck, 'skilful Women were hired to 'swaddle, rock, and carry him'. The poor child was 'wrapt, not according to his need' but with what his mother could afford.[88] The poor boy lived into adulthood, whereas the prince was constantly sick and overly sensitive to changes in weather and routine. The latter (who was swaddled more sparingly and loosely) lived into adulthood, while the prince was sickly. The religious author John Bunyan lamented how swaddling bands and clouts were like 'little winding sheets', in the way they hampered infant health.[89] In 1748, when William Cadogan, governor of

[86] Jones, *The Arte and Science*, 30. [87] *Ibid.*, 31.

[88] Peter Moulin, *Directions for the Education of a Young Prince till Seven Years of Age* (London: 1673), 203.

[89] John Bryan, *Harvest-home being the summe of certain sermons upon Job 5. 26: one whereof was preached at the funeral of Mr. Ob. Musson, an aged Godly minister of the Gospel in the Royally licensed rooms in Coventry: the other since continued upon the subject* (London, 1674), 7.

the London Foundling Hospital, established in 1739, in Bloomsbury, wrote *An Essay Upon Nursing*, he railed against swaddling. Too long 'this Business [of childcare]' had been 'left to the Management of Women, who cannot be supposed to have proper Knowledge to fit them for such a Task'. Women got their knowledge from 'Examples and transmitted Customs of their Great Grand-mothers'. This care was, in Cadogan's opinion, at best superstitious and parochial, and at worst murderous. The mother who 'has only a few rags to cover her child loosely, and little more than her own breast to feed it, sees it healthy and strong' while the 'puny insect' of a rich family languished under a 'load of finery' and 'dies a victim to the mistaken care and tenderness of his fond Mother'.[90] Cadogan justified this new care as part of a new genre of expert medical advice that 'finally' placed infant welfare above other concerns.[91] Perhaps he was more overtly pronatalist than other childbearing authors. However, this infant-centric concern was not new, and in fact was one of the key motivators behind the continuity of swaddling in the earlier period. In 1762, Jean-Jacques Rousseau also instructed parents not to 'confine' infants in 'tight wrappings' after birth; 'No cap, no bandages, nor swaddling clothes'.[92] Like Moulin and Cadogan's anecdotal evidence of the lustiness of the babies of poor women, Rousseau gestured to the long-standing trope in medical texts that non-European women gave birth more easily and raised their children effortlessly. The 'ancient Peruvians' supposedly clothed their infants loosely, meaning they were more independent than European toddlers at a mere two months old.[93] Referencing Buffon, he noted that the practice of swaddling was now 'obselete' in England. Some sixty years after Cadogan's text, the Scottish physician William Buchan professed in 1804 how much the *Essay on Nursing* had informed his own practice, and labelled swaddling bands as the 'cruel tortures', suggesting that actually the practice continued in homes far beyond the eighteenth century.[94] These new recommendations perpetuated the idea that the care an infant received was somehow symbolic of its parents' moral character and worth embedded in earlier works, whilst similarly affording little space to the difficulty of carrying out the activities needed to supposedly make babies healthy.

90 William Cadogan, *An Essay upon Nursing and the Management of Children, From their Birth to Three Years of Age* (London, 1748), 7.
91 Lisa Forman Cody, *Birthing the Nation: Sex, Science, and the Conception of Eighteenth-Century Britons* (Oxford: Oxford University Press, 2005).
92 Jean-Jacques Rousseau, *Emile, or On Education (1763)* (Garden City, NY: Dover Publications, 2013), 31.
93 *Ibid.*, 31.
94 William Buchan, *Advice to Mothers, on the subject of their own health, and on the means of promoting the health, strength, and beauty, of their offspring* (Edinburgh, 1804), 08.

Sleeping

After this regimen of crying, cutting the cord, searching, washing and clothing, and before feeding, babies had to sleep. 'A Child new born sleeps more than he wakes, because his brain is very moist, and he used to sleep in the womb', Culpeper explained.[95] Physicians opined in medical print and regimens that good restorative sleep was central to the maintenance of health and was central in soothing the passions of the soul. Medical writers became increasingly interested in sleep in the late and early eighteenth century as both a key part of regimen, but disturbed sleep as a symptom of bodily, emotional and religious malaise.[96] Sleeping for babies was even more important than for adults because it helped to concoct and digest their excessive moisture. Babies were free to sleep with abandon in their first days and weeks. Mauriceau explained 'There needs no certain limited time for his rest, for he may sleep at any time night or day'.[97] Guillemeau suggested that babies could sleep whenever they wanted, even whilst suckling, until they were two years old.[98] Crucially, sleeping kept the baby quiet and content, which was a key concern in managing health. Joan Ellyott echoed these words when she wrote to her sister Anne D'Ewes in Suffolk in the first half of the seventeenth century. She noted it was imperative that Anne's son should not 'be kept from sleepe or suck which I know has bin the way of very good docters in this case but let it have a full breast of new milke at command and all the quiet and content'.[99]

Only a soothed newborn would sleep and Guillemeau proposed there were three key tools the person caring for the baby, whether mother or nurse, had in their arsenal to procure this rest: 'giuing them the breast', 'rocking' and 'singing to them'.[100] Some nurses, Barret complained, were 'huffing and bounding about, and do not mind the poor Child'. A good nurse would 'sing with a soft voice to lull it to sleep, rocking gently all the while'.[101] Jones sung the praises of 'lullies' [lullabies] that would bring 'disquieted' children to 'reste'. It had the additional benefit of soothing and calming the nurse's emotions – 'light affections [that] may happen to annoy' the nurse could be uttered, alleviating her own distress.[102] People caring for the baby might also encourage it to look at pleasant things or carry them 'abroad', a phrase

95 Culpeper, *Directory for Midwives* (1662), 243.
96 Sasha Handley, *Sleep in Early Modern England* (New Haven, CT: Yale University Press, 2016).
97 François Mauriceau, *The Diseases of Women with Child, and in Child-bed: as also, the Best Directions How to Help Them in Natural and Unnatural Labours* (London, 1672), 369.
98 Guillemeau, *Child-birth,* 17
99 Joan Ellyott to Ann D'Ewes, 18 December c. 1620–1640, BL, MS Harleian 382, fol. 39.
100 Guillemeau, *Child-birth*, 18. 101 Barret, *A Companion for Midwives*, 91.
102 Jones, *The Arte and Science*, 13, 14. Leslie Herbert Daiken, *The Lullaby Book. Musical Research by Mary Hillis and Sebastian Brown. With Plates* (London: Ward, Lock & Co.,

meaning around the home or outside for short distances.[103] Rocking had to be gentle to facilitate digestion. If it was too vigorous, writers suggested it might 'hinder' concoction and cause the baby to vomit.[104] If the baby was 'swaithed too hard' or were 'pinched by the wrinkling of Linnen, or pricked by a pin' or if its clothes were too dirty ('for Children love to be clean'), it might not 'sleep quietly' until these things were rectified.[105]

If a baby was to be picked up and 'laye downe as ofte as neede shal require', however, families had to work out who would be on 'watch' duty.[106] This should not be the wet nurse or mother (if she was suckling) for it was vital that the person feeding the baby was well rested in order to produce good milk. Jones recommended hiring someone else to attend to the baby when it cried in the middle of the night and only disturb the nurse or mother if it was clear the infant needed feeding. Robert Delaval of Seaton Delaval Hall in Northumberland recommended his son, Ralph, do just this in 1600. He told him it was very important the family hire a 'watch woman in the nyght' to listen out for the child's cries. This was just after the birth of his first child. As well as potentially protecting the quality of the milk, getting an additional person to 'Ries to the Child' would ensure there were an additional pair of eyes watching the child lest it fall asleep with 'the papp' or breast in its mouth, which was 'wonderfull daungerous'.[107]

Once the child was two, however, many medical writers promoted a regimen of limiting and regulating the sleep of infants. Sleeping too much would cool and 'moisteneth the braine' harmfully, threatening to 'dull the infant's senses' and render 'their functions languishing and stupefied'.[108] Guillemeau thought it might 'besot the child's senses' and make them 'dull and lumpish'.[109] This regimen was to take into account the baby's condition and the seasons of the year.[110] This was the case for adults too. The 'prophylactic culture' of early modern regimens promoted moderating sleep, diet and behaviour in relation to the seasons, availability of light and individual constitutions.[111]

1959); Nicholas Tucker, 'Mothers, Babies and Lullabies', *History Today* 34, no. 9 (1984): 40–46.

103 Jones, *The Arte and Science*, 18. 104 Mauriceau, *The Accomplisht Midwife*, 368.

105 Pechey, *A General Treatise of the Diseases of Infants and Children*, 7.

106 Jones, *The Arte and Science*, 49.

107 Robert Delaval to Ralph Delaval, 4 October 1600, Northumberland Archives, Ashington, 1DE/5/20.

108 Mauriceau, *The Accomplisht Midwife*, 369. 109 Guillemeau, *Child-birth*, 15.

110 Pechey, *A General Treatise of the Diseases of Infants and Children*, 4.

111 Sasha Handley, 'Sleep-Piety and Healthy Sleep in Early Modern English Households', in *Conserving Health in Early Modern Culture: Bodies and Environments in Italy and England*, ed. Sandra Cavallo and Tessa Storey, Social Histories of Medicine (Manchester: Manchester University Press, 2017), 185–210, 203.

As well as debating when and for how long infants should sleep, medical writers were also concerned about how and in what position children should sleep. Most medical authors recommended laying babies on their backs with particular attention paid to raising the head on a pillow to help digestion. This was a long-standing recommendation in regimens to prevent regurgitation. Those who were ill or elderly were especially encouraged to elevate their heads above their stomach and feet.[112] It was important to alternate position during the night to support concoction to assist food in its descent to the pit of the stomach.[113] The cradle also ought to be shifted around the room lest the infant develop a squint from always staring in one direction. It was easy for young children to develop bodily asymmetries that were difficult to remove later in life because they were so impressionable. Pechey recommended also putting 'fine Pictures' in strategic spots to redirect the infant's gaze or making a mask so 'that the sight may be directed right'.[114] Babies ought to have their own separate cradles too and never sleep in the bed with their parents or nurses. Medical authors were very concerned about overlaying, or smothering, the infant.[115] Robert Delaval instructed his son to never let 'the child to be giuen to you in the bed', however tempting it was, for fear of lying on top of it.[116] Mauriceau explained placing a cradle 'close by the Bed-side' would prevent this tragedy and a mantle should be placed over the head of it to 'prevent the falling of dust on its Face, and that the Day-light, Sunshine, Cradle, or Fire in the Chamber may not offend' the baby.[117] Guillemeau described the way the infant should be 'laid in his cradle' with a little mattress placed deep in the bottom so the baby would not 'feare least he fall out of it'.[118] Strings might be tied around the baby so that when rocked, it would not all out.[119] Getting babies to sleep, like many other activities in the regimen of newborns, was important for settling their emotions, making them cheerful and correcting impediment. It also required vigilance and attentiveness from those caring for it.

112 *Ibid.*, 25–26. 113 *Ibid.*, 26.
114 Pechey, *A General Treatise of the Diseases of Infants and Children*, 82.
115 The Bills of Mortality reported infant deaths as 'overlaid' or 'smothered'. Craig Spence points out that death from overlaying presents particular interpretive difficulties, as it was often unclear whether this was a deliberate or accidental death, Craig Spence, *Accidents and Violent Death in Early Modern London, 1650–1750*, Studies in Early Modern Cultural, Political and Social History (Woodbridge: Boydell & Brewer, 2016), 125.
116 Delaval to Delaval, 4 October 1600, 1DE/5/20.
117 Mauriceau, *The Accomplisht Midwife*, 368.
118 Guillemeau, 'The Nursing of Children', 14–15.
119 Mauriceau, *The Accomplisht Midwife*, 368.

Feeding

Once the baby had been 'ordered as you have harde [heard], it shall be time to give it sucke'.[120] Religious and medical writers of the period were unequivocal that, if at all possible, mothers should breastfeed their own babies, and not get a wet nurse. Childbearing guides, however, often included instructions on how to select a good nurse, and as we have heard, often directed their advice to nurses in the assumption that they would be doing a significant amount of care. Elite families, however, often asked people who were not blood-related to feed their children. The term nurse was a capacious one that meant caring for elderly or other sick people as well as infants.[121] But despite the hazy linguistic usage of the term, wet nurses were often expected to take on considerable responsibility in addition to feeding. On top of the medical work they provided, they were also expected to remain abstinent while feeding, as sex and conception were thought to corrupt the milk.

Medical writers hoped that mothers would breastfeed their own children because breast milk was understood to be a purified form of the blood that had nourished the child in the womb. As we have seen, sudden changes were viewed as detrimental to babies' delicate bodies and constitutions. Continuity in their nutrition from within and then outside the womb helped ease their transition and adaptation to the outside world. Suckling immediately after birth was thought to be dangerous for babies because this milk had not yet been sufficiently purified.[122] You could discern that this milk was impure by the fact that it was not yet wholly white and thin (now commonly termed colostrum). Jones described how babies were very 'coueteth to sucke' as soon as they were born, but it would be 'vnholesome' and mothers should refrain.[123] Many authors, like Pechey, recommended giving infants a concoction of oil and sugar for the first three days of life or 'Order some other Woman' to feed the child 'till the Mothers milk be pure'.[124] Babies had supposedly been constantly nourished in the womb, and therefore fasting was good for them. The author of *Paidon Nosemata* explained that because babies had soft palates and were 'unaccustomed to meat', or food, they would suck 'more than they digest'.[125]

120 Jones, *The Arte and Science*, 39.

121 Mary E. Fissell, 'Women, Health and Healing in Early Modern Europe', *Bulletin of the History of Medicine* 82 (2008): 1–17; Deborah E. Harkness, 'A View from the Streets: Women and Medical Work in Elizabethan London', *Bulletin of the History of Medicine* 82, no. 1 (2008): 52–85; Margaret Pelling, 'Nurses and Nursekeepers: Problems with Identification in the Early Modern Period', in *The Common Lot: Sickness, Medical Occupations and the Urban Poor in Early Modern England*, 179–202 (London: Longman, 1998).

122 See, for example: Mauriceau, *The Diseases of Women with Child, and in Child-bed*, 365.

123 Jones, *The Arte and Science*, 8.

124 Pechey, *A General Treatise of the Diseases of Infants and Children*, 4.

125 J. S., *Paidon Nosemata*, 123.

Jones noted that the Roman writer Titus Pomponius Atticus believed children should not be fed until they were four days old, and Avicenna thought someone else should feed the child for two months after birth.[126]

Some parents followed this advice. When Simonds D'Ewes son, Clopton, was born, doctors advised that the 'child should not sucke any other till her [Simond's wife's] breasts were fully drawn and made fit for it'. This involved getting rid of the early milk, perceived to be corrupted. Simonds, however, felt that this advice, which was in keeping with that in printed medical literature, was responsible for Clopton's death. The 'cursed ignorance of such as were employed about my wife during her lying-in' made the baby 'so weakened as afterwards proved the cause of its ruin'.[127] The worry that breast milk was insufficiently purified or not old enough is also hinted at in a letter from Ralph Delaval to his son recommending the couple employ a nurse of 'second mylk' rather than 'furst mylk', meaning that the woman had already fed an infant before taking on the Delaval's child. Delaval asked his son to trust his expertise – he had 'good triall' of such situations – and insisted that babies of 'furst mylk' were often 'dull' and 'full of gript umours [humours]'.[128]

The second reason that medical writers were adamant that mothers ought to feed their own children was because breastfeeding fostered an emotional connection between mother and child that was perceived as unbreakable. Jones stated that breastfeeding led to an 'undoubted token of absolute kindnesse and friendshippe' between mother and child.[129] Guillemeau suggested this would mean that when the child became an adult, it would continue to be 'bound' to its mother both because 'she had borne him nine Moneths in her womb' and because 'shee hath nursed him, watched him, and often made him cleane'.[130] Thomas Moffett, for example, described how recently delivered women heaped 'labour upon labour' in 'suffering it to taste no other milk' because of the love they bore their children.[131] Affect was linked to parental effort: children would 'never love their parents so well; but that their fathers do often beare them in their armes, and mothers give them sucke at their owne breasts'.[132] Further still, affect was what drove parents to carry out this care in the first place. Barret supposed that if 'Nature had not oblig'd' mothers 'with stronger Tyes', they would never submit to breastfeeding.[133]

[126] Jones, *The Arte and Science*, 8.

[127] Simonds D'Ewes, *The Autobiography and Correspondence of Sir Simonds D'Ewes: During the Reign of James I and Charles I*, ed. James Orchard Halliwell, vol. 2 (London: Richard Bentley, 1845), 45. Clopton was born 24 June 1631. He died 9 July 1631.

[128] Delaval to Delaval, 4 October 1600, 1DE/5/20.

[129] Jones, *The Arte and Science*, 31.

[130] Guillemeau, 'The Nursing of Children', 8.

[131] Thomas Moffett, *Healths Improvement: or, Rules compromising and Discovering the Nature, Method and Manner of Preparing all sorts of Food used in this Nation* (London: 1655), 120.

[132] Guillemeau, 'The Nursing of Children', 9.

[133] Barret, *A Companion for Midwives*, 91.

The Countess of Lincoln, Elizabeth Clinton, similarly linked maternal breastfeeding to emotion in her 1622 Nurserie. A mother's love was 'so knit by natures law to her tender babe, as she finds no power to deny to suckle it', not even if her life were 'in hazard' by doing so. Clinton sorely regretted not breastfeeding her eighteen children. She was 'overruled by anothers authority', 'deceived by ill counsel' and at the time claimed she did not fully understand her 'godly duty'. She was sure, however, that the death of 'one or two of my little babes' was the fault of wet nurses she employed. She vowed to compensate for her perceived negligence and 'shew double loue to my children'.[134]

And yet, despite the plentiful pro-breastfeeding invectives, childbearing guides also offered considerable guidance on how to choose a 'good' nurse if a woman could not or would not suckle. The nurse had to be 'Young' and Healthy'. Barret criticised 'City Dames' who took the wet nurse into their own home and fed her 'high'. This made the 'Milk rampant' and instead, borrowing from Hippocrates, he proposed that the nurse should eat 'course Food as she gives to her own at Home', which would make the child brisk and hardy.[135] Culpeper instructed parents to use the 'temper' or complexion of the mother as a model for that of the nurse. Her breasts should be 'well fashioned with good Nipples, that the child may take them with pleasure' and she should be 'well bred, and peacable'.[136] Jones believed it was important to hire a woman who had recently given birth to a child that was the same sex as the baby to be fed.[137] Others suggested one should never hire a nurse with red hair because her milk would transfer traces of her 'fiery' personality.

Much of the scholarship on infant care and breastfeeding prior to the eighteenth century has assumed that wet nursing was the norm and first choice for the majority of middling- and upper-sort families. Stone understands this perceived trend as another symptom of lacklustre parental affection in the period before industrialisation. Breastfeeding in the sixteenth and seventeenth centuries was seen as a 'nuisance, interfering with sleep and the normal round of social engagements'.[138] Other scholars have pointed to a quantitative rise in maternal breastfeeding in the eighteenth century, concomitant with what is often termed the 'cult of motherhood'. They often draw on a very small sample size, meaning that it is difficult to know whether this statistical trend was simply the result of greater source survival in the later period or increased literacy, suggesting eighteenth-century parents were more likely to write about infant care.[139]

[134] Elizabeth Clinton, *The Countesse of Lincolnes Nurserie* (Oxford: 1622), 8, 15–16, 16.
[135] Barret, *A Companion for Midwives*, 77–78.
[136] Culpeper, *Directory for Midwives* (1651), 226. [137] Jones, *The Arte and Science*, 11.
[138] Stone, *The Family, Sex and Marriage in England 1500–1800*, 269–270.
[139] Linda Campbell, 'Wet-Nurses in Early Modern England: Some Evidence from the Townshend Archive', *Medical History* 33 (1989): 360–370; Valerie Fildes, *Breasts, Bottles, and Babies: A History of Infant Feeding* (Edinburgh: Edinburgh University Press, 1986), 158; Fildes, 'The

More importantly, within these accounts, the assumption that breastfeeding was fundamentally linked to affection or dedication of mothers to their infants remains intact. Lucinda Beier notes that Alice Thornton was 'uncommon for women of her social status' by wanting to 'give her younger five children the best possible start' by breastfeeding them herself.[140]

Early modern parents rarely seem to have chosen to hire a wet nurse out of convenience, let alone negligence or laziness, as Stone would assume. Indeed, like other medical choices, the selection of a nurse directly redounded to their social standing. Families sought 'good' nurses when mothers or infants became ill or when women simply did not produce enough milk. This does not mean, however, that families valued the care that wet nurses provided. Elite families consistently placed their own welfare above that of the nurse and her family, often demanding the nurse live in away from her own, possibly newborn, children.[141] Families also expected that nurses would engage with their babies in an affectionate and altruistic way, placing undue and unrealistic emotional expectations on those paid to do a difficult and exhausting job. Breastfeeding was a form of carework that involved parents ascribing and reinforcing social hierarchies, particularly with regard to the ways emotions were felt and expressed.[142] The tasks involved in being a wet nurse were ill defined, and the patterns of employment mirror what historians of work have described of early modern and eighteenth-century people having multiple and shifting occupations.[143] We learn much about the ways in which wet nursing was bound up with exploitative class and racial dichotomies from the long history of slaveholding communities, manipulating the generative bodies of slaves. In thirteenth- and fourteenth-century Aragon in Majorca, for example, wealthy urban women were encouraged to use enslaved Muslim women to feed their babies. This allowed elite women to continue their work as social

History of Infant Feeding 1500–1800'; Dorothy McLaren, 'Nature's Contraceptive: Wet Nursing and Prolonged Lactation: The Case of Chesham, Buckinghamshire, 1578–1601', *Medical History* 23 (1979): 426–441; Pollock, *Forgotten Children*, 212–213.

[140] Beier, *Sufferers and Healers*, 232.

[141] Marissa C. Rhodes has observed a similar trend in wet nursing advertisements placed by elite families in London and Philadelphia in the eighteenth century. See: Marissa C. Rhodes, 'Domestic Vulnerabilities: Reading Families and Bodies into Eighteenth-century Anglo-Atlantic Wet Nurse Advertisements', *Journal of Family History* 40, no. 1 (2014), 39–63.

[142] Alexandra Shepard, 'The Pleasures and Pains of Breastfeeding in England c. 1600–c. 1800: Narratives and Representations: A Collection to Honour Paul Slack', in *Suffering and Happiness in England 1550–1850*, ed. Michael J. Braddick and Joanna Innes, The Past & Present Book Series (Oxford: Oxford University Press, 2017), 229.

[143] Mark Overton, *Production and Consumption in English Households, 1600–1750* (London: Routledge, 2004), 74; K. Tawny Paul, 'Accounting for Men's Work: Multiple Employments and Occupational Identities in Early Modern England', *History Workshop Journal* 85 (2018): 26–46; Alexandra Shepard, *Accounting for Oneself: Worth, Status, and the Social Order in Early Modern England* (Oxford: Oxford University Press, 2015), 149–190.

networkers for their husbands, be sexually available and become pregnant again. The unfree woman's child was often removed from the house or neglected in preference for the master and mistress' child.[144] In eighteenth-century American colonies, it was a common practice for slaves to suckle their master's children. Enslaved, indentured and white women advertised their services as wet nurses (or in some instances sale) in newspapers in eighteenth-century Philadelphia.[145] This practice continued into the nineteenth century in the southern states of America, where slave-owning households relied on the milk and care of enslaved women to raise their own family.[146] This practice was common in colonial Jamaica, too. At the same time, there was a strong current in medical writing that warned white women about the dangerous and evil traits that their babies might imbibe from suckling black women. Lady Maria Nugent, wife of the governor of Jamaica from 1803 to 1804, opted to hire a white Irish woman instead of a black woman to suckle her two children while she resumed official public duties.[147] At the same time, doctors and planters in Jamaica and other parts of the Caribbean chastised enslaved mothers who 'got some of their friends to suckle their children for two or three days' after delivery instead of feeding themselves.[148] In such situations, it was convenient to draw on much longer notions of black bodies birthing, bearing and suckling children more easily than white ones.[149] This discourse bore similarities to the insistence of earlier writers that poorer or 'courser' women were better at procreating than elite ones.

The concern for the welfare of infants and lack of interest in the wellbeing of nurses is displayed in the ways in which early modern English families expressed the desire to get a 'good' nurse in their correspondence. Lord Broghill reassured his father-in-law in 1667 that they had got 'a verry good Nurse'.[150] Mary Browne wrote to Anne Le Neve in 1692 recommending a 'very tidy woman' that had a three-month-old child and had nursed another's infant previously. She was 'very much commended', but Browne noted if she was unable to 'under take it' or not to Anne's liking, she would 'endeavour to

[144] Rebecca Lynn Winer, 'Conscripting the Breast: Lactation, Slavery and Salvation in the Realms of Aragon and Kingdom of Majorca, c. 1250–1300', *Journal of Medieval History* 34, no. 2 (2012): 164–184.

[145] Rhodes, 'Domestic Vulnerabilities'.

[146] Emily West and R. J. Knight, 'Mother's Milk: Slavery, Wet-Nursing, and Black and White Women in the Antebellum South', *Journal of Southern History* 83, no. 1 (2017): 37–68.

[147] Sasha Turner, *Contested Bodies: Pregnancy, Childrearing, and Slavery in Jamaica*, Early American Studies (Pittsburg: University of Pennsylvania Press, 2017), 121.

[148] *Ibid.*, 121.

[149] Jennifer L. Morgan, '"Some Could Suckle over Their Shoulder": Male Travelers, Female Bodies, and the Gendering of Racial Ideology', in *Laboring Women: Reproduction and Gender in New World Slavery*, Early American Studies (Philadelphia: University of Pennsylvania Press, 2004), 12–49.

[150] Lord Broghill to Richard, fifth earl of Dorset, 7 January 1667, KHLC, U269/C18/12.

enquire up some other'.[151] Matthew Henry, a Presbyterian minister, described to his mother in a letter in 1697 how he and his wife, Katherine, had found an 'orderly lady' to breastfeed his daughter, Nancy, who was very ill. The family doctor thought the illness was a result of the 'badness' of Katherine's milk and was 'very apprehensive' the baby might die. He 'absolutely forbid' Katherine from feeding any longer and thankfully Nancy took to 'her breast very well'. Getting another woman to feed her child, however, put Katherine 'much adoe', especially because the nurse was in their own home.[152] The Henry family were vocal proponents of breastfeeding in other fora.[153] Matthew's father, Philip Henry, also a minister, afforded calls for mothers to breastfeed their own infants a prominent place in his sermons. In his sermon notes on Genesis, he scrawled 'Sarah gave suck to ye. child, ver. 7. Though a great woman, a rich woman, an aged woman, reproof to those out of nicenes & fineness refuse to doe that Office of love to their little ones, when no necessity.'[154] Alice Thornton similarly relied on a wet nurse when her baby, Betty, was unwell in 1655. She hired Dafeny Lightfoot, a former servant, for three months until she became pregnant herself. Then Thornton employed a 'stately louely girl' who lived several miles from the house.[155] Never did these families consider what would be done with the nurse's own child, or the toll of remaining abstinent for the months they were hired. In all of these cases, save Dafeny, we never learn the name of the wet nurse.

Families described wet nurses as 'good', orderly and, occasionally, pretty, in much the same way that midwives were framed in correspondence. Anne Conway's husband described a wet nurse they used to breastfeed their son Heneage as the 'prettiest' in contrast to the midwife who was one of the 'ugliest' women he had ever seen.[156] When Heneage was two months old, he was a healthy cheerful child, but Anne hoped that they could find way to divert him from 'sucking so much'.[157] After four months of nursing, however, the nurse became unwell. Edward wrote to his brother-in-law that Anne had been told by a doctor that 'to suck of such a woman is dangerous, and brings

[151] Mary Browne to Mrs Le Neve, 22 July 1692, Norfolk Record Office, Norwich, MC 44/20, 500 x1.

[152] Matthew Henry to Katherine Henry, 3 December 1697, BL, MS Add 42849, fol. 19.

[153] David Harley, 'From Providence to Nature: The Moral Theology and Godly Practice of Maternal Breast-Feeding in Stuart England', *Bulletin of the History of Medicine* 69, no. 2 (1995): 198–223.

[154] Philip Henry sermon book, 17 October 1658, Cambridge University Library, Cambridge, Add MS 7338, sermon on Gen. 21, unfoliated.

[155] Thornton, BL, Add MS 88897/1, 139.

[156] Lord Conway to Major Rawdon, 21 December 1658, Sarah Hutton and Marjorie Hope Nicolson, eds., *The Conway Letters: The Correspondence of Anne, Viscountess Conway, Henry More, and Their Friends 1642–1684* (Oxford: Oxford University Press, 1992), 154–155.

[157] Lady Conway to Lord Conway, 15 April 1659, *ibid.*, 156–157.

with it many diseases', and therefore Heneage was to be weaned 'much sooner than she intended'.[158] Several weeks later, Edward and Anne travelled to Ragley to find 'another nurse'. Edward noted that poor wet nurses had 'injured the child three times, we cannot think it possible to be borne any longer, and so all my wife's friends advise her'.[159]

This practice of employing a number of nurses in quick succession as a result of the infant or nurse being unwell was a common practice in elite families. When Penelope Mordaunt gave birth in summer 1702, her husband wrote to say 'I woul have you be enquireing after A wett Nurse'.[160] Just over two weeks later, Penelope had seemingly decided on a 'nurse from Wellsborn' but their daughter was unwell. Instead, Penelope was going to 'take' Mrs Lucas. Her husband, John, eagerly expected a letter in return, hearing 'what discourse hath pass'd betwixt yo[u]'. He sympathised with his wife, expressing 'how much trouble it must be to' her. He wondered whether getting a 'sucking Bottle' might improve the baby's condition (later letters suggest that the baby was not getting sufficient milk).[161] By the end of the month, the couple had had to replace Nurse Lucas too, which John imagined was going to make the nurse 'fall into great Passions about it'. The nurse's mother had expressed 'great complaints', wishing that her daughter had never nursed and protested that the child was unwell because of 'breeding teeth' rather than lack of milk.[162]

The anxiety around getting someone else to breastfeed a baby prompted parents to seek to have the wet nurse within their own home rather than allow the nurse to take the baby away with her. This echoed the more elite practice of asking midwives to travel to their estates for delivery, in order to ensure deliveries happened within the family home. When there were questions about the quality of Anne D'Ewes' milk, her sister insisted she get a nurse 'in the house where you may see the ordering of it yourself and feede the nurs at one of your one (sic) trenches'.[163] When Katherine Danby was heavily pregnant in 1632, there were problems with the wet nurse hired to feed and take care of her infant son, Tom. The nurse's husband was so 'covetous' that he was reluctant to let Tom go, along with the income he brought. Katherine's mother proposed in a letter to her husband that they should find a different woman to wean him and look after him, or if he was unable to be weaned, to have the original wet

158 Lord Conway to Major Rawdon, 14 June 1659, *ibid.*, 158–160.
159 Lord Conway to Major Rawdon, 5 July 1659, *ibid.*, 160–161.
160 Penelope Mordaunt to John Mordaunt, 8 September 1701/1702, Warwickshire Record Office, Warwick, CR 1368, vol. 1/14.
161 Mordaunt to Mordaunt, 24 September 1702, *ibid.*, vol. 1/18.
162 Mordaunt to Mordaunt, 29 September 1702, *ibid.*, vol. 1/21.
163 Ellyott to D'Ewes, 18 December c. 1620–1640, Harleian 382, fol. 39.

nurse in the house and 'in our power'.[164] A heavily pregnant Harriet, Lady Glenorchy, tried to circumvent the whole process of having another woman breastfeed her baby by hiring someone who would feed her baby 'without the breast'. She responded to a letter from her father encouraging her to breastfeed herself, saying that although her 'inclinatione to be nurs[e] my self', she found her 'constatution and my health much impared by the many troubles I have met'. She relayed how she had lost two 'fine boys' at wet nurses and one baby girl while feeding herself. She hoped that she could be 'excused complying with y[ou]r Lo[rdship]'s desire of nursing itt' and had got a woman 'whose buseness it has been for severell years in England to bring them up without the breast'. She refused to be drawn into imputing the death of her babyes 'to one way or an other' but rather insisted it was the will of God.[165]

When a wet nurse took her charge into her own home, parents or other family members regularly visited to check on the baby's health and happiness. When Elizabeth Freke left her infant son, Ralph, with a nurse while she travelled to Ireland with her husband, her father and sister visited regularly in her stead. The three of them collectively decided, in Elizabeth's absence, that the nurse was inadequate and took the baby away.[166] The lawyer and politician Bulstrode Whitelocke recorded in his autobiography that he was visited regularly by his mother while he was at nurse in 1605. On one occasion, his 'dyett' was judged 'not pleasing or thriving to the childe'. His mother discovered that the nurse had been feeding him pottage 'fattened' with 'rusty' bacon rather than breastfeeding. He was taken home immediately.[167] This kind of surprise visit was one recommended in medical texts to ensure parents had an accurate sense of the behaviour of the nurse.[168] Parents might also check up on nurses by visiting astrologers to ask whether the wet nurse had become pregnant, commonly thought to compromise the ability to feed or quality of the breast milk. Richard Napier's 'cousin' asked whether his nurse was pregnant in 1608.[169] Lady Anne Butler similarly asked Napier whether 'her nurce be with child' in 1626.[170] Here too these stories formed part of a family archive that attested to careful parenting and ongoing commitment to ministering and providing for household members. In these comments, family members also sought to reassure themselves and others that getting someone

[164] Alice Wandesford to Thomas Danby, 8 May 1632, North Yorkshire Record Office, Northallerton, MISC 2087/1229.

[165] Harriet, Lady Glenorchy, to Earl of Breadalbane, 23 January 1711, National Records of Scotland, Edinburgh, GD112/3/92/3.

[166] Elizabeth Freke, 8 January 1676, *The Remembrances of Elizabeth Freke*, ed. Raymond A. Anselment (Cambridge: Cambridge University Press, 2001), 48.

[167] Bulstrode Whitelock, 6 August 1605, 'Copy from my Father's George Whitelocke's Diary', BL, Add MS 5372, fol. 3.

[168] Barret, *A Companion for Midwives*, 79. [169] CASE34266, CB. [170] CASE1642, CB.

else to suckle their child would not alter the deep familial connection that the child had.

It was preferrable if elite families had two suckling children to place them together at the same nurse. At times, this was convenient for visiting, or perhaps because in the same way families valued recommendations with a personal connection – this meant the nurse had an existing bodily and emotional relationship with the family and household. A month after giving birth to a son in 1648, Lady Ann Fanshawe took him to Hartingfordbury to leave him 'at nurse with his brother'.[171] When Susan Lay, a servant, got pregnant by her master and then by her master's son in January and November 1649, respectively, both children were sent to the Beauty household to the same nurse, 'Richard Ballard's wife' in St Lawrence.[172] At other times, families seem to have sought out this prior connection because it provided a continuity of influence that might otherwise be fulfilled by mothers breastfeeding themselves. Bulstrode Whitelock's wet nurse was the daughter of the woman who had nursed his father, a fact so important it featured prominently in his father's diary and then, in turn, Bulstrode's own telling of his life.[173] Nurses were part of the family, often in a very real sense living in the household, during the time they were nursing, although they quite obviously did not have the same privileges as those who were blood related. Medical writers noted that wet nurses were bound to the family in perpetuity. The practice of hiring former servants to nurse children recurs frequently in correspondence. Dafeny Lightfoot had nursed Thornton's sister Catherine Danby after her birth and performed other kinds of work for the family over Alice's lifetime. Ralph Josselin asked Lydia, 'my former servant', to breastfeed his daughter in 1644.[174] It is no coincidence that there was considerable overlap between those who took on domestic labour as servants and those who were wet nurses. It was similar work both in terms of remuneration, social value and involved women working for the ascendancy of elite families.

Elite families were particularly unconcerned about the prospect of a wet nurse having to wean other children, including her own, in order to nurse their new charges. Alice Kenyon's sister wrote to her in 1667 'concerning a Nurss for you'. The trail of her enquiry reveals how many people might be involved in making recommendations for a wet nurse and the complexity of what made

171 Ann Fanshawe, *The Memoirs of Ann, Lady Fanshawe, Wife of Sir Richard Fanshawe, Bart. 1600–72, Reprinted from the Original MS. in the Possession of Mr Evelyn John Fanshawe of Parsloes* (London, 1907), 47.

172 Laura Gowing, 'The Haunting of Susan Lay: Servants and Mistresses in Seventeenth-Century England', *Gender & History* 14, no. 2 (2002): 183.

173 Whitelocke, 'Copy from my Father's George Whitelocke's Diary', MS Add 5372, fol. 3.

174 Ralph Josselin, 31 August 1646, *The Diary of Ralph Josselin, 1616–1683*, ed. Alan Macfarlane (Oxford: Oxford University Press, 1991), 68.

a good one. She had asked 'broth[e]r Parson' to 'get my Sist[e]r to inquire of that w[hi]ch was with her in the Moneth' but she could not yet 'giue you an account of her'. The day before she had heard from someone that one of Alice's neighbours 'now gives suck & her children is ould inough to weane', although she 'hath but on[e] brest' that was suitable. She directed Alice towards 'Ralph Horrids wife' who could give her an 'account' of this woman, who was herself John Partington's wife. If that 'will not fitt theres a very hansome & likely woman w[hi]ch is cosen [cousin] to them & Lives near Coliarst w[hi]ch will take yo[u]r childe if you cannot oth[e]r ways provid[e] better to your Likeing'. She reassured her, 'truly this I durst well put a childe to if I needed a Nurss'. She was the Kenyon's own 'Milk Woman', or wet nurse, and she promised that she would 'not come forth herself if she take yo[u]r child' – presumably meaning the nurse would ensure she did not get pregnant while feeding. Crucially the family were 'able people & doeth it not for Need', even though this woman had already nursed one or two children 'besides her own'. If Alice still wanted to have a nurse in her own home, she would have to keep enquiring.[175] For Alice it was preferrable if the nurse was not feeding out of financial need and therefore greedy or mercenary. This would mean the nurse would be more likely to engage with her charge or charges in an affectionate and loving manner.

Nurses were often employed for a matter of days or weeks, but sometimes they cared for babies for years. They were thus central actors in the upbringing of elite children and their medical care. The casebooks of Simon Forman and Richard Napier reveal that nurses often brought their charges with them when they received treatment, or when the infant itself was unwell. Goody Bette, for example, came to Napier in 1615 with the child she was nursing and its mother.[176] Eight-day-old Alexander Allen was taken to Simon Forman by his nurse in 1596.[177] The next day, he died of his unspecified illness. Robert Scrope's wet nurse came to Napier herself when the child was nineteen weeks old to inquire after his health.[178] A 'woman of Stratford' brought her eleven-week-old baby to Napier in 1622 because it was 'very unquiet & crying' and would 'sucke other bodyes teates but not hers'. Napier recorded in the margins that 'a woman' was suspected of bewitching the nurse or the child.[179] Ann Gale, a wet nurse, visited Napier on a number of occasions about a curse that she perceived had been placed on her by Ellen Warner; it seemed to have prevented her from suckling. She asked in 1621 'whether she must be nurse' to Lady Gosticke's 'sonne next child'. The Gostickes, we learn in a later

[175] Dorothy Lagoe [?] to Alice Kenyon, 7 November 1667, Lancashire Record Office, Preston, DDKe9/92/3/15

[176] CASE42419, CB. [177] CASE534, CB. [178] CASE13787, CB.

[179] CASE54777, CB.

consultation, were her landlords, and she returned five months later now nursing the new baby. The child had 'Drouped' for a fortnight since she 'chid' or disagreed with Warner.[180] In 1623, she was nursing another Gosticke child and asked on 24 March whether 'the child be likely to prosper', and again on 26 whether she ought to wean it, owing to her own poor health.[181] Gale's pattern of consultation reveals how taxing and time-consuming suckling a child as a wet nurse might be, even if this work was taken on to supplement or replace domestic work. Her initial question suggests a degree of trepidation about taking on the feeding of her landlords' child – perhaps not only was the baby's health and her reputation on the line, but her housing and current or future employment with the family too.

Elite families expected that the wet nurses they hired would prioritise their children but only in the ways they wanted, and like midwives, that they would uphold family secrets. The expectation that wet nurses would love their charges children but happily give them up when the parents decided to wean or shift the child points to the considerable emotional and bodily toll that this kind of caring took on the women who did it. These women in turn had to represent themselves as doing this job out of compassion rather than need, or face losing their livelihood. For Alice Kenyon's sister, it was barely notable that one of the women suggested would wean her own children in order to feed Alice's. Wet nursing must have defined women's lives and bodies for the time they were feeding whether they remained within their own home or moved to live with their employers. The example of Nurse Lucas in the Mordaunt correspondence suggests that the emotional tie between nurse and baby, although initially beneficial, could later become a nuisance to parents. Lucas' distress and her mother's insistence that she should keep nursing despite the difficulties she was experiencing highlights that this relationship was often seen as a purely financial one when it benefitted the parents to disregard the emotional ties of the wet nurse. At other times, as we have seen, elite parents went to great lengths to ensure such emotional ties between wet nurse and child as it clothed a commercial transaction in the veneer of familial love.

Hiring a wet nurse, at times, complicated the display of godly parenting. Breastfeeding was commonly used as an analogy in sermons and other religious writing for the ways a good Christian received and imbibed the word of God. Anne Bathurst described in her meditations how she was 'as pent milk in the breast ready to be poured forth & dilated into shee from whom my fullness flows with such fullnes & plentitude & pleas'd when eas'd'.[182] The labour and work of others sat uncomfortably alongside narratives about the family more

[180] CASE53375, CB. [181] CASE55844, CASE55880, CB.

[182] Anne Bathurst, 'Meditations and Visions 1693–1696', Bodleian Library, Oxford, MS Rawl D 1263, fol.1.

generally – both that generation would be difficult and that healthy lusty infants did not spring from their godliness and status. Although servants and other people paid to do work living in the household were considered 'family' in linguistic terms, they were not afforded the same consideration or status. The work of these individuals in making a healthy, lusty baby and perpetuating the family was rarely acknowledged, and serves as an extreme example of the ways in which medical bodywork when performed by women was largely invisible.

Conclusion

Although there were few detailed descriptions of the laborious and repetitive care that took place in the days, weeks and months after birth to foster newborn health in family paperwork, medical writers were thorough, didactic and inflexible in the care they suggested. A healthy baby was perceived as one that was large, active and initially loud. It should sleep plentifully, begin to resist being bound in swaddling clothes, and suck enthusiastically and plentifully. Medical writers often represented fulfilment of what appears to have been an exhaustive and all-encompassing regimen of care as simply 'good' motherhood or the bare minimum for nurses, midwives or servants. The lustiness of the infant had a bearing on stories that families told about their own ascendancy and godliness. The stakes then of securing infant survival and health after birth were high. Hiring others both complicated the view that childbearing was something mothers took on gladly, and allowed generation to appear and be less taxing. It is for this reason there is a quietness around these practitioners in medical texts, and in different ways, in family paperwork. This was no more obvious than in advice about breastfeeding. Clinton addressed those women who would not suckle their own children because 'it is troublesome; that it is noisome to ones clothes; that it makes one looke old'. These were 'uncomely, and unchristian' reasons and testament to 'unmotherly affection, idlenesse, desire to have liberty to gadd from home, pride, foolish finenesse, lust, wantonnesse, & the like evils'.[183] As we have seen, it was almost always infant or maternal illness that provoked families to seek a nurse, but when they did so, they did not afford these women the same spiritual and moral praise as they afforded elite mothers who fed their own children. Even the work of these mothers often proved uninteresting beyond proving a kind of sacrificial and bodily devotion to the family in these accounts.

Rocking, cleaning, clothing, settling, feeding and nursing infants into good health was laborious work. This work sat alongside the other kinds of

[183] Clinton, *The Countesse of Lincolnes Nurserie*.

domestic, bodily and medical labour that wives and other women took on within households. The emphasis on encouraging babies to lose heat and moisture points to the ways their bodies and futures were not secure until long after birth. As accounts of feeding indicate, weaning did not mark the end of this work or this period of uncertainty. Parents and nurses often chose to wean infants when they were unwell. Teething marked a particularly anxious moment – so much so that 'teeth' was listed as a disease or cause of death in Graunt's *Bills of Mortality.*[184] Bearing children was a fluid, complicated and family-driven experience that demanded quiet and intensive labour not just from mothers but also from other women who were not related to the family. It structured and conditioned everyday life for men and women, albeit often in ways that defied the strict boundaries of domestic labour and interests.

[184] John Graunt, *Natural and Political Observations Mentioned in a following Index, and Made upon the Bills of Mortality* (London: 1662).

Conclusion

As the judgement on the Earl of Macclesfield's bill to dissolve his marriage to Anne was read out in the House of Lords in 1698, it was not just the couple's friends, family members and servants that would have been waiting with baited breath for the result. The case and Anne's actions threatened to unpick the glue that upheld godly and elite society together: female procreative labour, and the push and pull between discretion and display. Even though the fact that the pair had been separated for ten years, the Earl and many of the peers who voted for the divorce bill including archbishops, bishops, marquises, earls, viscounts and barons thought that Anne still had a responsibility to appear to fulfil the role of a good wife and mother. This was despite the fact that servants had told the court repeatedly how the earl had often refused to speak to his wife when they did live together and had also refused to visit her chamber, let alone sleep next to her. Servants were frequently asked in the case to attest to whether the earl and his wife had behaved in ways that were honourable and fulfilled what were the perceived inviolable duties of spouses. This, however, was highly gendered. Servants were asked to comment on whether the earl had provided for his wife appropriately or whether he had spoken to his wife in ways that, as one long-time servant of the family, William Buckingham, commented, showed 'Respect' and him to be 'a Man of Quality'. Buckingham also told the court that he and all the fellow 'ffamily'(household including servants) had been ordered to 'shew her all the respect in the World and so We did'.[1] Another household servant, Mary Wethersby, told the court that Anne had lived in the Macclesfield's family estate 'in my Opinion as if she had bin the first subject of England, she had all things she Desired & never ask'd for anything but she had it'.[2] As one of several printed accounts of the case relayed, it was wholly unacceptable to many that because of 'his Wife's Fault he [Charles] should be deprived of the common Privilege of every Freeman in the World, to have an Heir of his own Body to inherit was he

[1] 'Earl of Macclesfield Divorce Act', 18 February 1697, Parliamentary Archives, HL/PO/JO/10/1/496/1197, fol. 88.

[2] *Ibid.*, 18 February 1697, fol. 84.

possesses either of Honour or Estate: Or that his only Brother should lose his Claim to both, and have his Birthright sacrific'd to the Lady Maclesfeld's Loose Life'. Not only would it be 'a most unreasonable hardship upon the Earl' but 'the greatest Wrong'.[3]

The case writ large the greatest fears that many middling and elite families had about generation: that as much as it was central to the perpetuation of the Church and the family, it also could bring profound and troubling domestic disorder. Having babies, this book finds, in a prescribed way, was fundamental not only to male status but the entire social apparatus of honour and estate in the period, across society at different levels but especially for the aristocracy and burgeoning middling sort. Anne's 'Loose Life' decimated not just her soon-to-be ex-husband's reputation but it reverberated right through the whole family and elite society more broadly. Anne's crime was not solely taking a lover, or even getting pregnant with his child, but behaving in a way that made this obvious to London society. A big part of this was keeping her pregnancy secret from her family, delivering the child in a way that excluded her and her husband's family, arranging the material aspects of her birth without recourse to her husband, and perhaps worst of all, naming her children after herself and her lover. These actions violated the idealised expectations of the household, godly maternity and the ways in which women ought to, as one seventeenth-century correspondent called it 'Multiplying in the World', or in a way that displayed and confirmed the family's ascendancy.[4] Anne's behaviour must have been a stark reminder to elite families of the ways that women's bodies could threaten their grasp on respectability with very little recourse to remedy. The successful dissolution of the marriage must have been a deeply comforting outcome for many.

But whilst Anne might have represented some kind of anti-mother in gossipy print of the period, we have heard in this book how easy it was for most women to transgress the restrictive model of godly and careful childbearing furthered in medical and religious prescriptive texts of the period. Ideally, early modern women would get pregnant easily and quickly; be constantly attentive to their bodies and minds; keep assiduous records; struggle through the discomfort and pain of pregnancy and birth with forbearance; accurately pinpoint when they would deliver; allow their husbands to coordinate the collection of things for birth but only items that were strictly necessary; travel a substantial distance to give birth in their or their husband's family's home; deliver a large, lusty (preferably male) baby painfully but without complication; and rest for a month and then wholly return to their normal lives and selves, including swiftly getting pregnant again. These normative perspectives

[3] *The Earl of Maclesield's Case* (London: 1697–1698), 4.
[4] Earl of Northampton to earl of Dorset, 12 January 1656, KHLC, U269/C86/3.

are also keen to point out that during this time babies had to be carefully watched, held, rocked, rubbed, bathed, changed and suckled, although one does not always have a sense from these texts who completed these tasks. Some of this work was meant to be done publicly with the regular intrusion of family members in this decision-making, and these labours were writ large in family paperwork, whilst other bits were deemed more favourable to be performed discreetly and without fuss.

Examining family archives as a whole has revealed many moments of tension in which the practice of making babies failed to live up to the expectations of prescriptive authors. So too has it also pointed to a profound anxiety that male and female family members felt about the process, the unknowability of procreation and people's attempts to impose order and understanding on it. Childbearing was habitually and almost exclusively represented as women's work in the letters, diaries, recipe books and almanacs that elite families compiled and were careful to keep for posterity. But this was often a fantasy. Male family members were everywhere in the experience of having babies, and they often put considerable physiological, emotional and financial efforts into securing positive procreative outcomes. This was in equal parts motivated by how central childbearing was to male status and honour in an individual sense, and by its prominence in larger familial narratives about godliness and fruitfulness.

The idea that men 'got' women pregnant and furnished them with material goods to 'bring' their conceptions to term that was often expressed in family correspondence is undermined by the substantial amount of medical work that men took on in households. This finding supports the work of historians who have pointed out that although it did not always meet prescriptive ideals of the division of domestic labour, medical practice and knowledge-gathering were often a collective exercise.[5] There are hints revealed in manuscript family archives of male family members desperately and secretly seeking treatment for their own perceived impotence and weak seed, of predicting when and how women might give birth, what babies might look like, who should feed the baby, and what had caused miscarriages. Many men were so interested and invested in procreation that they kept records of their wives' menstrual cycles, potential pregnancy symptoms and when (and where) they had sex. Many husbands, fathers, uncles and sons felt entitled and comfortable weighing in on important medical decisions with practitioners and were at home to facilitate

[5] Leah Astbury and Elaine Leong, 'Medical Knowledge and Practice' in Amanda Capern (ed.), *Routledge History of Women in Early Modern Europe* (Abingdon: Routledge, 2019); Elaine Leong, 'Collecting Knowledge for the Family: Recipes, Gender and Practical Knowledge in the Early Modern English Household', *Centaurus,* 55, no. 2 (2013): 81–103; Lisa Smith, 'The Relative Duties of a Man: Domestic Medicine in England and France, ca. 1685–1740', *Journal of Family History* 31, no. 3 (2006): 237–256.

the birth of healthy infants and maternal survival. They were well versed what a healthy, godly and ideal pregnancy should look and feel like, and authoritatively interpreted bodily signs such as large bellies or exuberant kicks from the baby within. Added to this, men were key negotiators in obtaining linens, clothes, alcohol, practitioners and other things in the months leading up to a woman's 'reckoning'. In this way, this book does not simply suggest that childbirth was important to men but that the medical and social rituals involved men in a very tangible and practical way, even if this did not always sit easily with the stories they wanted to tell about their effortless virility.

This book's findings also have implications for our understandings of the early modern family more broadly too. It suggests that within elite society particularly the importance of homosocial spaces and customs may have been overstated. Procreation continues to be a prime example of female friendship and solidarity in accounts of community and its centrality to life and status in early modern England. Bernard Capp thus notes that childbirth and child rearing represented effectively 'a semi-separate female domain, a subculture which existed uneasily and at times almost invisibly alongside the dominant, masculine culture of the age' that provided a 'refuge from patriarchal authority and a means to contain and accommodate it'.[6] Likewise, Tim-Reinke Williams suggests that motherhood 'brought women together since female friends, relatives and neighbours shared childcare duties'.[7] As we have heard, Linda Pollock and Laura Gowing have convincingly shown the ways in which female alliances, particularly during childbearing, were not always convivial and supportive.[8]

Making Babies n Early Modern England instead confirms that as historians of masculinity have pointed out, domesticity and domestic activities were intrinsic to male status. Childbirth and the medical work it demanded was no different, and as Joanne Begiato has commented, this co-dependency in which male status depended on household order often 'worked against male autonomy'.[9] Perhaps the greatest evidence of this instability and interleaving of masculinity and the family into childbirth practices is in the fact that it was

[6] Bernard Capp, 'Separate Domains? Women and Authority in Early Modern England', in *The Experience of Authority in Early Modern England* (Basingstoke: Macmillan, 1996), 117–145, 139.

[7] Tim Reinke-Williams, *Women, Work and Sociability in Early Modern London,* Genders and Sexualities in History (Basingstoke: Macmillan, 2014), 158.

[8] Laura Gowing, 'Secret Births and Infanticide in Seventeenth-Century England', *Past & Present* 156 (1997): 87–115; Laura Gowing, *Common Bodies: Women, Touch and Power in Seventeenth-Century England* (New Haven, CT: Yale University Press, 2003); Linda A. Pollock, 'Childbearing and Female Bonding in Early Modern England', *Social History* 22, no. 3 (1997): 286–306.

[9] Joanne Bailey, *Unquiet Lives: Marriage and Marriage Breakdown in England, 1660–1800* (Cambridge: Cambridge University Press, 2003), 199.

almost always men that kept records of women's bodies. Tawny Paul notes of the eighteenth century that although men frequently kept accounts of their wives', servants' and children's bodies and behaviours, the diaries and account books of women rarely fuss over the work of their husbands in the same way.[10] In drawing these conclusions, this book builds on the work of historians of the family who point to its fundamental instability in this period. Notably, examining familial paperwork reveals the many individuals like Mary Wethersby and William Buckingham, servants in the Macclesfields' household, who laboured to further wealthier and more ascendant families at the expense of their own. This is most poignantly apparent in the work of nurses who often kept middling and elite babies in their own homes or resided in their employers' home for years. Naomi Tadmor's work has been instrumental in pointing to the ways that wealthier households considered these employees part of the 'family' in affective and practical terms, albeit in unequal ways.[11] Considering the work of bearing and rearing children, this becomes an even more important intervention. Although family may have been central in the organisation and experience of daily life over and above community in the period, this was an invented category and had to be constantly remade, and by others who were not blood related.

Perhaps the most confronting and difficult take away from a deepened historical understanding of bearing children within households is the ways in which the contours of the cultural conversation in early modern England might not be too unfamiliar to a contemporary reader. While writing this book, it seemed everyday there was a new study or news article about how parental, but mostly maternal, behaviour might subtly secure poor outcomes for children, amounting to what has often been called 'intensive parenting'. Diet during pregnancy, sleep training and breastfeeding are, like in the seventeenth century, key topics that are also felt to have a bearing on one's own identity as well as the future wellbeing of one's child. Ironically for this book, one of the underpinning narratives of this style of parenting according to the sociologist Charlotte Faircloth is that this very period – the pre-modern one – represents a haven of natural birthing and parenting choices that we would do well to return to now. This is seen most powerfully in discussions about maternal breastfeeding and the ways in which many parents are made to feel inadequate, embarrassed and secretive about the need or the choice to bottle feed infants. The key to good practice in the present day is represented as being able to tap into one's intuition (of which women had greater access to in the seventeenth century),

[10] K. Tawny Paul, 'Accounting for Men's Work: Multiple Employments and Occupational Identities in Early Modern England', *History Workshop Journal* 85 (2018): 39.

[11] Naomi Tadmor, *Family and Friends in Eighteenth-Century England: Household, Kinship and Patronage* (Cambridge: Cambridge University Press, 2001).

which is additionally revealed through scientific findings and validated by evolutionary as well as historical 'facts'.[12] In contrast, we see that cultural norms profoundly conditioned what was perceived as correct medical and spiritual practice in the early modern period. In particular, what was 'natural' was similarly hotly contested in scientific literature and in familial correspondence. They too were confronted with the ways in which their bodies did not always map onto what medical professionals said they ought to be able to do in breastfeeding and ministering to their infants. In many ways, these values and normative models are inherited from the medieval and early modern period, and thus it might not be a surprise that these conversations have continued for hundreds of years. Other parts of the early modern experience, like understanding birth marks as the result of unsatisfied cravings or babies being gestated on the left or right side of the womb according to their sex, are alien to a modern reader. It is this mix of familiarity and unfamiliarity that might also help in understanding the modern impulse to tie reproductive experiences and labour to identity and in turn making it seem less inevitable or inimical.

This book has shown the ways that generation was central to family life. It was long, fluid and defied specificity despite the certainty that individuals sought to impose upon it. It demanded considerable financial, intellectual, practical and medical investment from family members, but the bulk of this labour fell on women. Family paperwork is forthcoming about some aspects of this process – namely the appearance of women's changing bodies, the outward signs of what the unborn child might be like, details of when and where women might give birth and the materials they might need to do so safely – and secretive about others. Men's generative failures, excessive pain, difficult and prolonged recoveries, the tedium of daily childcare, the emotional difficulties that men and women might feel after delivery or the death of mother or child were all left out at times because they were uninteresting and at other times because it was thought it reflected poorly on the family as a whole. As people made babies, they also made and remade favourable narratives about the family (their own or the one they worked for). Whilst this system benefited husbands, fathers and other male members of a given family, not everyone reaped the personal rewards of their labour.

[12] Charlotte Faircloth, *Militant Lactivism? Attachment Parenting and Intensive Motherhood in the UK and France* (Oxford: Berghahn Books, 2013).

Bibliography

Primary

Manuscripts

Bedfordshire and Luton Archives and Record Service, Bedford

Anne Burgoyne, 'Household account-book Burgoyne family 1679–1818', X143/1.

Blanch Hooker, 'Recipe book, 1690', GY7/2.

Elizabeth Danielle, 'Elizabeth Daniell her Booke of Reciepts 1660', LL17/270.

Elizabeth Welby, 'Her Booke 1682', GY7/1.

Hester Benyon, 'Hester Benyon Her Booke', c. 1701, GY7/3.

Lucy Wright, 'Recipe book c. 1700', LL17/271.

Mary, Baroness Lucas (?), 'Account book, 1678–1695', L31/122.

'Private letters of St John family of Bletsoe 1570–1699', J1400–1486.

'Symcotts family medical letters and case books 1628–92', X 125.

Beinecke Library, New Haven, CT

Anne Wentworth, 'Commonplace book', Osborn b285.

Anonymous, 'Commonplace book, 1599–1608', Osborn b106.

Anonymous, 'Midwife's Diary, 1694–1716', MS Rawl D 1141.

Dionys Fitzherbert, MS Bodl 154.

Dorothy Frances Feilding, 'Miscellany', Osborn b226.

E. Eyre and Lady Pakington, MS Add B 58.

Elizabeth Jekyll, 'Spiritual Journal', Osborn b221.

Jane Truesdale, 'Commonplace book of prose extracts and sermons', Osborn b188.

John Fairfax and Mary Hase, 'Sermons, c. 1650', Osborn b253.

Lady Anne Clifford, 'Account book, 1600–1602', Osborn b27.

Sarah Savage, 'Diary 1714–23', Ms Eng misc e 331.

Ursula Wyvill, 'Devotional Miscellany, 1662–1672', Osborn b222.

Bodleian Library, Oxford

Anne Bathurst, MS Rawl D 1262.
Anne Bathurst, 'Meditations and Visions, 1693–1696', MS Rawl D 1263.
Anne Bathurst, MS Rawl D 1338.
'Diary of an anonymous midwife, 1694–1716', MS Rawl D 1141.
Elizabeth and Anne Delaval, MS Rawl D 78.
Mary Arthington, 'Letter book c. 1680–1700', MS Add A 119.
Mary Honywood, MS Rawl D 102.
'Papers of the Herrick family of Leicestershire, 16th–19th century', MSS. Eng. hist. b. 216, c. 474–484.

Bristol Record Office, Bristol

Correspondence the Smyth Family of Ashton Court, 1548–1642, DD/PH.

British Library, London

Alice Thornton, 'Meditations', Add MS 88897/1–2.
'Copy from my Father's George Whitelocke's Diary', Add MS 5372.
'Correspondence with H. Oxenden and his wife, 1633–1639', Add MS 28003.
D'Ewes family correspondence, Harley 382.
Dering family correspondence Stowe 744.
Edward Poeton, 'The Midwives Deputie or a help for such as are not well furnished with knowledge concerning the misteries of that profession, gathered out of sundry authorized and authentict authors by Edward Poeton of Petworth Licentiate in physic and chyrurgery', Sloane MS 1954.
Elizabeth Egerton, 'Devotional Pieces by Elizabeth, Countess of Bridgewater', Egerton MS 607.
Gawdy family correspondence, MS Add 36989.
Hatton-Finch family correspondence 1600–1678, Add MS 29571.
Isabella Twysden almanacs, Add MS 34169–34172.
Jane Shrewsbury, 'Theological tracts', Harley MS 6826.
Joseph Binns, 'Medical Casebook, 1633–63', Sloane MS 153.
Lady Brilliana Harley, 'Medical recipes', Egerton MS 2214.
Mary Rich, 'Diary July 1666–March 1669', Add MS 27351.
Mary Rich, 'Some Specialities in the Life of M Warwicke', Add MS 27357.
Simonds D'Ewes, 'Account of his life by Symonds d'Ewes', Harley MS 646.
'Sir Philip Gawdy, letters to his family c. 1578–1617', Add MS 27395.
Trumbull papers 1672–1692, Add MS 72516.
Wentworth Correspondence, Add MS 22225.

Brotherton Library, Leeds

Dame Mary Lister, 'Household Book, 1623–1635', MS 621.
'Recipe book, c. 1651–1700, once in the possession of Gertrude Holcroft', MS 687.
'Recipe book eighteenth century', MS 485.

Cheshire Archives and Local Studies, Chester

City of Chester Assembly files, Mayors orders, ZAB/1/178.
Letters and papers relating to the Henry family, 1651–1733, DBASTEN 1–20.
Sarah Savage, 'Diary, 1686–88', Z/D/Basten/8.

Chetham's Library, Manchester
Edmund Harrold, 'Diary, 1712–16', Mun A.2.137.

Clark Library, University of California–Los Angeles
'Accounts and memoranda in Goldsmith's 1682 Almanac', t AY751. Z7 1682.
'Commonplace book', MS.1945.004.
'Commonplace book, ca. 1713–1740', MS.1982.001.
'Commonplace book 1636–1677', MS.1950.024.
'Cross family recipe book, 1724–1740', f MS.1986.002.
Elenor Poole and John Cobb, 'her Booke 1733', MS.2003.001.
Joanna Suddell, 'Recipe book, 1688–1751', MS.1950.023.
John Darracott, 'Diary, 1707–30', MS.1950.010.
Mariabella Charles, 'Cookery recipes and medical cures', MS.1950.009.
'Medical and culinary recipes, 1663', AY751.W55 1663.
Samuel Jeake, 'A diary of the actions and accidents of my life: tending partly to observe and memorize ye Providences therein manifested, and partly to investigate ye measure of time in astronomical directions and to determine the astral causes & c, 1694', MS.1959.006.

Cumbria Record Office, Kendal
Correspondence of Sir Daniel Fleming, WDRY/4 and 5.
Daniel Fleming, 'A Booke of my owne Receipts and Disbursem[en]ts 1656–1688', WDRY/Box 119.
Elizabeth Thompson, 'Diary', WDCR/11/60–61.
Elizabeth Tyndale, 'Recipe book, 1770', WDDF/Box 20/1.

Derby Record Office, Matlock
Chandos-Pole-Gell Correspondence, D258/.

Durham Cathedral Library and Archives
Alice Thornton, 'Thornton's Memoirs', Comber 7.

Firestone Library, University of Princeton, Princeton, NJ
'17th century recipe book', RTC01, MS 214.
Edmund Kershaw, 'Commonplace book concerning Law and Medicine in England', C0199 no. 553.
Elizabeth Isham, 'My Booke of Rememenberance', RTC01 no. 62.
'Lady Sandys her receipts', RTC01, no. 208.
Mary Whitelocke, 'Advice for Her Son Samuel, RTC01 MS 226.

Folger Shakespeare Library, Washington, DC
Cavendish Talbot Manuscripts 1333–1705, Cavendish-Talbot MS.
Rebeckah Winche, Receipt book c. 1666, V.b.366.

Gloucestershire Record Office, Gloucester
John Clifford, 'Account book', D149/A26.

Harris Manchester College, Oxford
Sarah Savage, 'Notebooks', MSS Savage 1–5.
Sarah Savage (transcriber), 'Notes on three sermons by Mr Dawson, 1737', Henry MS misc 4.

Hertfordshire Record Office, Hertford
Memorandum book of Sir William Cowper, Penshanger D/EP F25.
Penshanger family correspondence, D/EP F23.
Sarah Cowper, 'Commonplace book 1637–1710', D/EP F37.
Sarah Cowper, Diaries, D/EP F29–F35, vols 1–7.
Wittewronge Correspondence, DE/LwF28 and 29.

Huntington Library, San Marino, CA
Countess of Huntingdon, 'Commonplace book', HM15369.
Edmund Herbert, 'Expense Accounts, 1708–1733', msshe 100, 1–16.
Egerton family papers, EL.
'Godly Observations, With Maxims, Prayers, And other good Notions', mssHM 200.
Hastings family papers, HA.
Magdalen Coward, 'Booke of Reciepts, November 1695', MS 88.
Sir Edward Dering, 'Commonplace book 1656–1662', mssHM 41536.
Sir William Ashcombe, 'Memorable accidents, 1561–1625', HM 30665.
Thomas Brugis, Medical treatise describing illnesses and remedies, formerly laid into 'Vade Mecum or a companion for a Chirurgion', HM 59539.

The Keep, East Sussex Record Office, Brighton
Archive of the Ashburnham family, ASH.
Correspondence of the Roberts family, the Temple family, the Busbridge family, the Farnden family and other correspondence, DUN 51/62.
Papers of the Jeake family of Rye, 1558–c. 1700, FRE.
Roberts and Farnden families papers, DUN 52/10.

Kent History and Library Centre, Maidstone
Edward Dering, 'Diary, 1673–1675', U2981 F1.
Elizabeth James, 'Diary, 1750', U1961 F1.
Elizabeth Turner, 'Journal', U1015 F27.
Jeremiah Cliff, 'Surgeon and apothecary's diary, 1712–42', P362/28/4.
Leticia Child, 'Letters', U269 C108.
Rachel Fane, Notebooks, U269/F38/1–4.
Sackville family papers, U269/C12–C275.

Lambeth Palace Library, London
Talbot papers, 1506–1612, MS 3205.

Lancashire Record Office, Preston
Papers of the Hulton Family, DDHu 47.
Papers of the Kenyon family, DDKe/9.

Lincolnshire Archives, Lincoln

Family and estate papers of the Massingberg Mundy family, MASS 23–28.

Papers of the Monson family, MON 7–14.

Longleat House, Longleat

Thynne family papers, TH.

Magdalen College Library, Oxford

Bagot family correspondence, 1680–1754, MC: P287/C1–C5.

National Archives, Kew

State Papers, Sir John Gordon to Duke of Newcastle, 31 December 1746, SP 36/90/2/92.

National Library of Scotland, Edinburgh

Lady Anne Halkett, 'Meditations, prayers, and a mother's legacy, c. 1651–1656', MS 6489.

'Meditations 1659–1660', MS 6490.

'Meditations and prayers, 1660–1663', MS 6491.

'Meditations, 1667–1671', MS 6492.

'Meditations 1673–1675', MS 6493.

'Meditations 1676–1678', MS 6494.

'Meditations, 1679–1681', MS 6495.

'Meditations, 1683–1685', MS 6496.

'Meditations, 1686/7–1688', MS 6497.

'Meditations, 1688–1690', MS 6498.

Margaret Cunningham, 'The true copy of a letter yt Lady Margarett Cunningham wrote to her husband the Master of Evandale', MS 906.

National Records of Scotland, Edinburgh

Letters to Isabella, Lady Henderson of Fordell, from Jane Cochrane, her sister [later Countess of Dundonald], GD172/1330.

Papers of the Campbell Family, Earls of Breadalbane, GD112/3/92.

Papers of the Cunninghame Graham family of Ardoch, Dunbartonshire, 'Medical recipe for inducing conception', GD22/3/817.

Papers of the Leslie family, Earls of Leven and Melville, 'Letters from Margaret, Countess of Wemyss, to George, Earl of Melville, David, Earl of Leven, and her daughter, the Countess of Leven 1690–1698', GD26/13/401.

'Medical prescriptions for the Leven and Melville family, 1661–1702', GD26/6/207.

Papers of the Maule Family, Earls of Dalhousie, 'Notebook containing Roman Catholic prayers and notes for a nurse or midwife, eighteenth century, GD45/26/149.

Papers of the Oglivy family, Earls of Seafield, GD248/566/84.

Records of the Episcopal Church of Scotland, 'Note on Mrs Tulloch's pregnancy, and copy of a note sending her advice and shoes, 1721', CH12/12/795.

New York Public Library, New York
Abigail Rand, 'Her Book', v. 7.
'Book of cookery recipes', v. 6.
'Collection of household recipes, miscellaneous entries, 17th and 18th century', v. 9.
'Collection of medical and cookery recipes', v. 8.
Hester Denbigh, 'Cookery and medical recipes', v. 11.
Joanne Yate, 'Receipt Book ye 1st 1682', v. 3.
Lady Anne Morton, 'The Ladey Mortons Book of Receipts, most of which shee hath experimented her selfe and are uerey good 1693', b. 4.
Lady Anne Percy, 'Cookery book c. 1650', b.2.
Mary Bromehead, 'Her book given her by Aunt 1761', v. 13.
Mary Davies, 'Her booke 1684', v. 5.

Norfolk Record Office, Norwich
Campling family papers, MC 44.

North Yorkshire Record Office, Northallerton
Chaytor family correspondence, ZQH 9.
Danby family correspondence, MISC 2087.

Northamptonshire Record Office, Northampton
Correspondence of the Finch Hatton family, FH.
Correspondence of the Isham family, IC/1–2000.
Elizabeth Isham, 'Diary', IL 3365.

Northumberland Archives, Ashington
Delaval family papers, 1DE and 2DE.

Parliamentary Archives, Westminster
'An Act for dissolving ye Marriage between Charles Earle of Maclesfield and Anne his Wife and to Illegitmate the Children of the said Anne', HL/PO/JO/10/1/496/1197.

Somerset Heritage Centre, Taunton
Smyth family correspondence, DD/PH.

Staffordshire Record Office, Stafford
Jerningham family recipe book, D641/3/H/3/1.
Thomas Congreve, 'Commonplace book including diary entries, 1585–1611', D1057.
William Paget, Correspondence, Paget MS D603/K/2/1.

Sheffield Record Office, Sheffield
Strafford papers, Volume 22 b.
William Wentworth's advice to his son, WWM/StrP/40/1–2.

Sterling Library, New Haven, CT
Alice Thornton, Microfilm of 'A booke of remembrances of all the remarkable deliverances of my selfe, Husband & Children wth: theire

births, & other remarks conserning my selfe & Family beginning from the year 1625', FILM MISC 326.

University of Cambridge Library, Cambridge

Isaac Archer, 'Diary', Add 8499 G.

Philip Henry, 'Sermon Book', Add MS 7338.

University of Glasgow Library, Glasgow

Betty Maxwell, 'Account book', MS Murray 271.

Mary Harrison, 'Her Book 1692', MS Ferguson 61.

'Recipe book', MS Ferguson 15.

'Recipe book', MS Gen 575.

'Recipe book', MS Gen 831.

University of Nottingham Library, Nottingham

Portland Papers, PW1.

Warwickshire Record Office, Warwick

Elizabeth Barkham, 'Recipe book 10 June 1664', CR 2981/6/3/43.

Feilding of Newnham correspondence, CR 2017/c1–2.

Mordaunt family correspondence, CR 1368/vols 1–4.

Wellcome Library, London

'Boyle family recipe book, 1675–c.1710', MS 1340.

Elizabeth Okeover and others receipt book, MS3712.

'English Recipe Book, c.1675–c.1800', MS 7721.

Frances Springatt & others, 'Collection of cookery and medical receipts with later additions by several hands 1686–1824', MS 4683.

James Shrowl, 1625–c.1750, MS 749.

Jane Jackson, 'A very shorte and compendious Methode of Phisicke and Chirurgery Containeinge the Cures inwardly and also the Cureinge of all manner of woundes on the bodie together with remedies for the stone and the causes and signes thereof, etc. As also the making of Sirrups and all manner of oyles and waters whatsoever', MS 373.

Johanna St John, 1680, MS 4338/82.

'Johnson Family recipe book, 1694–1831', MS 3082.

Lady Ann Fanshawe, 'Recipe book, 1625–1680', MS 7113.

Matthey family, 'Receipts, 1750–1900?', MS 3498.

'Receipt book, late 17th century–mid 18th century', MS 7997.

Wiltshire and Swindon History Centre, Chippenham

Madam Arundell, 'Book of medicinal recipes, 1676', 2667/12/39.

'Letters, drafts and copies from Mary, Marchioness of Worcester, later Duchess of Beaufort, to her daughter Elizabeth Lady Bruce', 1300/724–748.

Whitby Museum, Whitby

Katherine Manley, 'Diary 1720–1764', WHITM:SOH170.

Printed Primary

Advice to Young Gentlemen; Or, An Answer to the Ladies of London, To the Tune of, The Ladies of London, EBBA 37687. London, 1685–1688.

The Amorous Lady's Garland, Shewing how a young lady going with her maid into St Jame's Market fell in Love with a young butcher, who desir'd him to walk with her into St James's Park, after some discourse they both agreed to be married the next morning, EBBA 34197. London, c. 1740.

An Answer to I Marry and thank ye too: Or, The Lass of Lyn's Sorrowful Lamentation for the Loss of her Maiden-head, EBBA 22080. London, 1657–1696.

Aristotle's Master-piece; Or, The Secrets of Generation Display'd in all the Parts thereof. London: 1684.

Aristotle's Master-piece; Or, The Secrets of Generation Display'd in all the Parts thereof. London, 1690.

Aristotle's Master-piece; Or, The Secrets of Generation Display'd in all the Parts thereof. London, 1697.

The Compleat Midwifes Practice. London, 1656.

A Copy of Verses of a Baker and a Mealman: Giving an Account of their subtle Intreagues with their Mistresses, and how the Mealman got his Maid with Child, EBBA 217071. London, 1690–1700.

The Cruel Mother; being a true relation of the bloody murther committed by M. Cook, upon her dearly beloved child. London, 1670.

Deeds Against Nature, and Monsters By Kinde Tried at the Goale Deliverie of Newgate, at the Sessions of the Old Bailey, the 18. And 19. Of July last, 1614. London, 1614.

A Discourse of the Married and Single Life Wherein, by Discovering the Misery of the One, is Plainely Declared the Felicity of the Other. London, 1621.

The Earl of Maclesield's Case. London, 1697–1698.

The English Midwife Enlarged. London, 1682.

Every Woman Her Own Midwife, or, A Compleat cabinet opened for child-bearing women furnished with directions to prevent miscarriages during the time of breeding. London, 1675.

The Female Doctress, or, Mothers Midnights Cure for Barrenness in Women, Being A True Relation of a Woman that pretended to Cure Women of Barrenness; Especially in the Mint in Southwark. London, 1685.

Fifteen Real Comforts of Matrimony being in requital of the late fifteen sham comforts, with satirical reflections on whoring and the debauchery of this age written by a person of quality of the female sex. London, 1683.

Fumblers-Hall kept and holden in Feeble-Court, at the sign of the Labour-in-vain, in Dee-little-Lane. London, 1675.

'An Homylee of the state of Matrimonie', in *Certaine sermons or homilies appointed to be read in churches in the time of the late Queene Elizabeth of famous memory and now reprinted for the use of private families, in two parts. The second Tome of Homilees, of such matters as were promised, and instituted in the former part of Homilees.* London, 1571.

A Lamentable Ballad of a Lady's Fall, EBBA 31270. London, 1720.

The Lass of Lynns New Joy For finding a Father for her Child. Being a Third Song of Marry and Thank ye too, EBBA 21315. London, 1682–1692.

A new Ballad, containing a communication between the carefull Wife, and the comfortable Husb. touching the common cares and charges of House-hold, EBBA 30031. London, 1640.

A New Ballad of the Midwives Ghost: Who appeared to several People in the House where she formerly lives in Rotten- Row in Holbourn, London, who were all afraid to speak unto her; but she growing very Impetuous, on the 16th of this Instant March, 1680, declarred her mind to the Maid of the said House, who with an Unanimous Spirit adhered to her, EBBA 20763. London, 1680.

Problemes of Aristotle with other Philosophers and Phisitions. Wherein are Contained Diuers Questions, with Their Answers, Touching the estate of Mans Bodie. London, 1595.

Reasons for the Earl of Maclesfeld's Bill in Parliament for Dissolving the Marriage between him and his wife, and illegitimating their spurious issue. 1697.

Scotch Moggy's Misfortune: Together With her cheerful Hops, that Shakum Guie will bury his Wife, and then make Moggy a happy Mother, EBBA 33786. London, 1683–1696.

Some observations made upon the maldiva nut shewing its admirable virtue in giving an easie, safe, and speedy delivery to women in child-bed written by a physitian in the country to Dr Hinton at London, 1663. London, 1694.

Strange Newes out of Kent, of a Monstrous and Misshapen Childe, Borne in Olde Sandwich, upon the 10 of Julie Last. London, 1609.

A True and Perfect Relation of A Horrible Murther, Committed by a Woman in Golden-Lane, on her Neighbour big with-Child, who had borrowed Thirty Shillings of her, who is since fled, EBBA 20741. London, 1678–1680.

A Warning for all Murderers. A Most Rare, Strange, and Wonderfull Accident, Which by Gods Just Judgement was Brought to Passe from Rithin in Wales, EBBA 30323. London, 1601–1640.

A Warning-Piece To All Married Men and Women. Being the Full Confession of Mary Hobry, The French Midwife, Who Murdered her Husband on the 27th January 1687/8. (As also the Cause thereof.) For which she receiv'd Sentence to be Burnt alive: And on Friday the Second Day of March, between the Hours of Ten and Eleven in the Morning, she was drawn upon a Sledge to Leicester-Fields, where she was burnt to Ashes, EBBA 34436. London, 1688.

A Womans Work is never done Here is a Song for Maids to sing, Both in the Winter and the Spring; It is such a pretty conceited thing, Which will much pleasure to them bring. Maids may sit still, go, or run, But a Womans work is never done, EBBA 30355. London, 1654–1663?

Womens Advocate: Or, Fifteen Real Comforts of Matrimony being in requital of the late Fifteen Sham-Comforts with Satyrical Reflections on Whoring, And the Debauchery of this Age Written by a Person of Quality of the Female Sex. London, 1683.

Abott, George. *The Case of Impotency As Debated in England, In that Remarkable Tryal An. 1613. Between Robert, Earl of Essex, and the Lady Frances Howard, who, after Eight Years Marriage, commenc'd a Suit against him for Impotency.* London, 1715.

Adams, Richard. 'How may Child-bearing Women be most encouraged, and supported against, in, and under the hazard of Travail?' In *Continuing of morning-exercise questions and cases of conscience practically resovled by sundry Ministers in October, 1682*. Edited by Samuel Annesley. London, 1683.

Barret, Robert. *A Companion for Midwives, Child-bearing Women, and Nurses Directing them how to Perform their Respective Offices: Together with an Essay, Endeavouring to Shew the Influence of Moral Abuses upon the Health of Children*. London, 1699.

Bentley, Thomas. *The Fift Lampe of Virginitie: Conteining sundrie forms of Christian praiers and meditations, to bee vsed onlie of and for all sorts and degrees of women, in their seuerall ages and callings; as namelie, of Virgins, Wiues, Women with child, Midwiues, Mothers, Daughters, Mistresses, maids, Widowes, and old women*. London, 1582.

Brathwaite, Richard. *The English Gentlewoman drawne out to the full Body: Expressing What Habilliments due best attire her, What Ornaments doe best adorne her, What Complements doe best adorne her, What Complements doe best accomplish her*. London, 1631.

Bright, Timothy. *A Treatise of Melancholie Containing the Causes thereof, & reasons of the Strange Effects it Worketh in Our Minds and Bodies*. London, 1586.

Bryan, John. *Harvest-home being the summe of certain sermons upon Job 5. 2: one whereof was preached at the funeral of Mr. Ob. Musson, an aged Godly minister of the Gospel in the Royally licensed rooms in Coventry: the other since continued upon the subject*. London, 1674.

Buchan, William. *Advice to Mothers, on the subject of their own health, and on the means of promoting the health, strength, and beauty, of their offspring*. Edinburgh, 1804.

Burroughs, Jeremiah. *The Rare Jewel of Christian Contentment. By Jeremiah Burroughs, preacher of the Gospel to two of the greatest congregations in England, viz. Stepney and Cripplegate, London*. London, 1648.

Cadogan, William. *An Essay upon Nursing and the Management of Children, From their Birth to Three Years of Age*. London, 1748.

Chamberlayne, Thomas. *The Complete Midwife's Practice Englarged, In the most Weighty and High Concernments of the Birth of Man Containing a perfect Directory, or Rules for Midwives and Nurses*. London, 1680.

Chevreau, Urbain. *The Mirror of Fortune, or, The true characters of fate and destiny*. London, 1676.

Cholmley, Hugh. *The Memoirs of Sir Hugh Cholmley, Knt. and Bart. Addressed to His Two Sons*. London, 1787.

Clerk, John. *Memoirs of the Life of Sir John Clerk of Penicuik, Baronet*. Edited by John M. Gray. Vol. 13. Scottish Historical Society. Edinburgh: Edinburgh University Press, 1892.

Clifford, Anne. *Anne Clifford's Autobiographical Writing, 1590–1676*. Edited by Jessica L. Malay. Manchester: Manchester University Press, 2018.

The Diaries of Lady Anne Clifford. Edited by D. J. H. Clifford. Stroud: The History Press, 2003.

Clinton, Elizabeth. *The Countesse of Lincolnes Nurserie*. Oxford, 1622.

Crooke, Helkiah. *Mikrokosmographia a description of the body of man*. London, 1615.

Culpeper, Nicholas. *A Directory for Midwives, or, A Guide for Women*. London, 1656.

A Directory for Midwives, or, A Guide for Women. London, 1662.

A Directory for Midwives, or, A Guide for Women. London, 1675.
Daffy, Anthony. *Elixir Salutis: The Choise Drink of Health*. London, 1674.
Dawkes, Thomas. *The Midwife Rightly Instructed*. London, 1736.
Dekker, Thomas. *The Bachelers Banquet: or, A Banquet for Bachelers*. London, 1604.
Denman, Thomas. *An Essay upon Natural Labours*. London, 1786.
D'Ewes, Simonds. *The Autobiography and Correspondence of Sir Simonds D'Ewes: During the Reign of James I and Charles I*. Edited by James Orchard Halliwell. Vol. 2. London: Richard Bentley, 1845.
D. R. *Matrimoniall Honour, or, The Mutuall Crowne and Comfort of Godly, Loyall, and Chaste Marriage*. London, 1642.
Evelyn, John. *Diary of John Evelyn: Vol 3: Kalendarium, 1650–1672*. Edited by E. S. de Beer. Oxford: Oxford University Press, 1955.
Fanshawe, Ann. *The Memoirs of Ann, Lady Fanshawe, Wife of Sir Richard Fanshawe, Bart. 1600–72, Reprinted from the Original MS. in the Possession of Mr Evelyn John Fanshawe of Parsloes*. London, 1907.
Fleming, Daniel. *The Estate and Household Accounts of Sir Daniel Fleming of Rydal Hall, Westmorland, from 1688–1701*. Edited by Blake Tyson. Record Series Volume 13. Lancaster: Cumberland and Westmorland Antiquarian and Archaeological Society, 2001.
Freke, Elizabeth. *The Remembrances of Elizabeth Freke*. Edited by Raymond A. Anselment. Cambridge: Cambridge University Press, 2001.
Giffard, William. *Cases in Midwifery Written by the late Mr William Giffard, surgeon and man-midwife. Revis'd and publish'd by Edward Hody*. London, 1734.
Gouge, William. *Of Domesticall Duties Eight Treatises*. London, 1622.
Graunt, John. *Natural and Political Observations Mentioned in a following Index, and Made upon the Bills of Mortality*. London, 1662.
Guillemeau, Jacques. *Child-birth or, The Happy Deliverie of Women Wherein is set downe the government of Women*. London, 1612.
Harrold, Edmund. *The Diary of Edmund Harrold, Wigmaker of Manchester 1712–1715*. Edited by Craig Horner. Aldershot: Ashgate, 2008.
Hoby, Margaret. *Diary of Lady Margaret Hoby 1599–1605*. Edited by Dorothy Meads. London: Routledge, 1930.
Hooke, Christopher. *The Child-birth or Womans Lecture*. London: 1590.
Jeake, Samuel. *An Astrological Diary of the Seventeenth Century: Samuel Jeake of Rye, 1652–1699*. Edited by Michael Hunter and Annabel Gregory. Oxford: Clarendon Press, 2002.
Jinner, Sarah. *An Almanack and Prognostication for the Year of Our Lord 1658*. London, 1658.
An Almanack and Prognostication for the Year of Our Lord 1659. London, 1659.
Jones, John. *The Arte and Science of preseruing Bodie and Soule in al Health, Wisedome, and Catholike Religion Phisically, Philosophically, and Diuinely deuised*. London, 1579.
Joscelin, Elizabeth. *The Mothers Legacie, to her Unborne Childe*. London, 1624.
Josselin, Ralph. *The Diary of Ralph Josselin, 1616–1683*. Edited by Alan Macfarlane. Oxford: Oxford University Press, 1991.
Diary of Rev. Ralph Josselin 1616–1683. Edited by E. Hockliffe. Vol. 15. Camden Third Series. London: Royal Historical Society, 1908.

J. S. *Paidon Nosemata. Or, Childrens Diseases, Both Outward and Inward. From the time of their Birth to Fourteen Years of Age. With their Natures, Causes, Signs, Presages and Cures*. London, 1664.

Leigh, Dorothy. *Mothers Blessing, or the Godly Counsel of a Gentlewoman Not Long Deceased Left Behind for Her Children*. Essex, 1616.

Markham, Gervase. *The English House-wife Containing the inward and outward Vertues which ought to be in a compleate Woman*. London, 1631.

Marsh, A. *The Ten Pleasures of Marriage Relating all the Delights and Contentments that are Mask'd Under the Bands of Matrimony*. London, 1682.

Mauriceau, François. *The Accomplisht Midwife, Treating of the Diseases of Women with Child, and in Child-bed*. London, 1673.

The Diseases of Women with Child, and in Child-bed: as also, the Best Directions How to Help Them in Natural and Unnatural Labours. London, 1672.

McMath, James. *The Expert Mid-wife a Treatise of the Diseases of Women with Child, and in Child-bed*. Edinburgh, 1694.

Middleton, Thomas. *A Chaste Maid in Cheapside*. Edited by Alan Brissenden. New Mermaids. London: Bloomsbury, 2002.

A Chaste Maid in Cheapside. Edited by Emma French. Drama Classics. London: Nick Hern Books, 2007.

Moffett, Thomas. *Healths Improvement: or, Rules compromising and Discovering the Nature, Method and Manner of Preparing all sorts of Food used in this Nation*. London, 1655.

Moody, Joanna, ed. *The Private Correspondence of Jane, Lady Cornwallis Bacon, 1613–1644*. London: Associated University Presses, 2003.

Moulin, Peter. *Directions for the Education of a Young Prince till Seven Years of Age*. London, 1673.

Newcome, Henry. *The Autobiography of Henry Newcome, MA*. Edited by R. Parkinson. Vol. 1. Remains Historical and Literary 26. Manchester: Chetham Society, 1852.

Oliver, John. *A present to be given to teeming women, by their husbands or friends Containing Scripture: Directions for women with child, how to prepare for the hour of travel*. London, 1663.

Pechey, John. *The Compleat Midwife's Practice Enlarged in the Most Weighty and High Concernments of the Birth of Man*. London, 1698.

A General Treatise of the Diseases of Infants and Children Collected from the Best Practical Authors by John Pechey. London, 1697.

A General Treatise of the Diseases of Maids, Bigbellied Women, Child-bed Women, and Widows together with the best methods of preventing or curing the same. London, 1696.

Pepys, Samuel. *The Diary of Samuel Pepys: A New and Complete Transcription*. Edited by Robert Latham. Vols 1–10. New York: Harper Collins, 1983.

Philalethes. *An Answer to Doctor Chamberlaines Scandalous and False Papers*. London, 1649.

Raynalde, Thomas. *Byrth of Mankynde. Newly translated out of Laten into Englysshe. In the which is entreated of all suche thynges the which chaunce to women in theyr labor, and all suche infyrmitees whiche happen unto the Infantes after they be delyuered*. London, 1540.

Rogers, Richard. *Seven Treatises: Containing Directions, Out of Scripture, Leading to True Happiness*. London: 1610.
Roeselin, Eucharius. *Byrth of Mankynde*. Edited by Richard Jonas. London, 1545.
Rüff, Jakob. *The Expert Midwife, or An Excellent and Most Necessary Treatise of the Generation and Birth of Man*. London, 1636.
Sadler, John. *The Sick Womans Private Looking-Glasse*. London, 1636.
Sennert, Daniel. *Practical Physick the Fourth Book Three Parts*. London, 1664.
Sermon, William. *The Ladies Companion, or, The English Midwife*. London, 1671.
Settle, Elkanah. *The New Athenian Comedy*. London, 1693.
Sharp, Jane. *The Midwives book. Or the whole Art of Midwifry Discovered. Directing childbearing women how to behave themselves*. London: 1671.
The Compleat Midwife's Companion: or, The Art of Midwifry Improv'd. London, 1724.
Stone, Sarah. *A Complete Practice of Midwifery. Consisting of Upwards of Forty Cases or Observations in that valuable Art, selected from many Others, in the Course of a very Extensive Practice*. London, 1737.
T. B. *The Bloudy Mother, Or, The Most Inhumane Murthers, Committed by Jane Hattersley vpon divers infants, the issue of her owne bodie & the priuate burying of them in an orchard with her arraignment and execution*. London, 1610.
T. C., I. D., M. S. and T. B. *The Compleat Midwifes Practice, In the most weighty and high Concernments of the Birth of Man*. London: 1656.
Thornton, Alice. *My First Booke of My Life: Alice Thornton*. Edited by Raymond A. Anselment. Lincoln: University of Nebraska Press, 2014.
Verney, Frances Parthenope, ed. *Memoirs of the Verney Family during the Civil War*. London: Longmans, 1892.
Walker, Antony. *Eureka, Eureka The Virtuous Woman found Her Loss Bewailed, and Character Exemplified in a Sermon Preached at Felsted in Essex, April 30 1678*. London, 1678.
The Virtuous Wife: or, the Holy Life of Mrs Elizabeth Wlaker, late wife of A. Walker, D. D. sometime Rector of Fyfield in Essex Giving a modest and short account of her exemplary piety and charity. Published in the Glory of God, and provoking others to be like graces and vertues. London, 1694.
Wallington, Nehemiah. *The Notebooks of Nehemiah Wallington, 1618–1654: A Selection*. Edited by David Booy. Aldershot: Ashgate, 2007.
Ward, Edward. *A Hue and Cry After A Man-Midwife, Who has Lately Deliver'd the Land Bank of Their Money*, EBBA 33185. London, 1699.
Watkins, Richard. *Newes from the Dead. Or A True and Exact Narration of the miraculous deliverance of Anne Greene*. Oxford, 1651.
Willughby, Percivall. *Observations in Midwifery by Percival Willughby*. Edited by Henry Blenkinsop. Warwick: H. T. Cooke, 1863.
Wolveridge, James. *Speculum Matricis Hypernicum, or, The Irish Midwives Handmaid*. London, 1670.
Woodford, Robert. *The Diary of Robert Woodford, 1637–1641*. Edited by John Fielding. Cambridge: Cambridge University Press, 2012.
Woolley, Hannah. *The Gentlewomans Companion; or, A Guide to the Female Sex Containing Directions of Behaviour, in all Places, Companies, Relations, and Conditions, from their Childhood down to Old Age*. London, 1673.

Yonge, James. *The Journal of James Yonge [1647–1721]: Plymouth Surgeon*. Edited by F. N. L. Poynter. London: Longmans, 1963.

Digital Editions and Tools

Alice Thornton's Books, Cordelia Beattie, Suzanne Trill, Joanne Edge and Sharon Howards, eds., https://thornton.kdl.kcl.ac.uk/.

The Casebooks Project, Lauren Kasell, Michael Hawkins, Robert Ralley, John Young, Joanne Edge, Janet Yvonne Martin-Portugues and Natalie Kaoukji eds., *The Casebooks of Simon Forman and Richard Napier, 1596–1634: a digital edition,* https://casebooks.lib.cam.ac.uk.

John Westover, 'The Casebook of John Westover of Wedmore, Surgeon, 1686', William Hall ed., www.tutton.org/.

National Archives Currency Converter, www.nationalarchives.gov.uk/currency-converter/.

The Proceedings of the Old Bailey online, www.oldbaileyonline.org/.

Secondary

Abala, Ken. *Eating Right in the Renaissance*. California Studies in Food and Culture. Berkeley: University of California Press, 2002.

Adair, Richard. *Courtship, Illegitimacy and Marriage in Early Modern England.* Manchester: Manchester University Press, 1996.

Aho, James. *Confession and Bookkeeping: The Religious, Moral, and Rhetorical Roots of Modern Accounting*. New York: State University of New York, 2005.

Alberti, Fay Bound. *Matters of the Heart: History, Medicine, and Emotion*. Oxford: Oxford University Press, 2010.

Al-Gailani, Salim. 'Hospital Birth'. In *Reproduction: Antiquity to the Present Day.* Edited by Nick Hopwood, Rebecca Flemming and Lauren Kassell, 553–566. Cambridge: Cambridge University Press, 2018.

Amussen, Susan D. 'The Contradictions of Patriarchy in Early Modern England'. *Gender & History* 30, no. 2 (2018): 343–353.

'Gender, Family and the Social Order, 1560–1725'. In *Order and Disorder in Early Modern England*. Edited by Anthony Fletcher and John Stevenson, 196–217. Cambridge: Cambridge University Press, 1985.

Angus, Douglas. *The Green and Burning*. London: Robert Hale, 1958.

Ariès, Philippe. *Centuries of Childhood: A Social History of Family Life*. Translated by Robert Baldick. Harmondsworth: Penguin, 1973.

Aspin, Richard. 'Illustrations from the Wellcome Library: Who Was Elizabeth Okeover?' *Medical History* 44, no. 4 (2000): 531–540.

Astbury, Leah. 'Being Well, Looking Ill: Childbirth and the Return to Health in Seventeenth-Century England'. *Social History of Medicine* 30, no. 3 (2017): 500–519.

'Eat, Sleep, Lust, Repeat: Bedtime Routine, Health and Herbals in Early Modern England'. *Cultural and Social History* 21, no. 2 (2024): 141–162.

'When a Woman Hates Her Husband: Love, Sex and Fruitful Marriages in Early Modern England'. *Gender & History* 32, no. 3 (2020): 523–541.

Astbury, Leah, and Elaine Leong. 'Medical Knowledge and Practice'. In *The Routledge History of Women in Early Modern Europe*. Edited by Amanda Capern, 181–198. The Routledge Histories. London: Routledge, 2020.

Atkinson, Colin. B., and Jo. Atkinson. 'Subordinating Women: Thomas Bentley's Use of Biblical Women in "The Monument of Matrones" (1582)'. *Church History* 60, no. 3 (1991): 289–300.

Atkinson, Colin B., and William P. Stoneman. '"These Griping Greefes and Pinching Pangs": Attitudes to Childbirth in Thomas Bentley's *The Monument of Matrones* (1582)'. *Sixteenth Century Journal* 2 (1990): 192–203.

Aveling, J. H. *The Chamberlens and the Midwifery Forceps: Memorials of the Family and an Essay on the Invention of the Instrument*. New Burlington Street, London: J. & A. Churchill, 1882.

English Midwives; Their History and Prospects. London: Churchill, 1872.

Baernstein, P. Renée, and John Christopoulos. 'Interpreting the Body in Early Modern Italy: Pregnancy, Abortion and Adulthood'. *Past & Present* 223, no. 1 (2014): 41–75.

Bailey, Joanne. '"Think Wot a Mother Must Feel": Parenting in English Pauper Letters, c. 1760–1834'. *Family and Community History* 13 (2010): 5–19.

Unquiet Lives: Marriage and Marriage Breakdown in England, 1660–1800. Cambridge: Cambridge University Press, 2003.

Barclay, Katie, and Nina Javette Koefoed. 'Family, Memory, and Identity: An Introduction'. *Journal of Family History* 46, no. 1 (2021): 3–12.

Barker, Hannah. *Family and Business During the Industrial Revolution*. Oxford: Oxford University Press, 2017.

'Soul, Purse and Family: Middling and Lower-Class Masculinity in Eighteenth-Century Manchester'. *Social History* 33, no. 1 (2008): 12–35.

Beattie, Cordelia. 'The Discovery of Two Missing Alice Thornton Manuscripts'. *Notes and Queries* 66, no. 4 (2019): 547–553.

Becker, Lucinda M. *Death and the Early Modern Englishwoman*. London: Routledge, 2003.

Beier, Lucinda McCray. *Sufferers and Healers: The Experience of Illness in Seventeenth-Century England*. London: Routledge & Kegan Paul, 1987.

Bell, Suzanne O., and Mary E. Fissell. 'A Little Bit Pregnant? Productive Ambiguity and Fertility Research'. *Population and Development Review* 47, no. 2 (2021): 505–526.

Ben-Amos, Ilana Krausman. 'Gifts and Favors: Informal Support in Early Modern England'. *Journal of Modern History* 72, no. 2 (2000): 295–338.

'Reciprocal Bonding: Parents and Their Offspring in Early Modern England'. *Journal of Family History* 25, no. 3 (2000): 291–312.

The Culture of Giving: Informal Support and Gift-Exchange in Early Modern England. Cambridge: Cambridge University Press, 2008.

Bennett, Judith M. *History Matters: Patriarchy and the Challenge of Feminism*. Philadelphia: University of Pennsylvania Press, 2006.

Berry, Helen. *Gender, Society and Print Culture in Late-Stuart England: The Cultural World of the Athenian Mercury*. Women and Gender in the Early Modern World. Aldershot: Ashgate, 2003.

Berry, Helen, and Elizabeth Foyster. 'Childless Men in Early Modern England'. In *The Family in Early Modern England*. Edited by Helen Berry and Elizabeth Foyster, 158–183. Cambridge: Cambridge University Press, 2007.

Biller, Peter. 'Birth-Control in the West in the Thirteenth and Early Fourteenth Centuries'. *Past & Present* 94, no. 1 (1982): 3–26.

Bittel, Carla, Elaine Leong and Christine von Oertzen, eds. *Working with Paper: Gendered Practices in the History of Knowledge*. Pittsburg, PA: University of Pittsburg Press, 2019.

Botonaki, Effie. 'Dissecting Bodies and Selves in the Early Modern Period'. In *Flesh Made Text Flesh: Cultural and Theoretical Returns to the Body*. Edited by Zoe Detsi-Diamanti, Katerina Kitsi-Mitakou and Effie Yiannopoulou, 75–86. New York: Lang Publishing, 2007.

'Seventeenth-Century Englishwomen's Spiritual Diaries: Self-Examination, Covenanting, and Account Keeping'. *Sixteenth Century Journal* 30, no. 1 (1999): 3–21.

Bouchard, Jack B., and Amanda E. Herbert. 'One British Thing: A Manuscript Recipe Book, ca. 1690–1730'. *Journal of British Studies* 59 (2020): 396–399.

Brady, Andrea. '"A Share of Sorrows": Death in the Early Modern English Household'. In *Emotions in the Household, 1200–1900*. Edited by Susan Broomhall, 185–202. Basingstoke: Palgrave, 2008.

Brammall, Kathryn M. 'Monstrous Metamorphosis: Nature, Morality, and the Rhetoric of Monstrosity in Tudor England'. *Sixteenth Century Journal* 27, no. 1 (1996): 3–21.

Bray, Alan. 'To Be a Man in Early Modern Society: The Curious Case of Michael Wigglesworth'. *History Workshop Journal* 41, no. 1 (1996): 155–165.

Homosexuality in Renaissance England. New York: Columbia University Press, 1995.

'Homosexuality and the Signs of Male Friendship in Elizabethan England'. *History Workshop Journal* 29 (1990): 1–19.

Braye, S. G., and G. Guy. 'Miraculous Deliverance of Anne Greene'. *British Medical Journal* 286 (1983): 556.

Breitenberg, Mark. *Anxious Masculinity in Early Modern England*. Cambridge Studies in Renaissance Literature and Culture. Cambridge: Cambridge University Press, 1996.

Broomhall, Susan, ed. *Emotions in the Household, 1200–1900*. Basingstoke: Palgrave, 2008.

Women's Medical Work in Early Modern France. Manchester: Manchester University Press, 2004.

Buck, Ann. *Clothes and the Child: A Handbook of Children's Dress in England 1500–1900*. Bedford: Ruth Bean Publishers, 1996.

Burns, Kathryn. *Into the Archive: Writing and Power in Colonial Peru*. Durham, NC: Duke University Press, 2010.

Butler, Sara M. 'Abortion Medieval Style? Assaults on Pregnant Women in Later Medieval England'. *Women's Studies* 40, no. 6 (2011): 778–799.

Cabré, Monserrat. 'Women or Healers? Household Practices and the Categories of Health Care in Late Medieval Iberia'. *Bulletin of the History of Medicine* 82 (2008): 18–51.

Cadden, Joan. *The Meanings of Sex Difference in the Middle Ages: Medicine, Science, and Culture*. Cambridge: Cambridge University Press, 1993.

Cambers, Andrew. 'Reading, the Godly, and Self-Writing in England, circa 1580–1720'. *Journal of British Studies* 46, no. 4 (2007): 796–825.

Campbell, Linda. 'Wet-Nurses in Early Modern England: Some Evidence from the Townshend Archive'. *Medical History* 33 (1989): 360–370.
Capp, Bernard. *Astrology and the Popular Press: English Almanacs 1500–1800*. London: Faber and Faber, 1979.
'Bigamous Marriage in Early Modern England'. *The Historical Journal* 52, no. 3 (2009): 537–556.
'The Double Standard Revisited: Plebian Women and the Male Sexual Reputation in Early Modern England'. *Past & Present* 162 (1999): 70–100.
'Separate Domains? Women and Authority in Early Modern England'. In *The Experience of Authority in Early Modern England*, 117–145. Basingstoke: Macmillan, 1996.
When Gossips Meet: Women, Family, and Neighbourhood in Early Modern England. Oxford: Oxford University Press, 2003.
Carlebach, Elisheva. 'Community, Authority, and Jewish Midwives in Early Modern Europe'. *Jewish Social Studies* 20, no. 2 (2014): 5–33.
Carlson, Eric Josef. 'English Funeral Sermons as Sources: The Example of Female Piety in Pre-1640 Sermons'. *Albion* 32, no. 4 (2000): 567–597.
Carter, Philippa. 'Childbirth, "Madness", and Bodies in History'. *History Workshop Journal* 91, no. 1 (2021): 29–50.
'Work, Gender and Witchcraft in Early Modern England'. *Gender & History* 37, no. 1 (2025): 91–108.
Cassidy, Tanya M. 'The Secrets of Touch and the Sexualities of Birth: A Queer Consideration of Early Modern European Midwifery'. In *Queering Motherhood: Narrative and Theoretical Perspectives*, 47–62. Ontario: Demeter Press, 2014.
Cavallo, Sandra. *Artisans of the Body in Early Modern Italy*. Manchester: Manchester University Press, 2007.
'Exhibit 17: Pregnant Stones as Wonders of Nature'. In *Reproduction: Antiquity to the Present Day*. Cambridge: Cambridge University Press, 2018.
Cavallo, Sandra, and Tessa Storey, eds. *Conserving Health in Early Modern Culture: Bodies and Environments in Italy and England*. Manchester: Manchester University Press, 2017.
Cavallo, Sandra, and Tessa Storey, *Healthy Living in Late Renaissance Italy*. Oxford: Oxford University Press, 2013.
Cavallo, Sandra, and Lyndan Warner, eds. *Widowhood in Medieval and Early Modern Europe*. Harlow: Longman, 1999.
Churchill, Wendy D. *Female Patients in Early Modern Britain: Gender, Diagnosis, and Treatment*. Farnham: Ashgate, 2012.
'The Medical Practice of the Sexed Body: Women, Men and Disease in Britain, circa 1600–1740'. *Social History of Medicine* 18, no. 1 (2005): 3–22.
Clark, Alice. *Working Life of Women in the Seventeenth Century*. Studies in Economics and Political Science. London: George Routledge & Sons, Ltd, 1919.
Clark, Gillian. 'Infant Clothing in the Eighteenth Century: A New Insight'. *Costume* 28, no. 1 (1994): 47–59.
Cockayne, Emily. *Hubbub: Filth, Noise and Stench in England*. New Haven, CT: Yale University Press, 2007.
'Who Did Let the Dogs Out?: Nuisance Dogs in Late-Medieval and Early Modern England'. In *Our Dogs, Our Selves: Dogs in Medieval and Early Modern Art,*

Literature, and Society. Vol. 6, 41–67. Art and Material Culture in Medieval and Renaissance Europe. Leiden: Brill, 2016.

Cody, Lisa Forman. *Birthing the Nation: Sex, Science, and the Conception of Eighteenth-Century Britons*. Oxford: Oxford University Press, 2005.

ed. *The Early Modern Englishwoman: A Facsimile Library of Essential Works. Printed Writings, 1641–1700: Part I. Writings on Medicine*. Series 2. Vol. 4. Aldershot: Ashgate, 2002.

Connell, Raewyn. *Masculinities*. Cambridge: Polity, 1995.

Cook, Harold J. *The Decline of the Old Medical Regime in Stuart London*. Ithaca, NY: Cornell University Press, 1986.

'Good Advice and Little Medicine: The Professional Authority of Early Modern English Physicians'. *Journal of British Studies* 33 (1994): 1–31.

Crawford, Patricia. 'Attitudes to Menstruation in Seventeenth-Century England'. *Past & Present* 91, no. 1 (1981): 47–73.

'Attitudes to Menstruation in Seventeenth-Century England'. In *Blood, Bodies and Families in Early Modern England*, 19–53. Women and Men in History. London: Routledge, 2004.

'Sexual Knowledge in England, 1500–1750'. In *Sexual Knowledge, Sexual Science. The History of Attitudes to Sexuality*. Edited by Roy Porter and Mikulas Teich, 82–106. Cambridge: Cambridge University Press, 1994.

'The Construction and Experience of Maternity in Seventeenth-Century England'. In *Blood, Bodies and Families in Early Modern England*, 79–112. Women and Men in History. London: Routledge, 2004.

Crawford, Patricia, and Laura Gowing, eds. *Women's Worlds in Seventeenth-Century England*. London: Routledge, 2000.

Crawshaw, Jane Stevens. 'Families, Medical Secrets and Public Health in Early Modern Venice'. *Renaissance Studies* 28 (2014): 597–618.

Cressy, David. *Birth, Marriage, and Death: Ritual, Religion, and the Life-Cycle in Tudor and Stuart England*. Oxford: Oxford University Press, 1997.

'Monstrous Births and Credible Reports: Portents, Texts, and Testimonies'. In *Travesties and Transgressions in Tudor and Stuart England: Tales of Discord and Dissension*, 29–50. Oxford: Oxford University Press, 1999.

'Purification, Thanksgiving and the Churching of Women in Post-Reformation England'. *Past & Present* 141 (1993): 106–146.

Travesties and Transgressions in Tudor and Stuart England: Tales of Discord and Dissension. Oxford: Oxford University Press, 2000.

Croft, Pauline, and Karen Hearn. '"Only Matrimony Maketh Children to Be Certain…": Two Elizabethan Pregnancy Portraits'. *The British Art Journal* 3, no. 3 (2002): 19–24.

Cunnington, Phillis, and Catherine Lucas. *Costumes for Births, Marriages and Deaths*. New York: Barnes & Noble, 1972.

Dabhoiwala, Faramerz. *The Origins of Sex: A History of the First Sexual Revolution*. London: Penguin, 1999.

Daiken, Leslie Herbert. *The Lullaby Book: Musical Research by Mary Hillis and Sebastian Brown. With Plates*. London: Ward, Lock & Co., 1959.

Dam, Fabiola I. W. M. van. 'Permeable Boundaries: Bodies, Bathing and Fluxes: 1135–1333'. In *Medicine and Space: Body, Surroundings and Borders in*

Antiquity and the Middle Ages. Edited by Patricia A. Baker, Han Nijdam and Karine van't Land, 117–149. Leiden: Brill, 2007.

Damme, Catherine. 'Infanticide: The Worth of an Infant under Law'. *Medical History* 22 (1978): 1–24.

Daston, Lorraine. 'The Sciences of the Archive'. *Osiris* 27, no. 1 (2012): 156–187.

Daston, Lorraine, and Katharine Park. *Wonders and the Order of Nature, 1150–1750*. Cambridge, MA: MIT Press, 1998.

Davis, Lennard J. *Bending over Backwards: Disability, Dismodernism, and Other Difficult Positions*. New York: New York University Press, 2002.

Daybell, James. *The Material Letter in Early Modern England*. Basingstoke: Palgrave, 2012.

'The Social Conventions of Women's Letter-Writing in England, 1540–1603'. In *Early Modern Women's Letter-Writing in England, 1450–1700*. Edited by James Daybell, 59–76. Basingstoke: Palgrave, 2001.

de Renzi, Silvia. 'Resemblance, Paternity, and Imagination in Early Modern Courts'. In *Heredity Produced: At the Crossroads of Biology, Politics, and Culture, 1500–1870*, 61–82. Cambridge, MA: MIT Press, 2007.

DeVun, Leah. *The Shape of Sex: Nonbinary Gender from Genesis to the Renaissance*. New York: Columbia University Press, 2021.

DiMeo, Michelle. 'Authorship and Medical Networks: Reading Attributions in Early Modern Manuscript Recipe Books'. In *Reading and Writing Recipe Books, 1550–1800*. Edited by Michelle DiMeo and Sara Pennell, 25–46. Manchester: Manchester University Press, 2013.

'Lady Katherine Ranelagh or Lady Margaret Orrery?: Reattributing Authorship for the Boyle Family Receipt Book. 2010 Prize for a Graduate Student Conference Presentation'. *Early Modern Women: An Interdisciplinary Journal* 6 (2011): 269–270.

DiMeo, Michelle, and Rebecca Laroche. 'On Elizabeth Isham's "Oil of Swallows": Animal Slaughter and Early Modern Women's Medical Recipes'. In *Ecofeminist Approaches to Early Modernity*. Edited by Jennifer Muroe and Rebecca Laroche, 87–104. Basingstoke: Palgrave, 2011.

DiMeo, Michelle, and Sara Pennell, eds. *Reading and Writing Recipe Books, 1550–1800*. Manchester: Manchester University Press, 2013.

Dobbie, B. M. Willmott. 'An Attempt to Estimate the True Rate of Maternal Mortality, Sixteenth to Eighteenth Centuries'. *Medical History* 26 (1982): 79–90.

Dolan, Frances E. *Marriage and Violence: The Early Modern Legacy*. Philadelphia: University of Pennsylvania Press, 2009.

Donnison, Jean. *Midwives and Medical Men: A History of the Struggle for the Control of Childbirth*. London: Historical Publications, 1988.

Donohoe, Róisín. '"Unbynde Her Anoone": The Lives of St. Margaret of Antioch and the Lying-in Space in Late Medieval England'. In *Gender in Medieval Places, Spaces and Thresholds*. Edited by Victoria Blud, Diane Heath and Einat Klafter, 139–156. IHR Conference Series. London: University of London Press, Institute of Historical Research, 2019.

Duden, Barbara. *The Woman beneath the Skin: A Doctor's Patients in Eighteenth-Century Germany*. Translated by Thomas Dunlap. Cambridge, MA: Harvard University Press, 1991.

Earle, Rebecca, ed. *Epistolary Selves: Letters and Letter-Writers, 1600–1945.* Aldershot: Ashgate, 1999.

Ehrenreich, Barbara, and Deirdre English. *Witches, Midwives, and Nurses: A History of Women Healers*. Oyster Bay, NY: Glass Mountain Pamphlets, 1971.

Evans, Jennifer. *Aphrodisiacs, Fertility and Medicine in Early Modern England.* Studies in History. Woodbridge: Boydell & Brewer, 2014.

'"Gentle Purges Corrected with Hot Spices, Whether They Work or Not, Do Vehemently Provoke Venery": Menstrual Provocation and Procreation in Early Modern England'. *Social History of Medicine* 25, no. 1 (2012): 2–19.

Men's Sexual Health in Early Modern England. Gendering the Late Medieval and Early Modern World. Amsterdam: Amsterdam University Press, 2023.

'Provoking Lust and Promoting Conception'. In *Aphrodisiacs, Fertility and Medicine in Early Modern England*, 87–130. Woodbridge: Boydell & Brewer, 2014.

'"They Are Called Imperfect Men": Male Infertility and Sexual Health in Early Modern England'. *Social History of Medicine* 29, no. 1 (2016): 311–332.

Evans, Jennifer, and Sara Read. '"Before Midnight She Had Miscarried": Women, Men, and Miscarriage in Early Modern England'. *Journal of Family History* 40, no. 1 (2015): 2–23.

Evenden, Doreen. *The Midwives of Seventeenth-Century London.* Cambridge History of Medicine. Cambridge: Cambridge University Press, 2000.

'Mothers and Their Midwives in Seventeenth-Century London'. In *The Art of Midwifery: Early Modern Midwives in Europe*. Edited by Hilary Marland, 9–26. London: Routledge, 1993.

Faircloth, Charlotte. *Militant Lactivism? Attachment Parenting and Intensive Motherhood in the UK and France*. Oxford: Berghahn Books, 2013.

Feroli, Teresa. '"Infelix Simulacrum": The Rewriting of Loss in Elizabeth Jocelin's *The Mother's Legacie*'. *English Literary History* 61, no. 1 (1994): 89–102.

Fildes, Valerie. *Breasts, Bottles, and Babies: A History of Infant Feeding*. Edinburgh: Edinburgh University Press, 1986.

ed. *Women as Mothers in Pre-Industrial England.* Wellcome Series in the History of Medicine. London: Routledge, 1990.

Fissell, Mary. 'Hairy Women and Naked Truths: Gender and the Politics of Knowledge in Aristotle's Masterpiece'. *The William and Mary Quarterly* 60, no. 1 (2003): 43–74.

'Man-Midwifery Revisited'. In *Reproduction: Antiquity to the Present Day.* Edited by Nick Hopwood, Rebecca Flemming and Lauren Kassell, 319–332. Cambridge: Cambridge University Press, 2018.

'The Marketplace of Print'. In *Medicine and the Market in England and Its Colonies, c. 1450–c.1850*, 108–132. Basingstoke: Palgrave, 2007.

Patients, Power and the Poor in Eighteenth-Century Bristol. Cambridge: Cambridge University Press, 1991.

'Remaking the Maternal Body in England, 1680–1730'. *Journal of the History of Sexuality* 26, no. 1 (2017): 114–139.

. *Vernacular Bodies: The Politics of Reproduction in Early Modern England.* Oxford: Oxford University Press, 2004.

. 'Women, Health and Healing in Early Modern Europe'. *Bulletin of the History of Medicine* 82 (2008): 1–17.

Flather, Amanda. *Gender and Space in Early Modern England.* Royal Historical Society Studies in History. Woodbridge: The Boydell Press, 2007.

Fletcher, Anthony. *Gender, Sex and Subordination in England, 1500–1800.* New Haven, CT: Yale University Press, 1995.

'Manhood, the Male Body, Courtship and the Household in Early Modern England'. *History* 84, no. 275 (1999): 419–436.

Fox, Adam. *Oral and Literate Culture in England 1500–1700.* Oxford: Clarendon Press, 2000.

Fox, Sarah. *Giving Birth in Eighteenth-Century England.* London: University of London Press, 2022.

Fox, Sarah, and Margaret Brazier. 'The Regulation of Midwives in England, c. 1500–1902', *Medical Law International* 20, no. 4 (2020): 308–338.

Foyster, Elizabeth. *Manhood in Early Modern England: Honour, Sex and Marriage.* London: Routledge, 1999.

Marital Violence: An English Family History, 1660–1857. Cambridge: Cambridge University Press, 2005.

French, Katherine. 'The Material Culture of Childbirth in Late Medieval London and Its Suburbs'. *Journal of Women's History* 28, no. 2 (2016): 126–148.

Froide, Amy M. *Never Married: Singlewomen in Early Modern England.* Oxford: Oxford University Press, 2005.

Fudge, Erica. *Quick Cattle & Dying Wishes: People and Their Animals in Early Modern England.* Ithaca, NY: Cornell University Press, 2018.

Fumerton, Patricia. 'Introduction: The New New Historicism'. In *Renaissance Culture and the Everyday.* Edited by Patricia Fumerton and Simon Hunt, 1–17. Philadelphia: University of Pennsylvania Press, 1999.

Furdell, Elizabeth Lane. *Publishing and Medicine in Early Modern England.* Rochester, NY: University of Rochester Press, 2002.

Galley, Chris, and Alice Reid. 'Sources and Methods: Maternal Mortality'. *Local Population Studies* 93, no. 1 (2014): 68–78.

Gennep, Arnold van. *The Rites of Passage.* Chicago: University of Chicago Press, 1960.

Gentilcore, David. *Healers and Healing in Early Modern Italy.* Manchester: Manchester University Press, 1998.

Giannetti, Laura. 'Of Eels and Pears: A Sixteenth-Century Debate on Taste, Temperance, and the Pleasures of the Senses'. In *Religion and the Senses in Early Modern Europe.* Edited by Wietse de Boer and Christine Göttler, 289–305. Intersections. Leiden: Brill, 2012.

Gowing, Laura. *Common Bodies: Women, Touch and Power in Seventeenth-Century England.* New Haven, CT: Yale University Press, 2003.

Domestic Dangers: Women, Words, and Sex in Early Modern London. Oxford: Oxford University Press, 1996.

'The Haunting of Susan Lay: Servants and Mistresses in Seventeenth-Century England'. *Gender & History* 14, no. 2 (2002): 183–201.

'Secret Births and Infanticide in Seventeenth-Century England'. *Past & Present* no. 156 (1997): 87–115.

Green, Monica H. 'From "Diseases of Women" to "Secrets of Women": The Transofrmation of Gynaecological Literature in the Later Middle Ages'. *Journal of Medieval and Early Modern Studies* 30 (2000): 5–39.

Making Women's Medicine Masculine: The Rise of Male Authority in Pre-modern Gynaecology. Oxford: Oxford University Press, 2008.

Grell, Ole Peter, and Andrew Cunningham, eds. *Medicine and the Reformation*. London: Routledge, 1993.

Grundy, Joan E. *History's Midwives Including a C17th and C18th Yorkshire Midwives Nominations Index*. Urmston: Federation of Family History Societies, 2003.

Hailwood, Mark. *Alehouses and Good Fellowship in Early Modern England*. Vol. 21. Studies in Early Modern Cultural, Political and Social History. Woodbridge: Boydell & Brewer, 2014.

Halbwachs, Maurice. *On Collective Memory*. Translated by L. Coser. Chicago: University of Chicago Press, 1992.

Hall, John. *John Hall Master of Physicke: A Casebook from Shakespeare's Stratford*. Edited by Greg Wells. Manchester: Manchester University Press, 2020.

Hammons, Pamela. 'Despised Creatures: The Illusion of Maternal Self-Effacement in Seventeenth-Century Child Loss Poetry'. *English Literary History* 66, no. 1 (1999): 29–49.

Handley, Sasha. 'Objects, Emotions and an Early Modern Bed-sheet'. *History Workshop Journal* 85 (2018): 169–194.

Sleep in Early Modern England. New Haven, CT: Yale University Press, 2016.

'Sleep-Piety and Healthy Sleep in Early Modern English Households'. In *Conserving Health in Early Modern Culture: Bodies and Environments in Italy and England*. Edited by Sandra Cavallo and Tessa Storey, 185–210. Social Histories of Medicine. Manchester: Manchester University Press, 2017.

Harkness, Deborah E. 'A View from the Streets: Women and Medical Work in Elizabethan London'. *Bulletin of the History of Medicine* 82, no. 1 (2008): 52–85.

Harley, David. 'Historians as Demonologists: The Myth of the Midwife-Witch'. *Social History of Medicine* 3, no. 1 (1990): 1–26.

'From Providence to Nature: The Moral Theology and Godly Practice of Maternal Breast-Feeding in Stuart England'. *Bulletin of the History of Medicine* 69, no. 2 (1995): 198–223.

Harol, Corrine. 'Misconceiving the Heir: Mind and Matter in the Warming Pan Propaganda'. In *Vital Matters: Eighteenth-Century Views of Conception, Life and Death*. Edited by Helen Deutsch and Mary Terrall, 130–147. UCLA Clark Memorial Library Series. Toronto: University of Toronto Press, 2012.

Harvey, Karen. 'The Body'. In *Early Modern Emotions: An Introduction*. Edited by Susan Broomhall, 165–167. London: Routledge, 2016.

'Epochs of Embodiment: Sex and the Material Body in the Eighteenth Century'. *Journal for Eighteenth-Century Studies* 42, no. 4 (2019): 455–469.

The Little Republic: Masculinity and Domestic Authority in Eighteenth-Century Britain. Oxford: Oxford University Press, 2012.

'"The Majesty of the Masculine-Form": Multiplicity and Male Bodies in Eighteenth-Century Erotica'. In *English Masculinities, 1660–1800*. Edited by Tim Hitchcock and Michelle Cohen, 193–214. London: Routledge, 1999.

'Men Making Home: Masculinity and Domesticity in Eighteenth-Century England'. *Gender & History* 21, no. 3 (2009): 520–540.

'Men of Parts: Embodiment and the Male Leg in Eighteenth-Century Britain'. *Journal of British Studies* 54, no. 4 (2015): 797–821.

'Rabbits, Whigs and Hunters: Women and Protest in Mary Toft's Monstrous Births of 1726'. *Past & Present* 238, no. 1 (2018): 43–83.

Reading Sex in the Eighteenth Century: Bodies and Gender in English Erotic Culture. Cambridge: Cambridge University Press, 2004.

'What Mary Toft Felt: Women's Voices, Pain, Power and the Body'. *History Workshop Journal* 80 (2015): 31–51.

Harvey, Karen, and Alexandra Shepard. 'What Have Historians Done with Masculinity?' *Journal of British Studies* 44, no. 2 (2005): 274–280.

Haycock, D. B., and Patrick Wallis, eds. 'Daffy's Elixir Pamphlet'. *Medical History* Supplement 25 (2005): 38–42.

eds. 'Quackery and Commerce in Seventeenth-Century London: The Proprietary Medicine Business of Anthony Daffy'. *Medical History* Supplement 25 (2005): 1–36.

Heal, Felicity. *The Power of Gifts: Gift-Exchange in Early Modern England*. Oxford: Oxford University Press, 2014.

Hearn, Karen. 'A Fatal Fertility? Elizabethan and Jacobean Pregnancy Portraits'. *Costume* 34, no. 1 (2000): 39–43.

Heller, Jennifer Louise. *The Mother's Legacy in Early Modern England: Women and Gender in the Early Modern World*. Farnham: Ashgate, 2011.

Hellwarth, Jennifer Wynne. '"I Wyl Wright of Women Prevy Sekenes": Imagining Female Literacy and Textual Communities in Medieval and Early Modern Midwifery Manuals'. *Critical Survey, Literacies in Early Modern Women* 14, no. 1 (2002): 44–63.

Herbert, Amanda. *Female Alliances: Gender, Identity and Friendship in Early Modern Britain*. New Haven, CT: Yale University Press, 2004.

'Gender and the Spa: Space, Sociability and Self at British Health Spas, 1640–1714'. *Journal of Social History* 43 (2009): 361–383.

'Queer Intimacy: Speaking with the Dead in Eighteenth-Century Britain'. *Gender & History* 31, no. 1 (2018): 1–16.

Hill Curth, Louise. *English Almanacs, Astrology and Popular Medicine, 1550–1700*. Manchester: Manchester University Press, 2007.

Hindle, Steve. 'The Problem of Pauper Marriage in Seventeenth-Century England: The Alexander Prize Essay'. *Transactions of the Royal Historical Society* 8 (1998): 71–89.

'The Shaming of Margaret Knowsley: Gossip, Gender and the Experience of Authority in Early Modern England'. *Continuity and Change* 9, no. 3 (1994): 391–419.

The State and Social Change in Early Modern England, c. 1550–1640. Basingstoke: Palgrave, 2000.

Hitchcock, James. 'A Sixteenth Century Midwife's License'. *Bulletin of the History of Medicine* 41, no. 1 (1967): 75–76.

Hitchcock, Tim. *English Sexualities, 1700–1800*. Social History in Perspective. New York: Macmillan Education, 1997.

'Sociability and Misogyny in the Life of John Cannon, 1684–1743'. In *English Masculinities, 1660–1800*. Edited by Tim Hitchcock and Michelle Cohen, 25–43. London: Routledge, 1999.

Hobby, Elaine. '"Secrets of the Female Sex": Jane Sharp, the Reproductive Female Body, and Early Modern Midwifery Manuals'. *Women's Writing* 8, no. 2 (2001): 201–212.

'"The World Was Never without Some Mad Men': Aphra Behn, Jane Sharp and the Body'. *Women's Writing* 19, no. 2 (2012): 177–191.

Hobgood, Allison P., and David Houston Wood. 'Ethical Staring: Disabling the English Renaissance'. In *Recovering Disability in Early Modern England*, 1–22. Athens: Ohio University Press, 2013.

Hodgkin, Katharine. 'Women, Memory and Family History in Seventeenth-Century England'. In *Memory before Modernity: Practices of Memory in Early Modern Europe*. Edited by Ericka Kuijpers, Judith Pollmann, Johannes Mueller and Jasper van der Steen, 297–313. Leiden: Brill, 2013.

Hoffer, Peter Charles, and N. E. H. Hull. *Murdering Mothers: Infanticide in England and New England 1550–1800*. New York: New York University Press, 1984.

Hopwood, Nick, Rebecca Flemming and Lauren Kassell, eds. *Reproduction: Antiquity to the Present Day*. Cambridge: Cambridge University Press, 2018.

Hopwood, Nick, Rebecca Flemming and Lauren Kassell, 'Reproduction in History'. In *Reproduction: Antiquity to the Present Day*, 3–18. Cambridge: Cambridge University Press, 2018.

Houlbrooke, Ralph A. *The English Family, 1450–1700*. Harlow: Longman, 1984.

Howard, Sharon. 'Imagining the Pain and Peril of Seventeenth-Century Childbirth: Travail and Deliverance in the Making of an Early Modern World'. *Social History of Medicine* 16, no. 3 (2003): 367–382.

Hubbard, Eleanor. *City Women: Money, Sex and the Social Order in Early Modern London*. Oxford: Oxford University Press, 2012.

Huet, Marie-Hélène. *Monstrous Imagination*. Cambridge, MA: Harvard University Press, 1993.

Hufton, Olwen. *The Prospect before Her: A History of Women in Western Europe, 1500–1800*. Vol. 1. London: Fontana Press, 1997.

'Women without Men: Widows and Spinsters in Britain and France in the Eighteenth Century'. *Journal of Family History* 9, no. 4 (1984): 355–376.

Huisman, Frank, and John Harley Warner. *Locating Medical History: The Stories and Their Meanings*. Baltimore: Johns Hopkins University Press, 2006.

Hull, Suzanne W. *Chaste, Silent, and Obedient: English Books for Women, 1475–1640*. San Marino, CA: Huntington Library, 1982.

Hunt, Margaret. *The Middling Sort: Commerce, Gender and the Family in England, 1680–1780*. Berkeley: University of California Press, 1996.

Hurl, Jenine. '"She Being Bigg with Child Is Likely to Miscarry": Pregnant Victims Prosecuting Assault in Westminster, 1685–1720'. *The London Journal* 24, no. 2 (1999): 18–33.

Hutton, Sarah, and Marjorie Hope Nicolson, eds. *The Conway Letters: The Correspondence of Anne, Viscountess Conway, Henry More, and Their Friends 1642–1684*. Oxford: Oxford University Press, 1992.

Ibbett, Katherine. 'Fellow-Feeling'. In *Early Modern Emotions: An Introduction*, 61–63. London: Routledge, 2017.

Ingram, Martin. *Carnal Knowledge: Regulating Sex in England, 1470–1600*. Cambridge Studies in Early Modern British History. Cambridge: Cambridge University Press, 2017.

Church Courts, Sex and Marriage in England, 1570–1640. Cambridge: Cambridge University Press, 1987.

'Reformation of Manners in Early Modern England'. In *The Experience of Authority in Early Modern England*. Edited by Paul Griffiths, Adam Fox and Steve Hindle, 47–88. Basingstoke: Palgrave, 1996.

Jackson, Mark. *New-Born Child Murder: Women, Illegitimacy and the Courts in Eighteenth-Century England*. Manchester: Manchester University Press, 1996.

'Suspicious Infant Deaths: The Statute of 1624 and Medical Evidence at Coroners' Inquests'. In *Legal Medicine in History*. Edited by Michael Clark and Catherine Crawford, 64–89. Cambridge: Cambridge University Press, 1994.

Jenner, Mark S. R., and Patrick Wallis. 'The Medical Marketplace'. In *Medicine and the Market in England and Its Colonies, c. 1450–c.1850*. Edited by Mark S. R. Jenner and Patrick Wallis, 1–23. Basingstoke: Palgrave, 2007.

Jenstad, Janelle Day. 'Lying-in Like a Countess: The Lisle Letters, the Cecil Family, and a Chaste Maid in Cheapside'. *Journal of Medieval and Early Modern Studies* 34, no. 2 (2004): 373–403.

Johnston, Archibald. *Diary of Sir Archibald Johnston of Wariston 1650–1654*. Vol. 2. Edited by David Hay Fleming. Publications of the Scottish History Society. Edinburgh: University of Edinburgh Press, 1919.

Jones, Ann Rosalind, and Peter Stallybrass. *Renaissance Clothing and the Materials of Memory*. Cambridge: Cambridge University Press, 2000.

Jordanova, Ludmilla. 'The Social Construction of Medical Knowledge'. *Social History of Medicine* 8, no. 3 (1995): 361–381.

Juel-Jenses, Bent. 'News from the Dead: The Remarkable Story of Anne Greene'. *Oxford Medical School Gazette* 14 (1962): 135–140.

Kadane, Matthew. *The Watchful Clothier: The Life of an Eighteenth-Century Protestant Capitalist*. New Haven, CT: Yale University Press, 2013.

Karim-Cooper, Farah, *Cosmetics in Shakespearean and Renaissance Drama*. Edinburgh: Edinburgh University Press, 2006.

Kassell, Lauren. 'Almanacs and Prognostications'. In *The Oxford History of Popular Print Culture: Cheap Print in Britain and Ireland to 1660*, 431–442. Vol. 1. Oxford: Oxford University Press, 2011.

'Exhibit 14: Jane Dee's Courses in John Dee's Diary'. In *Reproduction: Antiquity to the Present Day*, Cambridge: Cambridge University Press, 2018.

'Fruitful Bodies and Astrological Medicine'. In *Reproduction: Antiquity to the Present Day*, 225–240. Cambridge: Cambridge University Press, 2018.

Medicine and Magic in Elizabethan London: Simon Forman, Alchemist, Physician. Oxford: Oxford University Press, 2005.

'Paper Technologies, Digital Technologies: Working with Early Modern Medical Records'. In *The Edinburgh Companion to the Critical Medical Humanities*. Edited by Anne Whitehead, Angela Woods, Sarah Atkinson, Jane Macnaughton and Jennifer Richards, 120–135. Edinburgh: Edinburgh University Press, 2016.

Keller, Eve. *Generating Bodies and Gendered Selves: The Rhetoric of Reproduction in Early Modern England*. Seattle: University of Washington Press, 2007.

King, Helen. *The One-Sex Body on Trial: The Classical and Early Modern Evidence*. Farnham: Ashgate, 2013.

Klapisch-Zuber, Christiane. *Women, Family, and Ritual in Renaissance Italy*. Translated by Lydia G. Cochrane. Chicago: University of Chicago Press, 1985.

Knoppers, Laura, ed. *The Cambridge Companion to Early Modern Women's Writing*. Cambridge: Cambridge University Press, 2009.

Knott, Sarah. 'Theorizing and Historicizing Mothering's Many Labours'. *Past & Present* 246, no. Supplement 15 (2020): 1–24.

Kugler, Anne. 'Constructing Wifely Identity: Prescription and Practice in the Life of Lady Sarah Cowper'. *Journal of British Studies* 40, no. 3 (2001): 291–323.

Laqueur, Thomas. *Making Sex: Body and Gender from the Greeks to Freud*. Cambridge, MA: Harvard University Press, 1992.

'Orgasm, Generation, and the Politics of Reproductive Biology'. *Representations, The Making of the Modern Body: Sexuality and Society in the Nineteenth Century*, 14, no. Spring (1986): 1–41.

Laroche, Rebecca. *Medical Authority and Englishwomen's Herbal Texts, 1550–1650*. Aldershot: Ashgate, 2009.

Laslett, Peter. *Family Life and Illicit Love in Earlier Generations*. Cambridge: Cambridge University Press, 1977.

The World We Have Lost: Further Explored. London: Metheun, 1965.

Leavitt, Judith Walzer. *Brought to Bed: Childbearing in America, 1750–1950*. Oxford: Oxford University Press, 1986.

LeJacq, Seth Stein. 'The Bounds of Domestic Healing: Medical Recipes, Storytelling and Surgery in Early Modern England'. *Social History of Medicine* 26 (2013): 1–18.

Leong, Elaine. 'Collecting Knowledge for the Family: Recipes, Gender and Practical Knowledge in the Early Modern English Household'. *Centaurus* 55, no. 2 (2013): 81–103.

'"Herbals She Peruseth": Reading Medicine in Early Modern England'. *Renaissance Studies* 28, no. 4 (2014): 556–578.

'Making Medicines in the Early Modern Household'. *Bulletin of the History of Medicine* 82, no. 1 (2008): 145–168.

'Papering the Household: Paper, Recipes and Everyday Technologies'. In *Working with Paper: Gendered Practices in the History of Knowledge*. Edited by Carla Bittel, Elaine Leong and Christine von Oertzen, 32–45. Pittsburg, PA: University of Pittsburg Press, 2019.

Recipes and Everyday Knowledge: Medicine, Science, and the Household in Early Modern England. Chicago: University of Chicago Press, 2018.

'Writing the Family Archive: Recipes and the Paperwork of Kinship'. In *Recipes and Everyday Knowledge: Medicine, Science, and the Household in Early Modern England*, 124–146. Chicago: University of Chicago Press, 2018.

Leong, Elaine, and Sara Pennell. 'Recipe Collections and the Currency of Medical Knowledge in the Early Modern "Medical Marketplace"'. In *Medicine and the Market in England and Its Colonies, c. 1450–c. 1850*. Edited by Mark S. R. Jenner and Patrick Wallis, 133–152. Basingstoke: Palgrave, 2007.

Levene, Alysa. *Childcare, Health and Mortality at the London Foundling Hospital, 1741–1800: 'Left to the Mercy of the World'*. Manchester: Manchester University Press, 2007.

Lewis, Judith. '"Tis a Misfortune to Be a Great Ladie": Maternal Mortality in the British Aristocracy, 1558–1959'. *Journal of British Studies* 37, no. 1 (1998): 26–53.

Linton, Simi. *Claiming Disability: Knowledge and Identity*. New York: New York University Press, 1998.

Loftis, John, ed. *The Memoirs of Anne, Lady Halkett and Ann, Lady Fanshawe*. Oxford: Oxford University Press, 1979.

Long, Donna J. '"I, the Mother": Inscribing Maternal Right in Early Modern Mothers' Elegies'. In *The Literary Mother: Essays on Representations of Maternity and Child Care*. Edited by Susan C. Staub, 185–199. Jefferson, NC: McFarland & Company, Inc, 2007.

Longfellow, Erica. 'Public, Private, and the Household in Early Seventeenth-Century England'. *Journal of British Studies* 45, no. 2 (2006): 313–334.

Lord, Alexandra. '"The Great Arcana of the Deity" Menstruation and Menstrual Disorders in Eighteenth-Century British Medical Thought'. *Bulletin of the History of Medicine* 73, no. 1 (1999): 38–63.

Loudon, Irvine. 'Childbirth'. In *Western Medicine: An Illustrated History*. Edited by Irvine Loudon, 206–220. Oxford: Oxford University Press, 1997.

Lurie, S. 'Euphemia Maclean, Agnes Sampson and Pain Relief during Labour in 16th Century Edinburgh'. *Anaesthesia* 59, no. 8 (2004): 834–835.

Lyon, Harriet. 'The Fisherton Monster: Science, Providence, and the Politics in Early Restoration England'. *The Historical Journal* 60, no. 2 (2016): 333–362.

MacDonald, Michael. *Mystical Bedlam: Madness, Anxiety, and Healing in Seventeenth-Century England*. Cambridge: Cambridge University Press, 1981.

Macfarlane, Alan. *The Family Life of Ralph Josselin, a Seventeenth-Century Clergyman: An Essay in Historical Anthropology*. Cambridge: Cambridge University Press, 1970.

Mandelbrote, Scott. 'William Petty and Anne Greene: Medical and Political Reform in Commonwealth Oxford'. In *The Practice of Reform in Health, Medicine and Science, 1500–2000*. Edited by Margaret Pelling and Scott Mandelbrote, 125–151. Aldershot: Ashgate, 2005.

Mann, Catherine. 'Clothing Bodies, Dressing Rooms: Fashioning Fecundity in the Lisle Letters'. *Parergon* 22, no. 1 (2005): 137–157.

Mann, Jenny C. 'How to Look at a Hermaphrodite in Early Modern England'. *Studies in English Literature, 1500–1900* 46, no. 1 (2006): 67–91.

Mann, Sophie. 'A Dose of Physic: Confessional Identity and Medical Practice within the Family'. *Studies in Church History*. Edited by John Doran and Charlotte Methuen. Special issue: Religion and the Household 50 (2014): 282–293.

'Physic and Divinity: The Case of Dr John Downes M.D. (1627–1694)'. *The Seventeenth Century* 31, no. 4 (2016): 451–470.

Marland, Hilary, ed. *The Art of Midwifery: Early Modern Midwives in Europe*. London: Routledge, 1993.

Marland, Hilary, and Margaret Pelling, eds. *The Task of Healing: Medicine, Religion and Gender in England and the Netherlands, 1450–1800*. Rotterdam: Erasmus Publishing, 1996.

Maschuch, Michael. *Origins of the Individualist Self: Autobiography and Self-Identity in England, 1591–1791*. Cambridge: Cambridge University Press, 1996.

Matchinske, Megan. *Women Writing History in Early Modern England*. Cambridge: Cambridge University Press, 2009.

McClive, Cathy. 'The Hidden Truths of the Belly: The Uncertainties of Pregnancy in Early Modern Europe'. *Social History of Medicine* 15, no. 2 (2002): 209–227.

Menstruation and Procreation in Early Modern France. London: Routledge, 2015.

McLaren, Angus. '"Barrenness against Nature": Recourse to Abortion in Pre-Industrial England'. *The Journal of Sex Research* 17, no. 3 (1981): 224–237.

Reproductive Rituals: The Perception of Fertility in England from the Sixteeth Century to the Nineteenth Century. London: Routledge, 1984.

McLaren, Dorothy. 'Fertility, Infant Mortality, and Breast Feeding in the Seventeenth Century'. *Medical History* 22 (1978): 378–396.

'Nature's Contraceptive: Wet Nursing and Prolonged Lactation: The Case of Chesham, Buckinghamshire, 1578–1601'. *Medical History* 23 (1979): 426–441.

McShane, Angela. 'Ballads and Broadsides'. In *The Oxford History of Popular Print Culture: Cheap Print in Britain and Ireland to 1660*. Vol. 1, 339–361. Oxford: Oxford University Press, 2011.

McTavish, Lianne. *Childbirth and the Display of Authority in Early Modern France*. Women and Gender in the Early Modern World. Aldershot: Ashgate, 2005.

Mendelsohn, J. Andrew, and Annemarie Kinzelbach. 'Common Knowledge: Bodies, Evidence, and Expertise in Early Modern Germany'. *Isis* 108, no. 2 (2017): 259–279.

Moncrief, Kathryn M. '"Show Me a Child Begotten of Thy Body That I Am Father to": Pregnancy, Paternity and the Problem of Evidence in All's Well That Ends Well'. In *Performing Maternity in Early Modern England*. Edited by Kathryn M. Moncrief and Kathyrn R. McPherson, 29–44. Aldershot: Ashgate, 2007.

Moncrief, Kathryn M., and Kathryn R. McPherson, eds. *Performing Maternity in Early Modern England. Studies in Performance and Early Modern Drama*. Aldershot: Ashgate, 2007.

Morgan, Jennifer L. '"Some Could Suckle over Their Shoulder": Male Travelers, Female Bodies, and the Gendering of Racial Ideology'. In *Laboring Women: Reproduction and Gender in New World Slavery*, 12–49. Early American Studies. Philadelphia: University of Pennsylvania Press, 2004.

Mortimer, Ian. *The Dying and the Doctors: The Medical Revolution in Seventeenth-Century England*. Woodbridge: Boydell & Brewer, 2009.

Mueller, Judith C. 'Fallen Men: Representations of Male Impotence in Britain'. *Studies in Eighteenth-Century Culture* 28 (1999): 85–102.

Muldrew, Craig. *The Economy of Obligation: The Culture of Credit and Social Relations in Early Modern England*. Basingstoke: Palgrave, 1998.

Munkhoff, Richelle. 'Searchers of the Dead: Authority, Marginality, and the Interpretation of Plague in England, 1574–1665'. *Gender & History* 11, no. 1 (1999): 1–29.

Muri, Allison. 'Imagining Reproduction: The Politics of Reproduction, Technology and the Woman Machine'. *Journal of Medical Humanities* 31 (2010): 53–67.

Musacchio, Jacqueline Marie. *The Art and Ritual of Childbirth in Renaissance Italy*. New Haven, CT: Yale University Press, 1999.

Newall, Fiona. 'Wet Nursing and Child Care in Aldenham, Hertfordshire, 1595–1726: Some Evidence on the Circumstances and Effects of Seventeenth-Century Child Rearing Practices'. In *Women as Mothers in Pre-Industrial England. Essays in*

Memory of Dorothy McLaren. Edited by Valerie Fildes, 122–138. London: Routledge, 1990.
Newman, Karen. *Fetal Positions: Individualism, Science, Visuality*. Writing Science. Stanford, CA: Stanford University Press, 1996.
Newton, Hannah. *Misery to Mirth: Recovery from Illness in Early Modern England*. Oxford: Oxford University Press, 2018.
'"Nature Concocts and Expels": Defeating Disease'. In *Misery to Mirth: Recovery from Illness in Early Modern England*, 33–64. Oxford: Oxford University Press, 2018.
The Sick Child in Early Modern England, 1580–1720. Oxford: Oxford University Press, 2012.
Oakley, Ann. *The Captured Womb: A History of the Medical Care of Pregnant Women*. Oxford: Basil Blackwell, 1984.
Obladen, Michael. 'In God's Image? The Tradition of Infant Head Shaping'. *Journal of Child Neurology* 27, no. 5 (2012): 672–680.
O'Brien, Karen. 'Sexual Impropriety, Petitioning and the Dynamics of Ill Will in Daily Urban Life'. *Urban History* 43, no. 2 (2016): 177–199.
O'Day, Rosemary. *The Family and Family Relationships, 1500–1900; England, France & the United States*. Basingstoke: Macmillan, 1994.
O'Hara, Diana. '"Ruled by My Friends": Aspects of Marriage in the Diocese of Canterbury c. 1540–1570'. *Continuity and Change* 6, no. 1 (1991): 9–41.
Oosterwijk, Sophie. 'Chrysoms, Shrouds and Infants on English Tomb Monuments: A Question of Terminology?' *Church Monuments* 15 (2000): 44–64.
Oren-Magidor, Daphna. *Infertility in Early Modern England*. Early Modern History: Society and Culture. Basingstoke: Palgrave, 2017.
'Literate Laywomen, Male Medical Practitioners and the Treatment of Fertility Problems in Early Modern England'. *Social History of Medicine* 29, no. 2 (2016): 290–310.
O'Toole, Emma. 'Dressing the Expectant Mother: Maternity Fashion in Eighteenth- and Early-Nineteenth-Century Ireland'. *Women's History. The Journal of the Women's History Network* 2, no. 5 (2016): 26–32.
Ottway, Sheila. 'Autobiography'. In *A Companion to Early Modern Women's Writing*. Edited by Anita Pacheco, 231–247. Blackwell Companions to Literature and Culture. Oxford: Blackwell, 2002.
Overton, Mark. *Production and Consumption in English Households, 1600–1750*. London: Routledge, 2004.
Park, Katharine. *Secrets of Women: Gender, Generation, and the Origins of Human Dissection*. New York: Zone Books, 2010.
Park, Katharine, and Lorraine J. Daston. 'Unnatural Conceptions: The Study of Monsters in Sixteenth- and Seventeenth-Century France and England'. *Past & Present* 92, no. August (1981): 20–54.
Paster, Gail Kern. *The Body Embarrassed: Drama and the Disciplined of Shame in Early Modern England*. Ithaca, NY: Cornell University Press, 1993.
Paul, K. Tawny. 'Accounting for Men's Work: Multiple Employments and Occupational Identities in Early Modern England'. *History Workshop Journal* 85 (2018): 26–46.
Pears, Iain. *An Instance of the Fingerpost*. London: Jonathan Cape, 1997.

Pelling, Margaret. 'Child Health as a Social Value in Early Modern England'. *Social History of Medicine* 1, no. 2 (1988): 135–164.

'Compromised by Gender: The Role of the Male Medical Practioner in Early Modern England'. In *The Task of Healing: Medicine, Religion, and Gender in England and the Netherlands, 1450–1800*. Edited by Hilary Marling and Margaret Pelling, 101–109. Rotterdam: Erasmus, 1996.

'Nurses and Nursekeepers: Problems with Identification in the Early Modern Period'. In *The Common Lot: Sickness, Medical Occupations and the Urban Poor in Early Modern England*, 179–202. London: Longman, 1998.

The Common Lot: Sickness, Medical Occupations and the Urban Poor in Early Modern England. London: Longman, 1998.

'The Women of the Family? Speculations around Early Modern British Physicians'. *Social History of Medicine* 8, no. 3 (1995): 383–401.

Pelling, Margaret, and Frances White. *Medical Conflicts in Early Modern London: Patronage, Physicians, and Irregular Practitioners, 1550–1640*. Oxford Studies in Social History. Oxford: Oxford University Press, 2003.

Pennell, Sara. 'Perfecting Practice? Women, Manuscript Recipes and Knowledge in Early Modern England'. In *Early Modern Women's Manuscript Writing: Selected Papers from the Trinity/Trent Colloquium*. Edited by Victoria Burke and Jonathan Gibson, 237–258. Aldershot: Ashgate, 2004.

Perry, Ruth. 'Colonizing the Breast: Sexuality and Maternity in Eighteenth-Century England'. *Journal of the History of Sexuality* 2, no. 2 (1991): 204–234.

Peters, Christine. 'Single Women in Early Modern England: Attitudes and Expectations'. *Continuity and Change* 12, no. 3 (1997): 325–345.

Phillips, Sara E. K., Ann C. Celi, Alexandra Wehbe, Jasmine Kaduthodil and Chloe A. Zera. 'Mobilizing the Fourth Trimester to Improve Population Health: Interventions for Postpartum Transitions of Care'. *American Journal of Obsetrics and Gynecology* 229, no. 1 (2023): 33–38.

Pollock, Linda A. 'Childbearing and Female Bonding in Early Modern England'. *Social History* 22, no. 3 (1997): 286–306.

'Embarking on a Rough Passage: The Experience of Pregnancy in Early-Modern Society'. In *Women as Mothers in Pre-Industrial England*. Edited by Valerie Fildes, 39–67. London: Routledge, 1990.

Forgotten Children: Parent–Child Relations from 1500 to 1900. Cambridge: Cambridge University Press, 1983.

A Lasting Relationship: Parents and Children over Three Centuries. London: Fourth Estate, 1987.

Pomata, Gianna. *Contracting a Cure: Patients, Healers, and the Law in Early Modern Bologna*. Baltimore: Johns Hopkins University Press, 1998.

'Menstruating Men: Similarity and Difference of the Sexes in Early Modern Medicine'. In *Generation and Degeneration: Tropes of Reproduction in Literature and History from Antiquity to Early Modern Europe*. Edited by Valeria Finucci and Kevin Brownlee, 109–152. Durham, NC: Duke University Press, 2001.

Popiel, Jennifer J. 'Making Mothers: The Advice Genre and the Domestic Ideal, 1760–1830'. *Journal of Family History* 29, no. 4 (2004): 339–350.

Porter, Roy. *Health for Sale: Quackery in England, 1660–1850*. Manchester: Manchester University Press, 1989.

'The Patient's View: Doing Medical History from Below'. *Theory & Society* 14, no. 1 (1985): 175–198.

'The Secrets of Generation Display'd: Aristotles Master-Piece in Eighteenth-Century England'. In *'Tis Nature's Fault: Unauthorized Sexuality during the Enlightenment*. Edited by Robert Purks Maccubbin, 1–21. Cambridge: Cambridge University Press, 1985.

Purkiss, Diane. 'Women's Stories of Witchcraft in Early Modern England: The House, the Body, the Child'. *Gender & History* 7, no. 3 (1995): 408–432.

Radcliffe, Walter. *Milestones in Midwifery with a Foreword by David Brown*. Bristol: Wright, 1967.

Rankin, Alisha. 'Becoming an Expert Practitioner: Court Experimentalism and the Medical Skills of Anna of Saxony (1532–1585)'. *Isis* 98 (2007): 23–53.

Panaceia's Daughters: Noblewomen as Healers in Early Modern Germany/Alisha Rankin. Chicago: University of Chicago Press, 2013.

Rawcliffe, Carol. *Medicine and Society in Later Medieval England*. Stroud: Sutton, 1997.

Read, Sara. *Menstruation and the Female Body in Early Modern England*. Genders and Sexualities in History. Basingstoke: Palgrave, 2013.

'"Pregnant Women Gaze at the Precious Thing Their Souls Are Set On": Perceptions of the Pregnant Body in Early Modern Literature' In *Perceptions of Pregnancy from the Seventeenth to the Twentieth Century*. Edited by Jennifer Evans and Ciara Meehan, 133–159. Basingstoke: Palgrave, 2017.

'Thy Righteousness Is but a Menstrual Clout: Sanitary Practices and Prejudice in Early Modern England'. *Early Modern Women: An Interdisciplinary Journal* 3 (2008): 1–25.

Reinke-Williams, Tim. *Women, Work and Sociability in Early Modern London*. Genders and Sexualities in History. Basingstoke: Macmillan, 2014.

Rhodes, Marissa C. 'Domestic Vulnerabilities: Reading Families and Bodies into Eighteenth-Century Anglo-Atlantic Wet Nurse Advertisements'. *Journal of Family History* 40, no. 1 (2015): 39–63.

Rickman, Johanna. *Love, Lust, and License in Early Modern England: Illicit Sex and the Nobility*. Women and Gender in the Early Modern World. Aldershot: Ashgate, 2008.

Riddle, John M. 'Oral Contraceptives and Early Term Abortifacients during Classical Antiquity and the Middle Ages'. *Past & Present* 132, no. 1 (1991): 4–32.

Riello, Giorgio. '"Things Seen and Unseen": The Material Culture of Early Modern Inventories and Their Representation of Domestic Interiors'. In *Early Modern Things: Objects and Their Histories, 1500–1800*. Edited by Paula Findlen, 124–150. London: Routledge, 2012.

Roodenburg, Herman W. 'Maternal Imagination: The Fears of Pregnant Women in Seventeenth-Century Holland'. *Journal of Social History* 21, no. 4 (1988): 701–716.

Roper, Lyndal. 'Witchcraft and Fantasy in Early Modern Germany'. In *Oedipus and the Devil: Witchcraft, Sexuality and Religion in Early Modern Europe*, 199–225. London: Routledge, 1994.

Rousseau, Jean-Jacques. *Emile, or On Education (1763)*. Garden City, NY: Dover Publications, 2013.

Rublack, Ulinka. 'Pregnancy, Childbirth and the Female Body in Early Modern Germany'. *Past & Present* 150, no. 1 (1996): 84–110.

Ruhräh, John. *Pediatrics of the Past: An Anthology Compiled and Edited by John Ruhräh with a Foreword by Fielding H. Garrison*. New York: P. B. Hoeber, 1925.

Ryder, Dudley. *The Diary of Dudley Ryder 1715–1716*. Edited by William Matthews. London: Methuen & Co., 1939.

Ryrie, Alex. *Being Protestant in Reformation Britain*. Oxford: Oxford University Press, 2013.

Sánchez, Magdalena S. '"I Would Not Feel the Pain If I Were with You": Catalina Micaela and the Cycle of Pregnancy at the Court of Turin, 1585–1597'. *Social History of Medicine* 28, no. 3 (2015): 445–464.

Schmitz, Carolin. 'Travelling for Health: Local and Regional Mobility in Early Modern Rural Spain'. In *Connected Mobilities in the Early Modern World: The Practice and Experience of Movement*. Edited by Paul Nelles and Rosa Salzberg, 87–110. Amsterdam: Amsterdam University Press, 2023.

Schneider, Gary. *Culture of Epistolarity: Vernacular Letters and Letter Writing in Early Modern England, 1500–1700*. Newark: University of Delaware Press, 2005.

Scott, Joan. 'Gender: A Useful Category of Historical Analysis'. *American Historical Review* 91, no. 1986 (1986): 1053–1075.

Scott-Warren, Jason. 'Early Modern Bookkeeping and Life-Writing Revisited: Accounting for Richard Stonley'. *Past & Present* 230, no. Supplement 11 (2016): 151–170.

Sharp, Jane. *The Midwives Book Or the Whole Art of Midwifry Discovered*. Edited by Elaine Hobby. Women Writers in English 1350–1850. Oxford: Oxford University Press, 1999.

Sharpe, James. *Witchcraft in Early Modern England*. Harlow: Pearson Education, 2001.

Shepard, Alexandra. *Accounting for Oneself: Worth, Status, and the Social Order in Early Modern England*. Oxford: Oxford University Press, 2015.

'Manhood, Credit and Patriarchy in Early Modern England c. 1580–1640'. *Past & Present* 167, no. 1 (2000): 75–106.

Meanings of Manhood in Early Modern England. Oxford Studies in Social History. Oxford: Clarendon Press, 2003.

'The Pleasures and Pains of Breastfeeding in England c. 1600–c. 1800: Narratives and Representations: A Collection to Honour Paul Slack'. In *Suffering and Happiness in England 1550–1850*. Edited by Michael J. Braddick and Joanna Innes, 227–246. The Past & Present Book Series. Oxford: Oxford University Press, 2017.

Shepard, Alexandra, and Phil Withington, eds. *Communities in Early Modern England*. Manchester: Manchester University Press, 2000.

Sherman, William H. *Used Books: Marking Readers in Renaissance England*. Philadelphia: University of Pennsylvania Press, 2008.

Shorter, Edward. *Making of the Modern Family*. London: Collins, 1976.

Siebers, Tobin. 'Disability as Masquerade'. *Literature and Medicine* 23, no. 1 (2004): 22–65.

Siena, Kevin P. *Veneral Disease, Hospitals and the Urban Poor: London's 'Foul Wards', 1600–1800*. Rochester Studies in Medical History. Rochester, NY: University of Rochester Press, 2004.

Smith, Lisa W. '"An Account of an Unaccountable Distemper": The Experience of Pain in Early Eighteenth-Century England and France'. *Eighteenth-Century Studies* 41, no. 4 (2008): 459–480.

'The Body Embarrassed? Rethinking the Leaky Male Body in Eighteenth-Century England and France'. *Gender & History* 23, no. 1 (2010): 26–46.

'Imagining Women's Fertility before Technology'. *Journal of Medical Humanities* 31 (2010): 69–79.

'La Raillerie des Femmes? Les Femmes, La Stérilité Et La Société En France a L'époque Moderne'. In *Femmes En Fleurs, Femmes En Corps: Sang, Santé, Sexualités Du Moyen Age Aux Lumières*. Edited by Cathy McClive, 203–220. Saint-Étienne: Publications de l'Université de Saint-Étienne, 2010.

'Reassessing the Role of the Family: Women's Health Care in Eighteenth-Century England'. *Social History of Medicine* 16, no. 3 (2003): 327–342.

'The Relative Duties of a Man: Domestic Medicine in England and France, ca. 1685–1740'. *Journal of Family History* 31, no. 3 (2006): 237–256.

Smith, Charlotte Fell (ed.). *Mary Rich, Countess of Warwick (1625–1678): Her Family and Friends*. London: Longmans, 1901.

Smith, Sidonie, and Julia Watson. *Reading Autobiography: A Guide for Interpreting Life Narratives*. Minneapolis: University of Minnesota Press, 2010.

Smyth, Adam. 'Almanacs, Annotators, and Life-Writing in Early Modern England'. *English Literary Renaissance* 38, no. 2 (2008): 200–244.

Autobiography in Early Modern England. Cambridge: Cambridge University Press, 2010.

Snook, Edith. '"The Women Know": Children's Diseases, Recipes and Women's Knowledge in Early Modern Medical Publications'. *Social History of Medicine* 30, no. 1 (2017): 1–21.

Spence, Craig. *Accidents and Violent Death in Early Modern London, 1650–1750*. Studies in Early Modern Cultural, Political and Social History. Woodbridge: Boydell & Brewer, 2016.

Sperling, Jutta Gisela, ed. *Medieval and Renaissance Lactations: Images, Rhetorics, Practices*. Women and Gender in the Early Modern World. Farnham: Ashgate, 2013.

Spivack, Carla. 'To "Bring Down the Flowers": The Cultural Context of Abortion Law in Early Modern England'. *William & Mary Journal of Women and the Law* 14, no. 1 (2007): 107–151.

Stahnish, Frank W. 'The Tertium Comparationis of the Elementa Physiologiae: Johann Gottfriend von Herder's Conception of "Tears" as Mediators between the Sublime and the Actual Bodily Physiology'. In *Blood, Sweat and Tears: The Changing Concepts of Physiology from Antiquity into Early Modern Europe*. Edited by Manfred Hortsmanhoff, Helen King and Claus Zittel, 595–625. Intersections: Interdisciplinary Studies in Early Modern Culture 25. Leiden: Brill, 2012.

Stobart, Anne. *Household Medicine in Seventeenth-Century England*. London: Bloomsbury Academic, 2016.

Stolberg, Michael. *Experiencing Illness and the Sick Body in Early Modern Europe*. Basingstoke: Palgrave, 2011.

'An Unmanly Vice: Self-Pollution, Anxiety, and the Body in the Eighteenth Century'. *Social History of Medicine* 13, no. 1 (2000): 1–21.

Uroscopy in Early Modern Europe. Farnham: Ashgate, 2015.

'A Woman Down to Her Bones: The Anatomy of Sexual Difference in the Sixteenth and Early Seventeenth Centuries'. *Isis* 94 (2003): 274–299.

Stone, Lawrence. *The Crisis of the Aristocracy*. Oxford: Oxford University Press, 1965.

The Family, Sex and Marriage in England 1500–1800. London: Weidenfeld & Nicolson, 1977.

Strocchia, Sharon T. 'Women and Healthcare in Early Modern Europe'. *Renaissance Studies* 28 (2014): 496–514.

Suzuki, Mihoko. 'Anne Clifford and the Gendering of History'. *Clio* 30, no. 2 (2001): 195–229.

Tadmor, Naomi. 'Early Modern English Kinship in the Long Run: Reflections on Continuity and Change'. *Continuity and Change* 25 (2010): 15–48.

Family and Friends in Eighteenth-Century England: Household, Kinship and Patronage. Cambridge: Cambridge University Press, 2001.

Tague, Ingrid H. *Animal Companions: Pets and Social Change in Eighteenth-Century Britain*. Pennsylvania: Pennsylvania State University Press, 2015.

Thauvette, Chantelle. 'Sex, Astrology, and the Almanacs of Sarah Jinner'. *Early Modern Women: An Interdisciplinary Journal* 5 (2010): 243–249.

Thomas, Keith. 'Cleanliness and Godliness in Early Modern England'. In *Religion, Culture and Society in Early Modern Britain: Essays in Honour of Patrick Collinson*. Edited by Anthony Fletcher and Peter Roberts, 56–83. Cambridge: Cambridge University Press, 1994.

Man and the Natural World: Changing Attitudes in England 1500–1800. London: Allen Lane, 1983.

Religion and the Decline of Magic: Studies in Popular Beliefs in Sixteenth and Seventeenth Century England. London: Weidenfeld & Nicolson, 1971.

Thomas, Samuel S. 'Early Modern Midwifery: Splitting the Profession, Connecting the History'. *Journal of Social History* 43, no. 1 (2009): 115–138.

Thomson, Stephanie, and Katie Barclay. 'Religious Patronage as Gendered Family Memory in Sixteenth-Century England'. *Journal of Family History* 46, no. 1 (2021): 13–29.

Todd, Margo. 'Puritan Self-Fashioning: The Diary of Samuel Ward'. *Journal of British Studies* 31, no. 1992 (1992): 236–264.

Toomer, Heather. 'Seventeenth-Century Baby Clothes? The Problems of Identification'. *Costume* 55, no. 1 (2021): 24–48.

Tosh, John. 'What Should Historians Do with Masculinity? Reflections on Nineteenth-Century Britain'. *History Workshop Journal* 38 (1994): 179–202.

Toulalan, Sarah. '"The Act of Copulation Being Ordain'd by Nature as the Ground of All Generation": Fertility and the Representation of Sexual Pleasure in Seventeenth-Century Pornography in England'. *Women's History Review* 15, no. 4 (2006): 521–532.

Imagining Sex: Pornography and Bodies in Seventeenth-Century England. Oxford: Oxford University Press, 2007.

'"To[o] much eating stifles the child": Fat Bodies and Reproduction in Early Modern England'. *Historical Research* 87, no. 235 (2014): 65–93.

'"Unfit for Generation": Body Size and Reproduction'. In *The Secrets of Generation: Reproduction in the Long Eighteenth Century*. Edited by Raymond Stephanson and Darren Wagner, 299–318. Toronto: University of Toronto Press, 2013.

Travitsky, Betty S. 'The New Mother of the English Renaissance: A Descriptive Catalogue'. *Bulletin of Research in the Humanities* 82, no. 1 (1979): 63–89.

Trevor Hughes, J. 'Miraculous Deliverance of Anne Greene: An Oxford Case of Resuscitation in the Seventeenth Century'. *British Medical Journal* 285 (1982): 556.

Trumbach, Randolph. *The Rise of the Egalitarian Family: Aristocratic Kinship and Domestic Relations in Eighteenth-Century England*. Studies in Social Discontinuity. London: Academic Press Inc., 1978.

Tucker, Nicholas. 'Boon or Burden? Baby Love in History: Did Past Ages Care for, or Curse the Cradle and Its Occupant? Nicholas Tucker Sifts the Evidence'. *History Today* 43, no. 9 (1993): 28–35.

'Mothers, Babies and Lullabies'. *History Today* 34, no. 9 (1984): 40–46.

Turner, David. '"Nothing Is so Secret but Shall Be Revealed": The Scandalous Life of Robert Foulkes'. In *English Masculinities, 1660–1800*. Edited by Tim Hitchcock and Michelle Cohen, 169–192. London: Routledge, 1999.

Turner, Sasha. *Contested Bodies: Pregnancy, Childrearing, and Slavery in Jamaica*. Early American Studies. Philadelphia: University of Pennsylvania Press, 2017.

Tyers, Theresa L. '"In the Merry Month of May": Instructions for Ensuring Fertility in MS British Library, Lansdowne 380'. *Social History of Medicine* 29, no. 2 (2015): 267–289.

Vickery, Amanda. *Behind Closed Doors: At Home in Georgian England*. New Haven, CT: Yale University Press, 2010.

The Gentleman's Daughter: Women's Lives in Georgian England. New Haven, CT: Yale University Press, 1998.

'Golden Age to Separate Spheres? A Review of the Categories and Chronology of Women's History'. *The Historical Journal* 36, no. 2 (1993): 383–414.

Waddell, Brodie. 'Writing History from Below: Chronicling and Record-Keeping in Early Modern England'. *History Workshop Journal* 85, no. Spring (2018): 239–264.

Walker, Garthine. *Crime, Gender, and Social Order in Early Modern England*. Cambridge Studies in Early Modern British History. Cambridge: Cambridge University Press, 2003.

Wall, Alison D., ed. *Two Elizabethan Women: Correspondence of Joan and Maria Thynne 1575–1611*. Devizes: Wiltshire Record Society, 1983.

Wall, Wendy. 'Isabella Whitney and the Female Legacy'. *English Literary History* 58, no. 1 (1991): 35–62.

Wallis, Patrick. 'Consumption, Retailing, and Medicine in Early-Modern London'. *Economic History Review* 61, no. 1 (2008): 26–53.

Walsh, Katharine Phelps. 'Marketing Midwives in Seventeenth-Century London: A Re-examination of Jane Sharp's *The Midwives Book*'. *Gender & History* 26, no. 2 (2014): 223–241.

Walsham, Alexandra. *Providence in Early Modern England*. Oxford: Oxford University Press, 1999.

Reformation of the Landscape: Religion, Identity, and Memory in Early Modern Britain and Ireland. Oxford: Oxford University Press, 2011.

'The Social History of the Archive: Record-Keeping in Early Modern Europe'. *Past & Present* 230, no. 11 (2016): 9–48.

'"Tongues of Heaven": Prodigies, Portents, and Prophets'. In *Providence in Early Modern England*, 167–218. Oxford: Oxford University Press, 2001.

Waterhouse, Harriet. 'A Fashionable Confinement: Whaleboned Stays and the Pregnant Woman'. *Costume* 41, no. 1 (2007): 53–65.

Wear, Andrew. 'Epistemology and Learned Medicine in Early Modern England'. In *Knowledge and the Scholarly Medical Traditions*. Edited by Don Bates, 151–174. Cambridge: Cambridge University Press, 1995.

Knowledge and Practice in English Medicine, 1550–1680. Cambridge: Cambridge University Press, 2000.

'Puritan Perceptions of Illness in Seventeenth-Century England'. In *Patients and Practitioners: Lay Perceptions of Medicine in Pre-Industrial Society*. Edited by Roy Porter, 55–99. Cambridge: Cambridge University Press, 1985.

Weber, A. S. 'Women's Early Modern Medical Almanacs in Historical Context'. *English Literary Renaissance* 33, no. 3 (2003): 358–402.

Weil, Rachel J. 'The Politics of Legitimacy and the Warming-Pan Scandal'. In *Political Passions: Gender, the Family and Political Argument in England*, 65–82. Manchester: Manchester University Press, 1999.

Weisser, Olivia. 'Boils, Pushes and Wheals: Reading Bumps on the Body in Early Modern England'. *Social History of Medicine* 22, no. 2 (2009): 321–339.

'Grieved and Disordered: Gender and Emotion in Early Modern Patient Narratives'. *Journal of Medieval and Early Modern Studies* 43, no. 2 (2013): 247–273.

Ill Composed: Sickness, Gender, and Belief in Early Modern England. New Haven, CT: Yale University Press, 2015.

'Poxed and Ravished: Venereal Disease in Early Modern Rape Trials'. *History Workshop Journal.* 91, no. 1 (2021): 51–70.

Wells, Greg, trans. *John Hall Master of Physicke: A Casebook from Shakespeare's Stratford.* Manchester: Manchester University Press, 2020.

Wells, Marion A. '"Full of Rapture": Maternal Vocality and Melancholy in Webster's Duchess of Malfi'. In *Blood, Sweat, and Tears: The Changing Concepts of Physiology from Antiquity into Early Modern Europe*. Edited by Manfred Hortsmanhoff, Helen King and Claus Zittel, 685–713. Intersections: Interdisciplinary Studies in Early Modern Culture 25. Leiden: Brill, 2012.

West, Emily, and R. J. Knight. 'Mother's Milk: Slavery, Wet-Nursing, and Black and White Women in the Antebellum South'. *Journal of Southern History* 83, no. 1 (2017): 37–68.

Whiteley, Rebecca. *Birth Figures: Early Modern Prints and the Pregnant Body.* Chicago: Chicago University Press, 2023.

'Figuring Pictures and Picturing Figures: Images of the Pregnant Body and the Unborn Child in England, 1540–c.1680'. *Social History of Medicine* 32, no. 2 (2019): 241–266.

Whittle, Jane. 'The House as a Place of Work in Early Modern Rural England'. *Home Cultures* 8, no. 2 (2011): 133–150.

Whittle, Jane, and Mark Hailwood. 'The Gender Division of Labour in Early Modern England'. *Economic History Review* 73, no. 1 (2020): 3–32.

Whyman, Susan E. *Sociability and Power in Late-Stuart England: The Cultural Worlds of the Verneys 1660–1720*. Oxford: Oxford University Press, 1999.

Wilson, Adrian. 'The Ceremony of Childbirth and Its Interpretation'. In *Women as Mothers in Pre-Industrial England: Essays in Memory of Dorothy McLaren*. Edited by Valerie Fildes, 68–107. London: Routledge, 1990.

The Making of Man-Midwifery: Childbirth in England, 1660–1770. London: Routledge, 1995.

'Midwifery in the "Medical Marketplace"'. In *Medicine and the Market in Early Modern England*. Edited by Mark Jenner and Patrick Wallis, 153–174. Basingstoke: Palgrave, 2007.

'Participant or Patient? Seventeenth Century Childbirth from the Mother's Point of View'. In *Patients and Practitioners: Lay Perceptions of Medicine in Pre-Industrial Society*. Edited by Roy Porter, 129–144. Cambridge, 1985.

'The Perils of Early Modern Procreation: Childbirth with or without Fear?' *British Journal of Eighteenth Century Studies* 16 (1993): 1–19.

'Two Female Cultures'. In *The Making of Man-Midwifery: Childbirth in England, 1660–1770*, 185–196. Cambridge, MA: Harvard University Press, 1995.

Winer, Rebecca Lynn. 'Conscripting the Breast: Lactation, Slavery and Salvation in the Realms of Aragon and Kingdom of Majorca, c. 1250–1300'. *Journal of Medieval History* 34, no. 2 (2012): 164–184.

Winkel, Michiel de. 'The Interpretation of Dress in Vermeer's Paintings'. *Vermeer Studies*. Edited by Ivan Gaskell and Michiel Jonker. Symposium Papers, 55, no. 33 (1998).

Withey, Alun. *Physick and the Family: Health, Medicine and Care in Wales, 1600–1750*. Manchester: Manchester University Press, 2011.

Woodham, Anna, Laura King, Liz Gloyn, Vicky Crewe and Fiona Blair. 'We Are What We Keep: The "Family Archive", Identity and Public/Private Heritage'. *Heritage & Society* 10, no. 3 (2017): 203–220.

Woolf, Daniel. *The Social Circulation of the Past: English Historical Culture 1500–1730*. Oxford: Oxford University Press, 2003.

Wrightson, Keith. *English Society, 1580–1680*. New Brunswick, NJ: Rutgers University Press, 1982.

'Infanticide in Earlier Seventeenth-Century England'. *Local Population Studies* 15 (1975): 10–22.

Wrigley, E. A., and R. S. Schofield. *The Population History of England 1541–1871: A Reconstruction*. London: Edward Arnold, 1981.

Yale, Elizabeth. 'The History of Archives: The State of the Discipline'. *Book History* 18 (2015): 332–359.

Zuccolin, Gabriella. 'The Speculum Phisionomie by Michele Savonarola', in Universality of Reason, Plurality of Philosophies.16–22 September 2007, Palermo, Italy. Open Research Online, https://oro.open.ac.uk/, last accessed 27/03/2025.

Index

Note: page numbers in italic type indicate a figure.

For EU product safety concerns, contact us at Calle de José Abascal, 56–1°, 28003 Madrid, Spain or eugpsr@cambridge.org.

www.ingramcontent.com/pod-product-compliance
Lightning Source LLC
Chambersburg PA
CBHW060246290126
38964CB00004B/54